Geriatric Rehabilitation

Geriatric Rehabilitation

Edited by

Bryan Kemp, Ph.D.
Associate Clinical Professor, Departments of Psychiatry and Behavioral Science, and Family Medicine, University of Southern California School of Medicine, Los Angeles; Co-Chief, Clinical Gerontology Service, and Director, Rehabilitation Research and Training Center on Aging, Rancho Los Amigos Medical Center, Downey, California

Kenneth Brummel-Smith, M.D.
Associate Professor of Clinical Family Medicine, and Director, Section of Geriatrics, Department of Family Medicine, University of Southern California School of Medicine, Los Angeles; Co-Chief, Clinical Gerontology Service, and Training Director, Rehabilitation Research and Training Center on Aging, Rancho Los Amigos Medical Center, Downey, California

Joseph W. Ramsdell, M.D.
Adjunct Professor of Medicine, University of California, San Diego, School of Medicine, La Jolla; Acting Division Head, General Internal Medicine/Geriatrics, UCSD Medical Center, San Diego

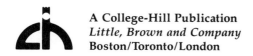

A College-Hill Publication
Little, Brown and Company
Boston/Toronto/London

College-Hill Press
A Division of
Little, Brown and Company (Inc.)
34 Beacon Street
Boston, Massachusetts 02108

Library of Congress Cataloging in Publication Data
Main entry under title:

Geriatric rehabilitation
  [edited by] Bryan Kemp, Kenneth Brummel-Smith, Joseph Ramsdell,
    p.   cm.
  "A College-Hill publication."
  Includes bibliographies and index.
  ISBN 0-316-48820-8
    1. Aged—Rehabilitation.   I. Kemp, Bryan.   II. Brummel-Smith,
  Kenneth.   III. Ramsdell, Joseph.
    [DNLM: 1. Chronic Disease—in old age.   2. Health Services for the
  Aged.   3. Rehabilitation—in old age.   4. Rehabilitation—
  organization & administration.   WT 30 G3696]
  RC952.5.G44344   1989
  618.97'03—dc20
  DNLM/DLC   89-9845
  for Library of Congress   CIP

ISBN 0-316-48820-8

Printed in the United States of America
EB

To Anne Kemp, Herbert Brummel, and
G. A. Ramsdell, M.D.

Contents

Preface

Geriatric Rehabilitation was written in the hope that it will add to a growing awareness of the need to provide improved health care to older persons who have chronic, disabling illness. The United States is fortunate to have one of the best systems, if not *the* best system, of acute health care available in the world. Our ability to diagnose and correct acute illnesses through advances in basic sciences, improved technology, and specialized procedures is unparalleled. Millions of people have benefited from these developments.

However, there is a growing portion of the population for which these advances are not the total answer. This portion includes persons who have sustained permanently disabling conditions. For these persons, a health care system focused on acute illnesses is incomplete and often even irrelevant.

There is a system of care that has developed over the last half century to help address the problems of chronic illness. It is termed *rehabilitation*. In essence, it is an approach to care that goes beyond the acute stages of illness. Unfortunately, many people have certain misconceptions about rehabilitation. For some, it is the provision of physical or occupational therapy. For others, it is seen as a medical specialty — physiatry. Actually, rehabilitation is neither of these. Rehabilitation is (1) a philosophy about how health care ought to be provided, (2) a set of principles governing health care delivery, and (3) a long-term (lifelong) commitment to providing services.

Philosophically, rehabilitation rests on several positions. First, the goals of rehabilitation are chiefly aimed at reducing disability, improving function, and eliminating handicap. Rehabilitation is not aimed at curing illness. Because of that, many physicians (and others) have not been interested in rehabilitation possibly because it lacks some of the excitement and prestige of "lifesaving," disease-oriented medicine. Disability is defined as diminished capacity to accomplish a necessary or desired task. Rehabilitation aims to improve such functioning. Second, rehabilitation aims to reduce handicap. A handicap is measured by the degree to which a person is excluded from participating in the physical or social environment. Clearly, both disability and handicap are *interactive* terms. They depend on the interaction of the person and the environment. The person with a chronic condition does not cause his or her disability or handicap. One is disabled or handicapped, or both, depending on the difficulties one has interacting with the environment. A disability can be reduced not only by increasing the person's abilities, but by reducing the environment's demands on the person. A handicap can be reduced not only by the person's becoming more comfortable with his or her condition and with others' reactions to it, but also by society's becoming more comfortable with, accepting of, and accommodating of the person with a disability.

Rehabilitation stresses a biopsychosocial approach to illness. Whether in its cause, in its consequences, or in its treatment, chronic illness (and probably acute illness as well) is *always* a mix of biologic, psychologic, and social phenomena. The degree to which a person regains functioning after a chronic illness depends on the adequacy of attention paid to all three realms. If any part of the biopsychosocial complex is not adequately addressed, chronic illness will result in diminished functioning and increased handicap.

In addition, rehabilitation stresses a "systems" approach to care. This means that the agents of care and improvement are not just the health professionals, but also include the family and the patient as part of the system. The *interaction* of these parts of the system, rather than the actions of any one of them, determines the adequacy of the outcome. Each part has its role and these roles change over the course of the person's improvement. Physicians may serve as technical experts early in the course of the illness but need to be good communicators and coaches with the patient as rehabilitation progresses. The family may need to be supportive and able to solve crises in the beginning but be able to be more realistic and even demanding as rehabilitation shifts to the home setting.

Rehabilitation is also a set of principles governing health care. These principles are clearly delineated in the chapters that follow. They are principles that all health professionals can and should learn. Rehabilitation, then, is not confined to the practice of physiatrists. It is a method of providing health care that should be incorporated into all health science training. This book provides substantial background for the eight basic principles of rehabilitation: stabilization of the underlying illness, prevention of secondary impairments, assessment and improvement of functional abilities, psychologic support and treatment, family education and support, home assessment and modification, long-term supportive services, and societal integration and acceptance.

This approach and these principles have great implications for structuring the training of medical and allied health science students. Too few students learn how to do a functional assessment, how to conduct a family interview, how to counsel a patient, or where to locate services in the community. Hopefully, a functionally oriented approach to health care will become a greater part of training.

Rehabilitation is particularly germane to aging. The most significant health care problem facing older adults is chronic, disabling illness. The prospects of diminished functioning, long-term care, and economic hardship, coupled with a health care system not geared to these kinds of problems, causes both individual hardships for older persons and dilemmas for health care financing.

The population over age 75 is the fastest growing segment of society. This age group has a disability rate that is 8 times that of the under-45 age group. Moreover, the older person is more likely to have multiple chronic illnesses and higher degrees of disability. Over 40 percent of all disabled persons in the United States are over age 60.

Historically, rehabilitation has focused on the young. It began with injured young workers and veterans. However, at that time life expectancy was only 50 to 55 years and what older disabled persons there were did not receive a lot of attention. Today, things are different. The older population has swelled to about 12 percent of the population and is still going up; disability rates are very high, and over 30 percent of all health care expenditures are for services to older persons. Rehabilitation offers one of the most viable alternatives to health care that can both improve functioning of disabled persons and better spend existing dollars.

This book is organized into five parts. Part I provides an overview of some of the broad issues in rehabilitation. Part II focuses on current concepts of care for some of the most prevalent physical conditions affecting the elderly population. Part III, which is rightfully the longest, addresses a number of ways in which functioning can be improved. These chapters range from developments in technology to assisting families. Part IV focuses on the issue of how rehabilitation-oriented services can be organized in a variety of different settings, from the private office to the rehabilitation hospital. Finally, Part V looks at special issues in rehabilitation, including ethics and policy concerns.

Geriatric rehabilitation is a two-way endeavor. Not only is it important to add rehabilitation to the mainstream of geriatric health care, but it is also important to bring more geriatrics into rehabilitation. It is hoped that this book will do some of each. Its intended audience is advanced students in the health and social service fields as well as practitioners in medicine, allied health sciences, and gerontology.

B.K.
K.B.-S.
J.W.R.

Acknowledgments

This book would not have been possible without the contributions of many people, whom we would like to acknowledge. First, credit goes to the National Institute of Disability and Rehabilitation Research, or NIDRR, (formerly the National Institute of Handicapped Research) for its support of the Rehabilitation Research and Training Center on Aging at Rancho Los Amigos Medical Center, Downey, California. At the time, Douglas Fenderson was Director of the NIDRR, and he provided understanding and support for the importance of geriatric rehabilitation. The foresight of NIDRR to fund centers on aging and rehabilitation is evidence of its role in helping the nation to care for people who have disabling conditions. In particular, Emily Cromar played a significant role in promoting and encouraging this effort. The University of California, San Diego, School of Medicine was instrumental in cohosting the national conference that preceded this text.

We also thank the many pioneers in rehabilitation and aging who have contributed, often unknowingly, to this book. Those include Howard Rusk, William Spencer, Bill Fordyce, Carolyn Vash, Stanley Brody, T. Franklin Williams, and Mary Switzer.

Finally, we thank those who helped prepare the text and turned it from a concept into a physical reality. These include the many chapter authors, Grace Farwell, Associate Training Director of the Rehabilitation Research Training Center, and Lynn Titus and her staff for the production of the manuscript.

Contributors

Dominick Addario, M.D.
Associate Clinical Professor, Department of Psychiatry, University of California, San Diego, School of Medicine, La Jolla; Medical Director, Behavioral Health Center, Mercy Hospital and Medical Center, San Diego

Lois A. Axtell, M.P.A., P.T.
Instructor, Health Occupations Division, Physical Therapist Assistant Program, Norwalk, California; Supervisor, Physical Therapy, Rancho Los Amigos Medical Center, Downey, California

Catherine E. Bannerman, M.D.
Clinical Assistant Professor, Department of Family Medicine, University of Southern California School of Medicine, Los Angeles; Director, Bay Shores Medical Group Senior Health Center, Torrance, California

Kenneth Brummel-Smith, M.D.
Associate Professor of Clinical Family Medicine, and Director, Section of Geriatrics, Department of Family Medicine, University of Southern California School of Medicine, Los Angeles; Co-Chief, Clinical Gerontology Service, and Training Director, Rehabilitation Research and Training Center on Aging, Rancho Los Amigos Medical Center, Downey, California

Helena Chang Chui, M.D.
Associate Professor, Department of Neurology, University of Southern California School of Medicine, Los Angeles; Attending Physician, Rancho Los Amigos Medical Center, Downey, California

Kenneth D. Cole, Ph.D.
Clinical Associate Professor, Department of Psychology, University of Southern California School of Medicine, Los Angeles; Program Director, Interdisciplinary Team Training in Geriatrics GRECC, Sepulveda Veterans Administration Medical Center, Sepulveda, California

Mark D. Corgiat, Ph.D.
Assistant Clinical Professor, Departments of Neurology and Family Medicine, University of Southern California School of Medicine, Los Angeles

William R. Freeman, M.D.
Assistant Professor, University of California, San Diego, School of Medicine, La Jolla; Administrative Director, Retina Service, Department of Ophthalmology, UCSD Medical Center, San Diego

Laurel E. Glass, M.D., Ph.D.
Professor of Anatomy and Psychiatry, University of California, San Francisco, School of Mediciné; Director, University of California Center on Deafness, San Francisco

Steven D. Hopson-Walker, Ph.D.
Assistant Professor of Criminology, California State University—Fresno, Fresno

Robert L. Kane, M.D.
Dean, University of Minnesota School of Public Health, Minneapolis

Joseph M. Keenan, M.D.
Assistant Professor, Department of Family Practice and Community Health, University of Minnesota Medical School—Minneapolis, Minneapolis

Jeremiah F. Kelly, M.D.
Assistant Professor, Evans Memorial Department of Clinical Research and Department of Medicine, Boston University School of Medicine; Director, Geriatric Evaluation Center, Evans Medical Group, University Hospital, Boston

Bryan Kemp, Ph.D.
Associate Clinical Professor, Departments of Psychiatry and Behavioral Science, and Family Medicine, University of Southern California School of Medicine, Los Angeles; Co-Chief, Clinical Gerontology Service, and

Director, Rehabilitation Research and Training Center on Aging, Rancho Los Amigos Medical Center, Downey, California

Dennis R. La Buda, M.A.
Director of Technology and Administrator, Stein Gerontological Institute, Miami Jewish Home and Hospital for the Aged, Miami

Bernard Lo, M.D.
Associate Professor of Medicine, University of California, San Francisco, School of Medicine, San Francisco

Lawrence S. Miller, M.D., F.A.C.P.
Clinical Associate Professor of Medicine, University of California, Los Angeles, School of Medicine, Los Angeles

Edward Mongan, M.D.
Associate Professor of Medicine, University of Southern California School of Medicine, Los Angeles; Chief of Medicine and Rheumatology, Rancho Los Amigos Medical Center, Downey, California

Dan Osterweil, M.D.
Assistant Professor of Medicine, University of California, Los Angeles, School of Medicine, Los Angeles

Michael Plopper, M.D.
Clinical Assistant Professor, Department of Psychiatry, University of Southern California School of Medicine, Los Angeles

Joseph W. Ramsdell, M.D.
Adjunct Professor of Medicine, University of California, San Diego, School of Medicine, La Jolla; Acting Division Head, General Internal Medicine/Geriatrics, UCSD Medical Center, San Diego

Andrew L. Ries, M.D.
Associate Professor of Medicine, University of California, San Diego, School of Medicine, La Jolla

Joan C. Rogers, Ph.D., O.T.R.
Assistant Professor of Psychiatry, University of Pittsburgh School of Medicine; Professor of Occupational Therapy, University of Pittsburgh School of Health Related Professions, Pittsburgh

Lori L. Rosenquist, M.S.G.
Doctoral Student, Heller School, Brandeis University, Waltham, Massachusetts

Marion B. Schoneberger, M.S., P.T.
Supervisor, Physical Therapy, Rancho Los Amigos Medical Center, Downey, California

William Selezinka, M.D., M.S.
Clinical Assistant Professor of Ophthalmology, University of California, San Diego, School of Medicine, La Jolla; Chairman, Department of Ophthalmology, Veterans Administration Medical Center, San Diego

Clifford W. Shults, M.D.
Assistant Professor of Neurosciences, University of California, San Diego, School of Medicine, La Jolla; Staff Neurologist, Veterans Administration Medical Center, San Diego

Hilary Siebens, M.D.
Assistant Medical Director, Department of Physical Medicine and Rehabilitation, Cedars-Sinai Medical Center, Los Angeles

Barbara A. Smith, M.A., R.N.C., C.R.R.N.
Clinical Coordinator, Southern California Alzheimer's Disease Diagnostic and Treatment Center, Rancho Los Amigos Medical Center, Downey, California

Fernando Torres-Gil, Ph.D.
Associate Professor of Gerontology and Public Administration, Leonard Davis School of Gerontology, Andrus Gerontology Center, University of Southern California, Los Angeles

Robert N. Weinreb, M.D.
Professor and Vice Chairman of Ophthalmology, University of California, San Diego, School of Medicine, La Jolla

Geriatric Rehabilitation

Notice

The indications and dosages of all drugs in this book have been recommended in the medical literature and conform to the practices of the general medical community. The medications described do not necessarily have specific approval by the Food and Drug Administration for use in the diseases and dosages for which they are recommended. The package insert for each drug should be consulted for use and dosage as approved by the FDA. Because standards for usage change, it is advisable to keep abreast of revised recommendations, particularly those concerning new drugs.

PART I

Overview

CHAPTER 1

Introduction

KENNETH BRUMMEL-SMITH

Developing a disability is not a normal part of aging. However, almost all conditions that cause disability are more frequently seen in the older population. Because of the high incidence of disabling conditions, geriatric patients must frequently be assessed for rehabilitation services. Such assessments should become routine to practitioners in geriatrics because in some respects the separation between rehabilitation and geriatrics is artificial. Since geriatrics promotes the "functional approach" in the care of the patient, it can be argued that rehabilitation is the foundation of geriatric care. Hence, it is incumbent upon geriatricians to provide a rehabilitation focus to all aspects of the care of the patient. For rehabilitation specialists the geriatric age group will provide the majority of their patients. This book is designed to satisfy both professional groups—to expand the knowledge of rehabilitation for those in geriatrics and to help those in rehabilitation deal more effectively with the special aspects of providing care to older patients.

Rehabilitation assists disabled persons in recovering lost physical, psychologic, or social skills so that they may be more independent, live in personally satisfying environments, and maintain meaningful social interactions. This type of care can be provided in many different health care settings, including the home, office, acute or rehabilitation hospital, or nursing home. An interdisciplinary team approach is required due to the complex nature of the various interventions. The process of rehabilitation also requires education of the patient and his or her family. Finally, rehabilitation is much more than a medical technique. Rather, it is a philosophic approach that recognizes that diagnoses are poor predictors of functional abilities,[52] that interventions directed to enhancing function are important, and that the "team" should always include the patient and his or her family.

DEFINITIONS OF DISABILITY

Part of the philosophic foundation of rehabilitation is an understanding of the meaning of disability. Three terms are often used when referring to alterations in a person's function: impairment, disability, and handicap. These words are often used interchangeably though their true meanings are quite distinct. A clearer understanding of these terms can be found in using the "systems approach." This approach is very useful in geriatric rehabilitation.[9]

In the systems approach a problem at the organ level (e.g., an infarct of the left hemisphere) must be viewed not only in terms of how it affects the brain but also how it affects the person, the family, the society, and ultimately, the nation (see Fig. 1-1). Using this approach we can define the terms impairment, disability, and handicap. *Impairment* refers to a loss of physical or physiologic function at the organ level. Many different types of impairments are found in older persons. Changes in renal function, nerve conduction velocity, or muscle strength are but a few. However, these "impairments" usually do not affect the person's ability to function and hence do not cause disability. On the other hand, if the impairment is so severe as to inhibit the person's ability to function, then it is termed a *disability*. Rehabilitation interventions are most often oriented toward adaptation to or recovery from a disability. With proper training or adaptive equipment the person with a disability can pursue an independent lifestyle. But

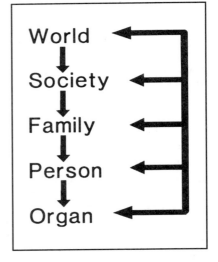

Figure 1-1. Feedback relationships when using the systems approach. The systems approach recognizes that changes in one part of the system impact upon all other parts of the system.

obstructions in the pursuit of independence can arise when the person with a disability confronts public buildings that are not accessible to wheelchairs, or policies that limit rehabilitation interventions. In this situation the person is *handicapped*. There are no handicapped persons, there are only handicapping societies. In this book we will be primarily concerned with approaches to reducing disability. It must be remembered though that the care of persons with a disability occurs in a societal context and it is this context that often creates the greatest stresses on our patients (Table 1-1).

Table 1-1. *Definitions of Disability*

Impairment—Organ level
Disability—Person level
Handicap—Society level

DEMOGRAPHICS OF DISABILITY

Most disabling conditions that require rehabilitation efforts disproportionally affect the elderly. The highest percentage of disabled older persons are in the "old-old" age group (>75 years).[50] Forty percent of all disabled persons are over age 65.[50] Three-fourths of strokes occur after age 65.[49] Most amputations occur in elderly people.[11] The average age of hip fractures is in the range of 70 to 78 years.[29] Eighty-six percent of those over 65 have at least one chronic condition and 52 percent of those over age 75 have some limitations in their daily activities.[15] But the simple presence of a disabling condition is not the most important factor to consider. Rather it is the impact that the condition has on the person's state of independence.

Disabilities, particularly in old age, are associated with higher mortality, increased health problems, shorter life span, and increased health care costs. Certain disabilities, such as decreased ability to walk, feed, or make one's toilet strongly predict dependency on others and increase the burden on caregivers.[14] Higher levels of disability create a greater burden of illness, thereby stressing the caregivers and increasing the risk of institutionalization. Rehabilitation interventions that enhance functional abilities have been shown to be cost-effective, and are associated with fewer hospitalizations later, greater levels of independence, and lower mortality.[31,39]

THE PROCESS OF REHABILITATION

STEPS IN REHABILITATION

Rehabilitation is often conceptualized as a series of steps. These steps are summarized in Table 1-2.

Table 1-2. *Steps in Rehabilitation*

Stabilize the primary problem(s)
Prevent secondary complications
Restore lost functional abilities
Promote adaptation of the person to his/her environment
Adapt the environment to the person
Promote family adaptation

When dealing with geriatric patients it may not always be possible to follow these steps in chronologic order. For instance, complete stabilization of the primary problem may not be possible in that there may be more than one "primary problem." An 80-year-old with a recent amputation may have underlying cardiac disease, hypertension, and peripheral neuropathy necessitating the close supervision of a primary physician during an inpatient rehabilitation stay. Preventing secondary complications is more difficult in the elderly due to the relative ease with which they develop and the great risk of such complications. Many types of secondary complications are encountered in older patients. These are summarized in Table 1-3.

Table 1-3. *Secondary Complications Seen in Rehabilitation*

Anorexia	Incontinence
Confusion	Pneumonia
Contractures	Pressure sores
Deconditioning	Psychologic dependency
Depression	Venous thrombosis

Most of these complications are more frequently seen in older persons. With decreased subcutaneous fat, poor capillary function, and low blood volumes, the geriatric patient is particularly prone to develop pressure sores. A sacral pressure sore, besides adding great costs to the care of the patient, may necessitate a period of cessation of wheelchair training in the person who is not ambulatory, thereby increasing the risk of the development of other secondary complications such as deconditioning or psychologic dependence. The all-too-common "cascade of disasters" seen in older hospitalized patients often can be traced to the development of a number of secondary complications (see Fig. 1-2).

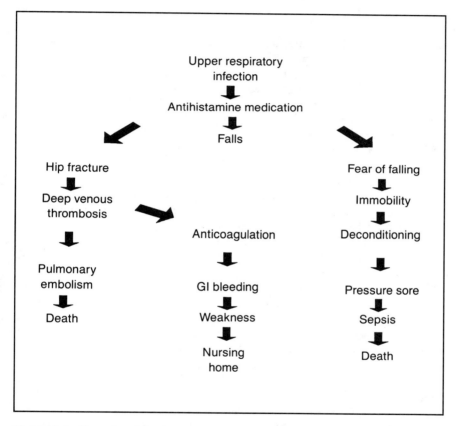

Figure 1-2. Cascade of disasters. A common problem, such as an upper respiratory infection, can lead to a series of "disasters" that can affect the person's physical, psychologic, or functional health.

Contractures, the shortening of muscles about the joints causing a decrease in the functional range of motion, begin to develop within 24 hours of the cessation of activity.[42] If the contracture has been longstanding or severely limits activity, recovery of lost motion may take weeks or may even be impossible. Strength is lost rapidly when people are immobilized or when they reduce their activity level. Younger persons may lose muscle strength at the rate of 5 percent per day when immobilized.[40] The rate of recovery of lost strength is much slower than the rate of loss. Studies evaluating the older person's loss of strength with bed rest need to be conducted but it is likely that the rate of loss would at least equal that of the younger person and recovery would likely be lower. Finally, it appears that the type of "help" given may affect the development of secondary complications. Patients who are encouraged to maintain activities of daily living (ADLs) may lose abilities less rapidly than those for whom all activities are assisted.[5] Therefore, a concerted effort by the team and the patient is needed to prevent the development of secondary disabilities.

The crux of rehabilitation interventions is the restoration of lost functional abilities. Often the simplest daily activity, such as dressing, can be a major impediment to independent living. Through the use of directed exercises, usually carried out by physical, occupational, and often communication therapists, the patient can "relearn" how to carry out these activities. Relearning may involve using a new way of dressing or the use of specialized aids such as a sock-donor.

The process of adapting to the environment, or of adapting the environment to the person, is especially important in geriatrics. With decreased physiologic reserves the older person may not be able to continue an activity that is extremely demanding. For instance, some younger paraplegics can learn ambulation techniques using canes and braces. The older person with a stroke and underlying cardiac insufficiency will usually need to learn wheelchair mobility skills. Therefore the environment will need significant modification. Doors may need to be widened, ramps installed, and counters lowered. Opportunities for obtaining new housing or adapting the present home may be restricted by financial concerns and personal preferences.

Finally, the family needs assistance in adapting as well. Eighty-five percent of all care given to dependent elders is provided by the family system.[8] Many of the family caregivers are also elderly spouses and older children. Training of family caregivers is basically an educational program. They will need to expand their knowledge of the problems of the older person and be taught skills needed for safe and effective caregiving. Their attitudes toward caregiving will need to be clarified because caregiving can be stressful to the family. The family's ability to function as a team is crucial to good rehabilitation outcomes. When necessary, family therapy may need to be provided to deal with problems and prevent burnout.

As stated above, the various steps are not necessarily addressed chronologically. In geriatrics the window of opportunity for an intervention may be rather limited. Rehabilitation teams may find themselves promoting adaptation, providing family training, and recurrently trying to stabilize the primary problems all at one time. Such is the challenge of geriatric rehabilitation.

REHABILITATION TEAMS

Rehabilitation teams are usually either multidisciplinary or inter-disciplinary. Multidisciplinary teams work in consulting relationships with one another, usually seeing the patient individually and then communicating with other team members by written notes or telephone contacts. Interdisciplinary teams usually work in the same setting and meet periodically as a group to discuss the patient's problems and progress. Each team member has a specific area of expertise but in geriatrics there is often considerable overlap in roles. Interdisciplinary teams are particularly effective when dealing with more complex problems such as inpatient or long-term care rehabilitation.

During team meetings members discuss their assessments, establish goals, provide updates on progress toward those goals, and estimate the length of time needed to meet the patient's goals. If possible, the patient should attend these meetings or at least his or her input and response to the team treatment plan should be obtained. A written summary of the meeting should be placed in the patient's record. It is also advisable to give a copy of the summary to the patient (and the family after obtaining the patient's permission).

SPECIAL ASPECTS OF REHABILITATION AND THE OLDER PATIENT

The care of geriatric persons differs in many ways from the care of younger persons. Similarly, in geriatric rehabilitation there are some fundamental differences which are commonly encountered. It is important for the clinician to recognize these differences and adapt the rehabilitation program accordingly. These differences belong to four categories: those that are (1) patient-specific, (2) provider-specific, (3) environment-specific, and (4) goal-specific.

PATIENT-SPECIFIC DIFFERENCES

Those differences that relate to the patient can be further divided into those that are age-related and those that are disease-related. Because geriatrics recognizes that the patient's abilities are a function of the interplay among the biologic, psychologic, and social realms of life, these areas are discussed specifically (Fig. 1-3).

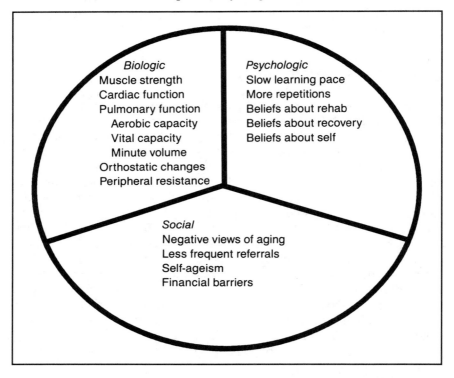

Figure 1-3. Age-related changes that may affect rehabilitation. Normal changes of age, or common problems faced by elderly persons, may affect their performance in a rehabilitation program.

Age Related Changes

Biologic. There is some controversy over the degree of physiologic change that is expressly age-related as opposed to disease-related. Most investigators agree, however, that certain changes in muscle strength, and in cardiac and pulmonary function are so common that they may be thought of as typical. Because rehabilitation often involves intense exercise programs these changes are likely to affect the older person. Aerobic capacity (VO_2 max) decreases with advancing age.[43] Declines in aerobic capacity are probably even greater in the patient who has become deconditioned during a recent hospital stay or had poor exercise habits prior to developing a disability. Exercise capacity may be further affected by decreases in vital capacity and minute volume.[28] With age, lean muscle mass decreases as does muscle strength.[44] Orthostatic hypotension is frequently seen, particularly in those recently bed-bound. Lastly, peripheral vascular resistance rises with age, increasing the risk of developing hypertensive episodes with new exercise programs.

Psychologic. Functionally significant changes in cognitive function are not normal. However, certain normal changes may affect the older person's participation in a rehabilitation program. A slower pace of learning may need to be provided and more repetitions of the activity may be necessary to "strengthen" learning.[21] The patient may have strong ideas concerning the place of exercise in his or her life. Personality remains rather stable throughout age.[13] A person's negative viewpoint regarding the ability to recover from major losses may impede the learing process. Older persons are less likely to believe that they will be able to recover from a disabling condition and are more likely to believe that they do not have enough time left to adjust.[27]

Social. Perhaps the most significant age-related social phenomenon is the existence of ageism. As Abdellah notes, "Chronological age in and of itself can be a factor that causes a person not to meet criteria of eligibility for rehabilitation services."[1] Health care professionals may mistakenly try to protect older persons by not referring them for rehabilitation services due to fears of their failing or being harmed. In spite of the high prevalence of disability in this population, less than 5 percent of the caseloads of departments of rehabilitation are persons over the age of 65.[6]

Unfortunately, these ageist views may even be held by older persons. They may feel they don't deserve rehabilitation services or that the money should be spent on younger persons. Older persons may be on fixed incomes and may not be able to purchase rehabilitation services that are not covered by Medicare.

Disease-Related Changes

Types of disease-related changes are given in Figure 1-4.

Biologic. Unlike younger persons seen in rehabilitation, older persons are much more likely to have multiple diseases. In a study of community-dwelling elderly Hispanics, 40 percent had more than four medical

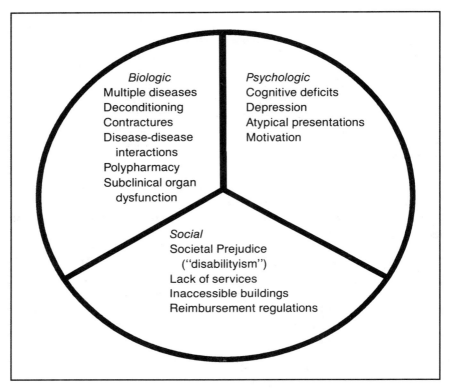

Figure 1-4. Disease-related changes that may affect rehabilitation. Underlying or premorbid conditions will affect the person's rehabilitation program.

problems.[34] Inpatient rehabilitation programs often receive their referrals from acute hospitals where the older person may have been bedbound for many days, becoming severely deconditioned, losing strength, or developing contractures. A 20-degree knee flexion contracture increases the energy costs of walking by 35 percent.[30] This level of increased demand may be enough to tax the reserve of a person with subclinical coronary insufficiency. The person with underlying pulmonary disease may be significantly stressed during a poststroke gait training program. Because oxygen consumption increases with the use of upper extremity walking aids, or even the use of a wheelchair, such a person may decompensate if not closely followed. Following a stroke the older person will have approximately twice the normal energy expenditure when walking with a hemiparetic gait.[30] Preexisting upper extremity osteoarthritis may limit the use of a cane following a hip fracture. It is a rare patient in geriatric rehabilitation that has only his or her disabling disease with which to contend. Hence, the potential for disease interactions is great. Similarly, multiple diseases are treated with multiple medications, further increasing the chance for adverse developments.

Psychologic. Both cognitive and affective problems often go undetected in medical and rehabilitation settings.[18,35] Their cognitive deficits may go unnoticed in the acute hospital because they are not taxed intellectually in that setting. In fact, quiet, nonassertive patients are often deemed to be "good" patients. Depression is frequently found in patients being evaluated for or provided with rehabilitation services. Such patients may state that they don't want to be a "bother" to others or may present more subtly with decreased energy, lack of interest in activities, or decreased participation in therapeutic exercises. As many as 50 percent of patients develop depression following a stroke.[12] In another study 28 percent of all rehabilitation patients were clinically depressed and half of these had depressive histories which antedated their disability.[17] All geriatric patients being evaluated for rehabilitation should have their cognitive and affective states assessed. Periodic reevaluations are also recommended.

Practitioners of rehabilitation frequently encounter the person with "low motivation." In rehabilitation settings low motivation often means that the patient won't do what the clinician wants him or her to do. True motivation refers to what the patient wants (or doesn't want) to do. The person who refuses to exercise may simply be more motivated to stay in bed. In other words, the patient is actually quite motivated!

Motivation can be evaluated in a comprehensive fashion by looking at the various components of decision making that influence a person's choices and effort.[26] These components can be illustrated by the following equation:

$$\text{Motivation} = \frac{W \times B \times R}{C}$$

Where in order to understand a person's motivation one must know what the individual really wants (W), what he or she believes (B) will occur if their goal is to be achieved, and what rewards (R) are likely to be garnered. These factors are in turn influenced by the costs (C), physically, economically, emotionally, or socially. Thus motivation is highest when the person clearly wants the intervention, believes that it will be of benefit, receives a modicum of positive rewards (the sooner the better), and has relatively low costs.

Aging may affect motivation. Older persons often make choices that tend toward the status quo, avoid taking risks in new situations, require more time to make decisions, and try to avoid the cost of failure.[26] Because of these changes the older person may appear less motivated. The clinician can help by providing explanations as to the reasons for a particular activity, by projecting a nonjudgmental attitude, and by allowing for more time to practice.

Social. As defined above, when society prevents people from functioning at their highest level they are handicapped. Many disabled people feel that the major impact of a disability is social.[19] Adjustment to the social consequences of a disability may be the most difficult task faced by the older person. This area requires the greatest degree of adaptation. Much of the physical and psychologic adaptation to a disability is accomplished in the first 2 years after the disabling problem begins. But social adaptation must continue throughout a person's lifetime. Every time the person with a stroke confronts a set of steps without a rail, or the person who uses a wheelchair encounters a curb without a ramp, or the deconditioned patient is refused rehabilitation services, the social consequences of disability are felt more strongly. Reimbursement regulations that limit availability of rehabilitation interventions due to a person's age or place of residency (e.g., a nursing home) have the effect of erecting a handicapping barrier that prevents achievement of the person's full potential.

PROVIDER-SPECIFIC DIFFERENCES

The providers of rehabilitation must also function differently when working with geriatric clients. Some of these differences include the overlap of roles, the emphasis on not missing opportunities to intervene on the patient's behalf and the need to be aware of ageist attitudes that affect decision making.

The roles of providers often overlap in geriatric settings. An example of such an overlap is seen when both a geriatrician and a physiatrist are caring for the patient. In some settings, geriatricians are called upon to coordinate rehabilitation interventions in outpatient settings or in areas where there are no physiatrists. In other settings the geriatrician may have to advocate for the patient to receive services. A solution that emphasizes both disciplines is seen when the geriatrician manages the complex, multiple medical problems while the physiatrist coordinates the interventions of the rehabilitation team.

Other providers' roles may overlap as well. Nurses may provide counseling services to the patient or family,[20] psychologists may make recommendations regarding psychotropic medication, and occupational or speech therapists participate in cognitive evaluations. These kinds of experiences have both positive and negative effects. On the one hand, the sharing of divergent views and the opportunity to provide interventions from different orientations offers a greater chance of meeting the patient's needs. This diversity may also help the providers from experiencing burnout. On the other hand, the team must provide an open forum for discussion so that the other providers can be aware of the treatments that the patient is receiving from other professionals. These forums take time and create the possibility that discord over "turf" encroachments will surface. The most effective rehabilitation team is the one that encourages the expression of the full potential of individual team members. This type of interchange is crucial in geriatric rehabilitation where patients have multiple problems and psychosocial issues predominate.

One must be careful to not miss opportunities to enable the patient to make even small gains in independence. The process of adjusting to a disability is made more difficult with the addition of advanced age, loss of family members, or preexisting medical problems. Enjoyable games and fun, physical activities done in a group setting, may be more acceptable and accomplish more in regaining range of motion or strength than a rigorous training program. Recreational therapy can sometimes enable a patient to remove attention from his or her "performance" and progress and still accomplish worthwhile goals. During an inpatient stay a therapeutic pass may offer the patient a chance to feel independent and become more aware of the value of hospital-based therapies. A prosthetic limb used for cosmetic purposes may allow the amputee to feel more comfortable in the community, thereby promoting a sense of self-respect.

Finally, each provider must prevent potentially ageist attitudes from influencing decisions regarding rehabilitation. For some, age itself is a deterrent to rehabilitation. Yet there is little evidence supporting this bias. Age has not been shown to be detrimental in stroke rehabilitation,[3] and even those over age 85 can benefit from rehabilitation interventions.[36] Rehabilitation is cost-effective in the elderly.[7] Unfortunately, negative attitudes toward elderly persons are common in the rehabilitation fields.[10,37] Therefore the team leader must assess all decisions regarding cessation (or refusal) of therapy as to the possibility that "therapeutic hopelessness" is developing.

ENVIRONMENT-SPECIFIC DIFFERENCES

The interaction between the person and his or her environment becomes potentially more precarious as one ages. These interactions are affected by the person's underlying physical status, his or her living surroundings, and the social systems. Of course, all persons interact with their environment. As one ages, however, the physiologic reserves, underlying medical problems, affective states, and a host of other factors complicate the relationship between the person and his or her environment.

The response of rehabilitation providers is to manipulate the environment to make it "safer." Assistive walking devices or modifications of the home may be recommended. But even these interventions are subject to differences when dealing with aging persons. The older person with a disability may view such aids as unattractive or demeaning. Unlike eyeglasses, where the "disabled" person can choose a pair that enhances his or her appearance, walkers or chrome-plated grab bars may project an image of illness and disability. The older person may have difficulty finding family members or friends who can install home modifications. Some retired senior volunteer programs (RSVPs) have carpenters available for this purpose,[24] but many communities are without such support services.

Another "environment" where personal conflicts may arise is in the area of reimbursement policies. Currently Medicare reimbursement guidelines require those undergoing acute rehabilitation to receive 3 hours per day, 6 days a week, of combined physical, occupational, or speech therapies. Some geriatric patients are physically taxed by such a demanding program and could benefit from a less intensive schedule. Of interest is the evidence that persons receiving the 3-hour intervention don't improve significantly over those receiving less and the costs are higher![23] A 2-week trial of rehabilitation is often provided to geriatric patients when completely accurate predictions of recovery are impossible. However, the hospital may not be reimbursed if the patient is discharged to a nursing home despite an improvement in functional status. It is more difficult to obtain funding to equip a geriatric patient's car with hand controls than in the case of younger patients. These problems may lead to a decision not to provide rehabilitation services based on the likelihood of being reimbursed rather than on the likelihood of improvement.

GOAL-SPECIFIC DIFFERENCES

There are also differences seen in deciding upon the goals of rehabilitation when working with geriatric patients. Patients may have difficulty establishing their own goals because of beliefs that persons their age cannot recover or adapt to a disability. Family members may be quite elderly themselves and be uncertain about their capacity to carry out the goals of the home program. Providers also experience goal modifications when working with older persons. For instance, the concern of the physical therapist working with an older person with a gait disturbance is often centered on the patient's safety. Yet for some older person it may be better to walk "incorrectly" than to not walk at all. Such decisions are heavily value-laden. The older person may be willing to take the risk of a fall rather than be placed in a nursing home. Many older persons fear the loss of independence more than they fear death. Another example is seen when the geriatrician advocates for the patient with a fractured hip to receive a more aggressive surgical intervention that will promote early ambulation rather than one that is associated with prolonged immobility or non–weight bearing. The ultimate goal in geriatric rehabilitation is to promote independence, as defined by the patient.

REHABILITATION IN DIFFERENT CARE SITES

Rehabilitation interventions can be provided in a multitude of sites. These include the home, outpatient or inpatient settings, and the nursing home.

An ideal site for providing rehabilitation is the patient's home. Transportation problems are minimal and services can be rendered at lower costs than in hospitals.[22] Medicare reimburses for some in-home services provided by nursing, physical, and occupational therapies. In the home one can assess the patient's ability to function with available equipment, the supportiveness of the environment, and the degree of carryover of techniques learned. Patients treated in a home program obtain the greatest degree of functional improvement from home modifications, the next best improvement from instruction in the proper use of assistive aids, and the least from exercises.[32] The ideal patient for home care is one judged to be able to benefit from rehabilitation in outpatient settings but unable to attend clinics due to transportation difficulties, limited endurance, psychologic reasons, or personal preference.

Outpatient rehabilitation centers take a variety of forms: physician's offices, private physical (and occupational) therapy practices, certified outpatient rehabilitation facilities (CORFs), day health centers, and hospital-affiliated facilities. The advantages of such facilities are easier access to a wider variety of practitioners and technology, stimulation of being around other people (a disadvantage to some patients), and more patients are able to be served by fewer practitioners. The disadvantage of needing to provide transportation to the clinic is often a major problem when dealing with the very old.

The potential negative effects of acute hospitalization on the elderly person are well-known.[45] Functional disability is often overlooked. Over 50 percent of patients in the acute hospital setting have difficulties with

ADLs, and the hospital environment may interfere with functional recovery.[49] Hence, the potential for rehabilitation may go unrecognized. Some hospitals have begun to provide a free one-time rehabilitation consultation for older patients to help "case-find" those with modifiable disabilities. It is important to obtain early allied health consultation as well as discharge planning so that the patient in need of rehabilitation receives preventive interventions while awaiting more intensive interventions. Except when absolutely necessary patients should spend a large portion of time out of their beds, walk to the bathroom or to diagnostic studies, and receive encouragement to dress and feed themselves.

The rehabilitation hospital may be freestanding or affiliated with an acute hospital. In this type of facility the team, as described above, is composed of the full complement of rehabilitation specialists. A physiatrist (or in the case of some geriatric rehabilitation units, a geriatrician) is usually the team leader. In order to receive Medicare reimbursement, patients must undergo 3 hours per day of physical, occupational, or speech therapy. As of 1988, most of these units are not subject to the Diagnostic Related Group (DRG) prospective payment system. However, documentation requirements are strict and to receive reimbursement patients must make regular progress toward specific goals. Regular team meetings are used to document progress. Some rehabilitation centers are beginning to specialize with the creation of geriatrics, geriatric-ortho,[41] stroke,[16] and assessment units.[4] The effectiveness of geriatric rehabilitation,[25,33,46] as well as the fact that age need not be a deterrent to providing rehabilitation, has been documented.[3,36]

The nursing home is an important site for rehabilitation. For patients requiring physical or occupational therapy Medicare funding can be obtained. In selected patients the costs are less than those of acute care or intensive rehabilitation and the results are encouraging.[47] In a study by Reed and Gessner, 17 percent of patients were able to return home.[38] Some patients in the community may be unable to take part in the rigorous training schedule required in intensive rehabilitation facilities. The nursing home offers the opportunity for community-based patients to receive rehabilitation. Adelman reported that 57 percent of the patients that came from their homes to the nursing home for rehabilitation were able to return home.[2]

SUMMARY

Rehabilitation is a process that is not determined by the specific diagnosis nor the type of facility where services are provided. The prime goal of rehabilitation is to promote independent living, as defined by the patient. When working with older persons rehabilitation specialists need to be aware of a number of factors which make caring for the elderly more complex, challenging, and fulfilling.

REFERENCES

1. Abdellah, F.G. (1986). Public health aspects of rehabilitation of the aged. In S.J. Brody and G.E. Ruff (Eds.), *Aging and rehabilitation. Advances in the state of the art* (pp. 47–61). New York: Springer.
2. Adelman, R.D. et al. (1987). A community-oriented geriatric rehabilitation unit in a nursing home. *Gerontologist,, 27,* 143.
3. Adler, M.K., Brown, C.C., and Acton, P. (1980). Stroke rehabilitation—is an age determinant? *J. Am. Geriatr. Soc., 28,* 499.
4. Applegate, W.B., et al. (1983). A geriatric rehabilitation and assessment unit in a community hospital. *J. Am. Geriatr. Soc. 31,* 206.
5. Avorn, J. (1982). Induced disability in nursing home patients. *J. Am. Geriatr. Soc. 30,* 397.
6. Benedict, R.C., and Ganikos, M.L. (1981). Coming to terms with ageism is rehabilitation. *J. Rehabil., 47,* 19.
7. Bennett, A.E. (1980). Cost-effectiveness of rehabilitation for the elderly: Preliminary results from the community hospital research program. *Gerontologist, 20,* 284.
8. Brody, E. (1986). Informal support systems in the rehabilitation of the disabled elderly. In S.J. Brody and G.E. Ruff (Eds.), *Aging and rehabilitation: Advances in the state of the art* (pp. 87–104). New York: Springer.
9. Brummel-Smith, K. (1988). Family science and rehabilitation. *Top. Geriatr. Rehabil., 4,* 1.
10. Burdman, G.D.M. (1974). Student and trainee attitudes on aging. *Gerontologist, 14,* 65.
11. Clark, G., Blue, B., and Bearer, J. (1983). Rehabilitation of the elderly amputee. *J. Am. Geriatr. Soc., 31,* 439.
12. Collin, S.J., and Lincoln, N.D. (1987). Depression after stroke, *Clin. Rehabil., 1,* 27.
13. Costa, P.T., and McCrae, R.R. (1984). Concurrent validation after 20 years: The implications of personality stability for its assessment. *Adv. Pers. Assess., 4,* 2.
14. Enright, R.B., and Friss, L. (1987). Employed care-givers of brain-damaged adults: An assessment of the dual role. Unpublished, 1987.
15. Federal Council on the Aging. (1981). *The need for long-term care. A chartbook of the Federal Council on Aging.* U.S. Dept. of Health and Human Services publication No. (OHDS) 81-20704, 29, Government Printing Office.
16. Feigenson, J.S., Gitlow, H.S., and Greenberg, S.D. (1979). The disability oriented rehabilitation unit—a major factor influencing stroke outcome. *Stroke, 10,* 5–8.
17. Gans, J.S. (1981). Depression diagnosis in a rehabilitation hospital. *Arch. Phys. Med. Rehabil. 62,* 386.
18. Garcia, C.A., Tweedy, J.R., and Blass, J.P. (1984). Underdiagnosis of cognitive impairment in a rehabilitation setting. *J. Am. Geriatr. Soc. 32,* 339.

19. Gill, C. (1984). Social aspects of disability. Geriatric rehabilitation grand rounds presentation, Rancho Los Amigos Medical Center, Downey, CA.
20. Hamberger, S.G., and Tanner, R.D. (1988). Nursing intervention with families of geriatric patients. Top. Geriatr. Rehabil., 4, 32.
21. Huyck, M.H., and Hoyer, W.J. (1982) Memory. In Adult development and aging (pp. 134–159). Belmont, CA; Wadsworth.
22. Jarnlo, G.B., Ceder, L., and Thorngren, K.G. (1984). Early rehabilitation at home of elderly patients with hip fractures and consumption of resources in primary care. Scand. J. Primary Health Care, 2, 105.
23. Johnston, M.V., and Miller, L.S. (1986). Cost-effectiveness of the Medicare three-hour regulation. Arch. Phys. Med. Rehabil. 67, 581.
24. Johnston, R.B., Director, Humboldt County Retired Senior Volunteer Program. Personal communication, 1987.
25. Keith, R.A., Breckenridge, K., and O'Neil, W.A. (1977). Rehabilitation hospital patient characteristics from the hospital utilization project system. Arch. Phys. Med. Rehabil., 58, 260.
26. Kemp, B. (1986). Psychosocial and mental health issues in rehabilitation of older persons. In S.J. Brody and G.E. Ruff (Eds.), Aging and rehabilitation; Advances in the state of the art (pp. 122–158). New York: Springer.
27. Kemp, B. (1986). Psychosocial and mental health issues in rehabilitation of older persons. In S.J. Brody and G.E. Ruff (Eds.), Aging and rehabilitation; Advances in the state of the art (pp. 122–158). New York: Springer.
28. Kohn, R. (1978). Principles of mammalian aging, (p. 169). Englewood Cliffs, NJ: Prentice Hall.
29. Kumar, V.N., and Redford, J.B. (1984). Rehabilitation of hip fractures in the elderly. Am. Fam. Physician, 29, 173.
30. Lehman, J.F. (1971). Gait analysis: Diagnosis and management. In F.J. Kotke (Ed.), Krusen's handbook of physical medicine and rehabilitation (pp. 86–101). Philadelphia, Saunders.
31. Lehman, J.F., et al. (1975). Stroke: Does rehabilitation affect outcome? Arch. Phys. Med. Rehabil. 56, 375.
32. Liang, M.H., et al: Evaluation of comprehensive rehabilitation services for elderly homebound patients with arthritis and orthopedic disability. Arthritis Rheum., 27, 258.
33. Liem, P.H., Chernoff, R., and Carter, W.J. (1986). Geriatric rehabilitation Unit: A 3 year outcome. J. Gerontol. 41, 44.
34. Lopez-Aqueres, W., Kemp, B., Plopper, M., Staples, F., and Brummel-Smith, K. (1984). Health needs of Hispanic elderly. J. Am. Geriatr. Soc. 32, 191.
35. McCartney, J.R., and Palmateer, L.M. (1984). Assessment of cognitive deficit in geriatric patients. J. Am. Geriatr. Soc. 33, 467.
36. Parry F. (1983). Physical rehabilitation of the old, old patient. J. Am. Geriatr. Soc., 31, 482.
37. Rasch, J.D., Crystal, R.M., and Thomas, K.R. (1977). The perception of the older adult: A study of trainee attitudes. J. Appl. Rehabil. Counseling, 8, 121.
38. Reed, J.W., and Gessner, J.E. (1979). Rehabilitation in the extended care facility. J. Am. Geriatr. Soc., 27, 325.
39. Rubenstein, L.Z., Josephson, K.R., and Gurland, B. (1984). Effectiveness of a geriatric evaluation unit: A randomized trial. N. Engl. J. Med. 311, 1664.
40. Ryback, R.S., Lewis, O.F., and Lessard, C.S. (1971). Physiologic effects of prolonged bed rest (weightless) in young, health/volunteers (Study 11). Aerospace Med., 42, 529.

41. Sainsbury, R., et al. (1986). An orthopedic geriatric rehabilitation unit: the first two years experience. *N.Z. Med. J., 99,* 583.
42. Sharpless, J.W. (1982). *Mossman's problem oriented approach to stroke rehabilitation.* Springfield, IL, Thomas.
43. Shepard, R.J. (1966). World standards of cardiorespiratory performance. *Arch. Environ. Health, 13,* 664.
44. Shock, N.W., and Norris, A.H. (1970). Neuromuscular coordination as a factor in age changes in muscular exercise. In D. Brunner and E. Jokl (Eds.), *Physical Activity and Aging* (pp. 166–179). Karger, Basel.
45. Steel, K., et al. (1981). Iatrogenic illness on a general medical service at a university hospital. *N. Engl. J. Med., 304,* 638.
46. Strax, T.E., and Ledebur, J. (1979). Rehabilitating the geriatric patient: Potential and limitations. *Geriatrics, 34,* 99.
47. Sutton, M.A. (1986). "Homeward bound": a minimal care rehabilitation unit. *Br. Med. J., 293,* 319.
48. *National survey of stroke.* U.S. Dept. of Health, Education, and Welfare publication No. (NIH) 80-2064, 6–7, 1980.
49. Warshaw, G, et al. (1982). Functional disability in the hospitalized elderly. *JAMA, 248,* 847.
50. Wedgewood, J. (1985). The place of rehabilitation in geriatric medicine: An overview. *Int. Rehabil. Med. 7,* 107.
51. Williams, T.F. Keynote speech, Aging and Rehabilitation Conference, Philadelphia, PA, Dec. 2, 1984.

CHAPTER 2

A Rehabilitation Orientation in the Workup of General Medical Problems

JOSEPH W. RAMSDELL

The prevalence of disability increases with advancing age such that 60 percent of the population 85 years and older have disabilities which impose some limitations on their daily activities.[9] Furthermore, the nature of assistance that people 65 and older need to deal with these limitations falls into categories not commonly included in the traditional medical model. Physicians do not routinely think in terms of homemaking, administrative, legal assistance, or transportation problems when assessing elderly patients. But these are among the major types of help required by the elderly in their daily lives.[1] The problem of dealing with disability in the elderly is going to be even more important as the number of people 85 and older continues to grow. Primary care physicians are increasingly going to be required to deal with elderly patients who have disabilities.[20]

It is important for primary care physicians to understand and utilize rehabilitation principles and methods when caring for the elderly. It is equally important that rehabilitation specialists understand the primary care perspective and work closely with primary care physicians in the care of patients in their rehabilitation programs. Differences between these approaches may be more apparent than real but ignorance or misunderstanding of the relative roles of these disciplines can lead to therapeutic nihilism or neglect, thereby depriving many elderly patients of optimal treatment of their impairments. This chapter explores the similarities and differences between the primary care and rehabilitation models and the ways in which an integrated approach applies to the care of the geriatric patient. Since primary care practice is largely outpatient, this chapter highlights the ambulatory aspects of these issues.

ELEMENTS OF PRIMARY CARE

Primary care is composed of several key elements. Ideally, it is the primary care physician who is the individual patient's point of contact with the healthy care system. The main thrust of primary care goes beyond assisting patients with acute problems to focus on continuity of medical care. The dimensions of continuity have been defined and include the following:[8,16]

1. Chronologic—Primary care involves following patients over time with repeated assessment of the patient's condition.
2. Geographic—The primary care doctor-patient relationship continues regardless of the setting in which it occurs, that is, home, clinic, hospital, nursing home, day care center, or day hospital.
3. Interdisciplinary—Primary care often crosses traditional medical disciplines and the primary care physician must understand and relate to those professions appropriate to the patient's needs.
4. Interpersonal—Primary care involves understanding and maintaining relationships, that is, doctor-patient, family, interprofessional.
5. Informational—Primary care is concerned with the availability and completeness of the record of patient care and a smooth flow of information between the patient, primary physician, and others on the health care team.
6. Accessibility—Primary care is responsive to patient needs at all hours.
7. Stability—Primary care fosters a stable home and community environment for patient care.

The second major feature of primary care is comprehensiveness, that is, attending to the full spectrum of patient needs. Comprehensive care includes preventive and curative care; it is concerned with psychologic, social, economic, family, and other factors which impact on the patient's well-being.[15] This means that the primary care physician continues to maintain an active role as the health care manager for patients as they move through the different phases of their illness and through different care settings. It also implies a recognition of factors beyond the usual medical parameters which can impact on a patient's well-being. This approach is especially important when dealing with older patients.

In a simplistic model that defines health as the absence of disease, the physician's traditional goals center on diagnosis and cure. The primary care paradigm likewise recognizes the importance of a cure, when possible, but moves away from the binary concept of either sickness or health and considers an individual's state of well-being along a continuum with the theoretical state of perfect health, free of any disease or impairment, at one extreme and death at the other. During most of their lives normal people are functioning in the good health domain, but the body is constantly adjusting to internal and external perturbations. When these perturbations lead to significant impairment, illness results and, usually, a physician is consulted.

This model recognizes the importance of health maintenance, and the diagnosis and treatment of self-limiting and chronic illness in a person's daily existence. It places high value on an organized and thorough evaluation of presenting complaints, but also emphasizes case-finding and health maintenance as part of the doctor-patient encounter. This view of health and the principal of continuity of care means that primary care physicians must be adept at the management of chronic disease. In this paradigm, cure is not always an end in and of itself and the management of persistent and recurrent problems becomes increasingly important. The goals of management in chronic disease are to minimize distress, optimize function, and avoid impairment. In this respect, the primary care approach is consistent with the realities of both geriatric medicine and rehabilitation.

THE REHABILITATION APPROACH IN PRIMARY CARE

Rehabilitation can be viewed from several perspectives, but the unifying concept in all interpretations is the importance of a functional orientation.[13] Indeed, the preservation of function is the ultimate goal of any rehabilitation effort. The second major consistent principle is a comprehensive approach to patient disabilities incorporating a team approach.[13] Both of these concepts are also central to primary care of geriatric patients.

Function is the key to this approach. Function is determined by a number of factors, no one of which is usually predominant.[21] Physical factors clearly define certain functional limitations. Psychologic factors can play a predominant role in functional disability in a number of patients. Social and economic issues, likewise, play a profound role in determining the patient's ability to function. It is the interaction of these factors which ultimately determines the patient's functional status.

Because the elements of function subsume the expertise of many disciplines, rehabilitation is built on the team model to achieve comprehensive care. While some aspects of a rehabilitation approach to primary care can be implemented by the physician and patient working together, most of the benefits result from the concerted application of skills of several other disciplines. As discussed in Chapter 24, rehabilitation programs routinely utilize interdisciplinary teams and the primary care physician may access these skills by referring patients to an interdisciplinary team or build a multidisciplinary team on an ad hoc basis depending on the patient' needs. Either way a clear understanding of the training, skills, and objectives of the rehabilitation professions is critical.

The rehabilitation disciplines include the following:

Physiatrist: The physiatrist has had special training in the area of physical medicine and rehabilitation including diagnosis, assessment, and treatment of musculoskeletal impairments; pain evaluation; mobility defects; and muscle weakness. The physiatrist's experience in physical treatment modalities such as the use of heat and cold, hydrotherapy, electrical stimulation, traction, exercise, and biofeedback can be very helpful in the management of chronic musculoskeletal problems.

Physical therapist: The physical therapist is trained to evaluate and treat musculoskeletal disorders using physical treatment modalities. This training enables the therapist to assess physical capabilities in a systematic fashion and administer treatments designed to address physical impairments and improve or maintain function.[12] The physical therapist's main orientation is toward restoration or maintenance of mobility and deals with problems affecting major joints, the back, and overall conditioning issues.

Occupational therapist: The occupational therapist is trained to assess and treat functional impairments in activities of daily living (ADLs). This includes working on fine motor activities, especially in the upper extremities. The occupational therapist works on exercises and devices which allow patients to relearn lost skills or master new ones. The occupational therapist is familiar with adaptive equipment (e.g., one-hand shoe tie, modified eating utensils) and splints or other supports which allow patients to accomplish skilled activities in spite of physical impairments. Finally, occupational therapists are skilled at using the various scales and instruments available for formally assessing ADLs.

Nurse: Whether on an inpatient rehabilitation service or in the home, the nurse plays a central role in the rehabilitation process. It is the nurse who usually oversees the rehabilitation program and reviews it in the context of the patient's other medical and functional problems. Assessing the home is of critical importance in addressing functional issues in outpatients, and the visiting nurse is in a key position to carry out home evaluations. The nurse's initial assessment is the starting point for organizing in-home rehabilitation and his or her continuing assessments chart the patient's progress. On the inpatient service the nurse's ongoing contact with inpatients provides the most constant opportunity for reinforcement of rehabilitation goals and techniques and the nurse is responsible for assessing postdischarge home care needs.

Social worker: The social worker's training in community resources, human behavior, and family dynamics allows him or her to evaluate the patient's social and psychologic situation, living arrangements, family structure, financial resources, mental abilities, social skills, values, and expectations. The social worker can then provide counseling or suggest financial resources and community services, and work with the patient, the patient's family, the primary care physician, and other members of the health care team to implement the management plan.

Clinical psychologist: The clinical psychologist usually has a Ph.D and is trained to assess intelligence, personality, cognitive skills, and perceptual-motor skill. This may include administering and analyzing standard neuropsychologic tests. He or she can then proceed to work with patients to help them adjust to illness or disability.

Home health aides and homemakers: These health care professionals are generally available from home health agencies and can be invaluable in providing supportive services in the patient's home. They perform a range of services from home management and personal hygiene to simple housecleaning.[34] Home health aides provide personal care and simple household chores. Their training usually involves at least 40 hours of classwork and in-service training. Homemakers assist with household tasks only and have no training in personal care.

Nutritionist: The nutritionist should play an important role in both inpatient and outpatient rehabilitation programs. He or she can assess the patient for nutritional adequacy and plan corrective diets which are palatable and consistent with the patient's capabilities. The nutritionist may also suggest ways to deal with the impact of disabilities on grocery shopping, cooking, eating in restaurants, etc.

Speech therapist: The speech therapist or language pathologist is trained to evaluate and treat mechanical or neurologic problems with speech, hearing, and swallowing.

A number of other professionals may be required in dealing with an individual patient's impairments. Neurologist, psychiatrist, ophthalmologist, urologist, and other physicians, as well as the prosthetist, orthotist, vocational counselor, podiatrist, audiologist, and others all play a role in developing and implementing a rehabilitation plan. By using a constant set of consultants the primary care physician can develop shared values and consistent approaches to patient problems that will ensure both continuity of care and a comprehensive approach to the problem.

REHABILITATION TERMINOLOGY

It is important for primary care physicians to understand the nuances of language associated with rehabilitation medicine and the nature of the problems. These have been described in detail in Chapter 1 and are summarized below:

Impairment refers to any loss or abnormality of psychologic, physiologic, or anatomic structure or function independent of etiology or activity of disease process. Impairment, therefore, is the difficulty in organ functioning that results directly from the illness.

Disability refers to any restriction or lack of ability to perform an activity in the manner or within the range considered normal for a person of the same age, culture, and education. This may be temporary or permanent and is independent of type of impairment. The concept of a disability moves beyond psychologic or physiologic dysfunction and considers the effect of the dysfunction in terms of more integrative aspects of behavior and of the individual compared to his or her prior functional status and to normal persons in his or her peer group.

Handicap is a disadvantage for a given individual that limits or prevents the fulfillment of a role in society that is normal for a person of his or her age, sex, social status, etc. This is a societal issue which may or may not relate directly to true impairment or disability. A handicap is a social disadvantage.[14]

A rehabilitation approach to geriatric primary care incorporates a focus on the ability to function effectively in the various aspects of life. Implicitly, the primary care model addresses not only the illness but also the impaired function. The concept of health as a relative position along a continuum is compatible with the disability model popular in rehabilitation. This model views disability as a continuum from pathology through impairment and functional limitation to disability.[31] Patients can move in either direction along either of these continua and the purpose of medical treatment is to minimize the effects of disease (i.e., impairment) in each. Each phase of the disability model reflects a position on the primary care continuum. If the pathologic condition can be addressed and eliminated (i.e., cured), then the disability is eliminated. That failing, the primary care geriatrician focuses on the other phases of the disability model, and rehabilitation principles become important. Both the primary care model and the rehabilitation model, therefore, do not limit themselves to dealing with the cause and management of physical problems but also seek to contend with the functional impact of the problem(s).

In summary, the major changes that a rehabilitation approach brings to primary care is a more explicit focus on the patient's ability to function in various aspects of his or her life regardless of the underlying problem and on an intrinsic reliance on the interdisciplinary or multidisciplinary health care team.

ASSESSMENT OF GERIATRIC PATIENTS IN PRIMARY CARE

The scope of responsibilities that flow from the primary care model are encompassed in the major elements of health maintenance, diagnosis, and treatment. Augmenting the primary care approach with a strong orientation to functional outcomes can impact on every phase of primary care practice.

HEALTH MAINTENANCE IN THE ELDERLY

Prevention of functional limitation begins with classic preventive medicine and health maintenance in the elderly, both traditional aspects of primary care. Safety counseling, attention to hypertension, cholesterol level, and so forth are perfectly rational extensions of the concept of maintaining function and are activities that the primary care physician is uniquely positioned to accomplish. These issues have been reviewed in detail elsewhere[25] and a comprehensive discussion is beyond the scope of this chapter.

DIAGNOSTIC ASSESSMENT

It is important to differentiate the signs of aging from the signs of disease when assessing patients. Age-related changes do not lead to illness. Physiologic reserves diminish with advancing age but remain adequate, and normal persons are able to function at a very effective level unless disease intervenes.

Accurate diagnosis of the primary complaint remains central to a functionally oriented primary care approach. It is absolutely critical that the patient's medical problems be clearly defined and well understood. But the introduction of a functional orientation brings new meaning to the assessment routine of primary care. Because functional ability is determined by a number of factors, the assessment process must go beyond simply making an etiologic diagnosis. Coexisting problems that may limit the ability to deal directly with the principal complaint or which dictate options for treatment or rehabilitation must be carefully evaluated through an organized system of case-finding. Both primary and coexisting problems need to be assessed from several different perspectives. The cause of the problem must be determined, the level of physiologic or biologic impairment evaluated, and the possibilities of cure or control assessed. The functional approach recognizes, however, that there are other parameters which need to be defined. The social, environmental, and psychologic aspects of the principal and coexisting problems should be considered and evaluated as required.

A careful medical assessment should establish the probable cause of the patient's problem(s). This should include an objective delineation of the degree of physiologic impairment and an estimate of the rate of change. Disability is usually a subjective concept and the physician's perception of disability may differ from that of the patient. An objective estimate of the level of physiologic impairment can help the physician reconcile differences between the physician's and patient's impressions of the level of disability. This type of medical evaluation will also permit prediction as to whether the patient's current level of impairment is likely to improve or not, either on the basis of the natural history of the disease or after treatment.

An equally careful approach to case-finding should accompany the diagnostic evaluation of the principal complaint. Primary care physicians must be familiar with diseases that are prevalent in the elderly and which are the major targets of the medical assessment. The elderly have a disproportionate burden of hypertension, coronary heart disease, other forms of arteriosclerosis, other heat diseases, obstructive lung disease, arthritis, diabetes, urinary problems, visual impairment, hearing impairment, and dental problems. Impairments or treatments of these problems will usually affect management of the principal complaint.

The last three types of impairment deserve special mention. Sensory decline associated with aging is important, but often seems to be beneath the attention of a physician. This attitude is not only improper but potentially dangerous. Age-related impairment of the senses has a direct impact on the quality of life of elderly patients and presents a risk of further disability. A normally functioning elderly person with cataracts may be unable to see potential hazards in his path and fall. It doesn't make any difference that this patient's medical diagnoses are correct and perfectly managed; if he falls because of an unseen impediment in his path and breaks his hip he is likely to be disabled and possibly die as a result of his vision impairment.

The problem of recognizing coexistent illness is difficult in many elderly patients. Unapparent illnesses, usually attributed to age-related changes by patients, their families, or physicians, are common in the elderly and can have an important effect on functional outcomes. It is vital to recognize depression, incontinence, musculoskeletal problems, drug abuse, hearing loss, and dementia because these illnesses can all impair the ability to rehabilitate the patient.

Dementia may be especially elusive in the elderly. Primary care physicians should screen all elderly patients for evidence of cognitive dysfunction during the course of an initial visit. It is important to verify normal mental status in patients who deny thinking or memory problems. This may require only a few simple questions aimed at cognitive status during the course of the history, but should be part of the physician's routine. Often patients develop very successful techniques for hiding cognitive impairment, which becomes apparent only after a careful, but not necessarily extensive, evaluation.

When patients complain of thinking or memory problems, the presence or absence of cognitive impairment must be verified by specific inquiries during the medical history regarding the nature of the problem and by more formal mental status testing. Some patients concerned about memory problems have a normal level of intellectual functioning, and this group deserves identification and cautious reassurance. Structured mental status examinations such as the simple but useful test devised by Kahn and colleagues,[19] the more elaborate Mini-Mental State examination of Folstein, Folstein, and McHugh,[11] and several others listed in Table 2-1 can be helpful in documenting and quantifying cognitive impairment. Such tests are quite useful in the hands of primary care physicians and should be employed with all patients suspected of cognitive impairment. Sophisticated tests of cognitive function, more suitably administered by a psychologist, neurologist, or psychiatrist, may be needed in highly functioning individuals who complain of thought or memory disorders (see Table 2-1).

Table 2-1. *Psychometric Tests Commonly Used to Evaluate Cognitive Function*

SCREENING TESTS USEFUL IN PRIMARY CARE

Blessed Mental Fuld
Mini-Mental State
Goldfarb Modified Kahn
Ward Modified Kahn

PSYCHOMETRIC TESTS WHICH REQUIRE SPECIALIZED TRAINING
TO ADMINISTER AND INTERPRET

Dementia Rating Scale (Mattis)
Boston Naming Test
Wisconsin Card Sorting Test
Bushke Selective Reminding Task
Verbal Fluency Test
Number Information Test
Moss Recognition Span Test
WAIS-P Subtests
WISC-R Blocks
Grip Strength Test
Grooved Pegboard
Clock Drawing Test
Clock Setting Test
Draw-A-Cross Test
Trailmaking Test (A & B)
Copy-A-Cube

Some intellectually gifted patients may have a real decline in cognitive function yet still score in the normal range on screening and more extensive tests (J.W. Ramsdell, H.W. Ward, E. Rockwell, and J.E. Jackson, unpublished observation.). The presence of cognitive impairment in such patients can only be verified prospectively, but their complaints should always be taken seriously. They should be evaluated completely, even if their scores are normal, to rule out treatable causes of preclinical impairment, and followed with repeated testing at appropriate intervals if one wishes to identify the advent of measurable impairment.

ASSESSMENT OF FUNCTION

Functional status is not synonymous with the degree of physical impairment. When the primary care physician assesses functional ability, it is important to determine the degree of impairment posed by individual diseases, to look at the patient's unique assets and liabilities in terms of dealing with that disease process, to understand the impact of these nonmedical factors on the patient's disability, and to recognize handicaps, that is, societal impediments, which result from the patient's disability.[21]

The importance of social and environmental factors in the care of the elderly has led to the development and testing of an array of instruments which assess functional status for use in health care and social research[10,28–30] It has been noted, however, that such instruments are of uncertain value in understanding the problems of an individual patient for the purpose of that patient's care.[36] This problem has been highlighted by a leading expert in the field who suggests that the challenge currently before us is to "assess conveniently and accurately those aspects of social functioning *relevant* to medical care."[22]

Nonetheless, it is important for every primary care physician to be familiar with scales and techniques for assessing various aspects of ADLs and other approaches to assessing functional status. These methods have been reviewed[3,21] and are summarized in Table 2-2. In spite of their weaknesses for patient care purposes, it is important that primary care geriatricians understand the concepts involved in these instruments and be able to apply the concepts and forms when needed in the course of a comprehensive clinical assessment of functional status.

Table 2-2. *Summary of Functional Assessment Scales and Indices* *

Self-care measures	Domains	Assessors	Report Mode	References
Katz ADL (Original)	Eating Bathing Dressing Transfer Continence Toileting	Professional	Performance (subsequently, self-report)	21,23

(continued)

Table 2-2. *(continued)*

Self-care measures	*Domains*	*Assessors*	*Report Mode*	*References*
Modified ADL Scales	Eating Ambulation Bathing Dressing Transfer Personal grooming Continence Toileting	Lay	Self, performance	4,21,23
Barthel Index Performance	Feeding Grooming Transfer Toileting Bathing Walking, locomotion Continence	Professional	Performance	21,27b,33a,38
Rapid Disability Rating Scale	Eating Diet Medication Speech Hearing Sight Ambulation Bathing Dressing Continence Shaving Safety Bedfastness Confusion Cooperation Depression	Professional	Performance	21,27a

ADL = activities of daily living.
Source: From Branch L.B. and Meyers, A.R. (1987). Assessing physical function in the elderly. *Clin. Geriatr. 3*, 29–51.

The clinical assessment of functional status can be compared to the classic diagnostic process used to evaluate disease, that is, the elicitation and analysis of symptoms, signs, and laboratory-derived information.

Functional assessment also makes use of interviewing the patient, observing or examining a patient, and testing a patient using standard scales or instruments. With a transition from evaluating the disease to evaluating impairment and disability, however, the focus shifts. The initial evaluation of the patient's complaints should determine the cause and quantify the physiologic or biochemical ramifications of the disease. The evaluation of disability places this information in a lifestyle context. Performance, rather than cause, is the focus and it is the impact of impairment on the patient's life that is in question. Because of this, the clinical functional assessment goes beyond the physical ability to carry out a procedure or a certain task, and considers the patient's ability to function in the context of his or her home and community.

The actual performance of isolated physical tasks in a laboratory setting may be less important than the patient's perceived capability — how the patient feels he or she can perform in real-life situations. Integrated functional skills define lifestyle and are more important than isolated physical skills, for it is the loss of functional skills which defines disability. History, physical examination, and more sophisticated and integrative approaches to laboratory "tests" such as an occupational (OT) or physical therapy (PT) assessment, home visits, social work assessment, and input from family and community sources are important in assessing the disability that accompanies a patient's medical complaint and in understanding the patient's ability to carry out a task regardless of physical capability.

Minimal social assessment should include the patient's pattern of daily life, abilities and activities of daily living, suitability and safety of the home, attitudes of caregivers and neighbors, availability of emergency health services, transportation, occupational history, and so forth. Financial status must be understood; financial limits can seriously limit the approach to medical treatment.

A careful assessment of the home environment can provide information central to understanding disabilities and developing appropriate management plans. This information may be difficult to obtain during the course of a visit to a clinic or physician's office.[37] A visit to the patient's home, however, offers the opportunity to acquire such information and home visits have been employed for this purpose by geriatric assessment programs in this country and abroad.[7,17,33,35] The home visit has been shown to yield unique information regarding drug history and results in the recognition of new, clinically significant problems and recommendations during the course of geriatric assessment.[18,32]

Social and home evaluations may be especially useful for determining the ability of the patient's caregivers to support a rehabilitation plan and can uncover signs of caregiver stress.[32]

ASSESSING PATIENTS FOR REHABILITATION

When considering a patient for referral to a formal rehabilitation program, there are several points the primary care physician should consider. A good rehabilitation outcome is associated with recent onset of the impairment; less severe disability; an assertive, goal-oriented personality; good family supports; and adequate economic support. A poor prognosis is suggested by a more chronic course, poor patient motivation, cognitive impairment, and a paucity of family or economic support. These factors represent statistical associations and should be considered in evaluation for rehabilitation referral, but may not preclude a good response in individual patients.[5]

Before referring a patient for formal rehabilitation, a comprehensive medical and functional assessment should be completed. In general, the primary care physician should optimize the patient's medical regimen prior to referral. Factors that will influence rehabilitation potential need to be clearly defined. Goals and realistic expectations of the rehabilitation program should be understood by the primary care physician and discussed with the patient prior to referral. It should be stressed that these are preliminary discussions, but patients and their families must have realistic expectations of rehabilitation and agree to the effort and cost involved in the program. These goals may change as the rehabilitation team becomes involved, but a general, informed commitment from the patient at the outset is desirable. Finally, the primary care physician should communicate clearly and concisely the results of the initial assessment and the patient's expectations at the time of referral.

Once the patient has begun the rehabilitation program the primary care physician should continue to be involved and communication becomes a two-way street as the rehabilitation team keeps the referring physician abreast of progress and involved in management decisions.

THE REHABILITATION TEAM AND THE PRIMARY CARE PHYSICIAN

Just as it is imperative for the primary care geriatrician to understand rehabilitation principles and the benefits of interdisciplinary rehabilitation programs, so it is important for rehabilitation programs to understand primary care principles and respect the role of the primary care physician in the overall rehabilitation process. Continuity of care and comprehensive care are as important to the primary care geriatrician as a functional orientation and team approach are to the rehabilitation specialist. The approaches of these disciplines are not only complementary, they are indispensible to each other. The primary care physician must refer patients to rehabilitation programs in a timely and appropriate fashion. On the other hand, the rehabilitation team must work closely with the primary care physician, building on his or her knowledge of the patient and respecting the need for informed, two-way communication and consultation. The primary care physician is an equal partner with the patient and the rehabilitation team in establishing goals and objectives. He or she should be kept abreast of important changes in patient status or treatment approaches. In most situations changes in medications should be supervised by the primary care physician unless responsibility for this has been explicitly transferred to the rehabilitation team. This is not a one-point-in-time process. The importance of careful follow-up and reassessment at given intervals cannot be overstated.

A rehabilitation approach can apply to almost every aspect of primary care. The importance of health maintenance and preventive medicine in maintaining functional status has been discussed. The rehabilitation approach should be applied to most chronic and many acute medical conditions in the elderly. The appropriate disease for the rehabilitation approach in primary care geriatrics is literally any disease that has the potential to become chronic. Taken to its extreme, it can be applied to any patient who is actively aging. Indeed, many of the characteristics of physiologic decline with age mimic those of deconditioning[2] and can be ameliorated by an appropriate exercise program.[6] Health maintenance should include advice or encouragement to avoid deconditioning as a result of inactivity. The techniques and concepts that are embraced by rehabilitation medicine can help many normal elders to lead a more vigorous, satisfying lifestyle.

In elderly patients the rehabilitation approach is also helpful in cases of acute, treatable illness where the chance of lasting disability would seem low. If the patient can be moved quickly from acute disability associated with illness to a normal functioning state by curing that disease, then rehabilitation *may* be a moot point. But even patients with acute, potentially curable illness and convalescence lie on the disability continuum during the acute illness and convalescence. Although the implications for care are less obvious, the application of a functional orientation in the management of such problems in elderly patients can hasten convalescence and prevent the development of complications associated with the illness or treatment. For example, in the management of most pulmonary infections in the elderly, antibiotics can lead to a cure, but functional considerations may require hospitalization or in-home assistance for infections which could be simply treated with antibiotics in younger patients. Likewise, the period of convalescence is likely to be prolonged in elderly patients, a factor which must be considered when arranging for patient support. Striving for cure is always important, but rehabilitation techniques may limit disability associated with convalescence and facilitate prompt return of function.

When prompt or complete cure is not likely, the virtue of a rehabilitation orientation is more apparent and rehabilitation assessment principles should be invoked early in order to plan for the appropriate level of rehabilitation for each phase of the illness, anticipating actions early in the disease that might facilitate later, more formal, rehabilitation. During the acute phase the assessment must be aimed at identifying preexisting impairments or disabilities, risk factors for significant disability associated with the acute illness, and the proper point for the implementation of various rehabilitation techniques. Classic rehabilitation techniques are not likely to be utilized when a patient is acutely ill and the degree or activity of the disease is such that the patient cannot actively participate in a formal rehabilitation program. On the other hand, a concern for maintaining function and preventing complications while treating the acute illness will facilitate rehabilitation when that level of impairment has stabilized. Other chapters in this book address the precise approaches to timing of rehabilitation assessment and techniques in different diseases, but the primary care physician, who is usually the first to see and manage patients in this situation, must be familiar with the approaches to acute management that will lead to optimal functional outcome.

Finally, a rehabilitation approach may prove helpful when dealing with "failure to thrive" in the frail elderly. Here the insidious onset of multisystem disease may render specific disease-oriented therapy useless. A generalized approach combining optimal medical management with rehabilitation principles may be the only way to achieve meaningful gains in functional status and quality of life.

In summary, it is not enough to address the cause and physiologic consequences of a disease in older patients. The primary care physician must also strive to preserve and enhance functional ability. By integrating a rehabilitation approach into the primary care paradigm, one can enable a patient to function effectively within the limitations of his or her illness, despite its cause. It is imperative that primary care physicians understand and use this approach and thereby avoid discriminating against patients in need of rehabilitation because of their age.

REFERENCES

1. Allen, C.A., and Brotman, H. (compilers). (1981). *Chartbook on aging in America.* The 1981 White House Conference on Aging.
2. Bortz, W. (1982). Disease and aging. *JAMA, 248,* 1203.

3. Branch, L.B., and Meyers, A.R. (1987). Assessing physical function in the elderly. *Clin. Geriatr. Med., 3*, 29–51.
4. Branch, L.G., et al. (1984). A prospective study of functional status among community elders. *Am. J. Public Health, 74*, 266.
5. Brummel-Smith, K. (in press). Geriatric rehabilitation. In Cassel, C. (Ed.), *Geriatric medicine* in press.
6. Council on Scientific Affairs. (1984). Exercise programs for the elderly. *JAMA, 252*, 544.
7. Currie, C.T., et al. (1981). Assessment of elderly patients at home: A report of fifty cases. *J. Am. Geriatr. Soc., 29*, 398.
8. Curtis, P., and Rodgers, J. (1979). Continuity of care in a family practice residency program. *J. Fam. Pract. 8*, 1029–1030.
9. Federal Council on the Aging. (1981). *The need for long-term care: A chartbook of the Federal Council on the Aging.* U.S. Dept. of Health and Human Services publication No. (OHDS) 81–20704. Washington, DC: Government Printing Office.
10. Fillenbaum, G.G. (1984). *The wellbeing of the elderly: Approaches to multidimensional assessment.* Geneva: World Health Organization, WHO Offset Publication No. 84.
11. Folstein, M.F., Folstein, S.E., and McHugh, P.R. (1975). Mini-mental state: A practical method for grading the cognitive state of patients for the clinician. *J. Psychiatr. Res., 12*, 189–198.
12. Goldenson, R.M., Dunham, J.R., and Dunham, C.S. (Eds.). (1978). *Disability and rehabilitation handbook* (p. 37). New York: McGraw-Hill.
13. Granger, C.V. (1986). Goals of rehabilitation of the disabled elderly: A conceptual approach. In S.J. Brody and G.E. Ruff (Eds), *Aging and rehabilitation: Advances in the state of the art* (pp. 27–35). New York: Springer.
14. Granger, C.V., Selzer, G.B., and Fishbien, C.F. (1987). *Primary care of the functionally disabled: Assessment and management* (pp. 6–7). Philadelphia: Lippincott.
15. Haggerty, R. (1971). Does comprehensive care make a difference? Introduction: Historical perspectives. *Am. J. Dis. Child., 122*, 467–468.
16. Hennen, B.K. (1975). Continuity of care in family practice. Part 1: Dimensions of continuity. *J. Fam. Pract., 2*, 371–372.
17. Hodes, C. (1973). Care of the elderly in general practice. *Br. Med. J., 4*, 41.
18. Jackson, J.E., Ramsdell, J.W., Renvall, M., Swart, J., and Ward, H. Reliability of drug histories in a specialized geriatric outpatient clinic. *J. Gen. Intern. Med. 4*, 39, 1989.
19. Kahn, R.L., et al. (1960). Brief objective measures for the determination of mental status in the aged. *Am. J. Psychiatry, 117*, 326–328.
20. Kane, R.L., Solomon, D.H., Beck, J.C., Keeler, E., and Kane, R.A. (1981). *Geriatrics in the United States: Manpower projections and training considerations,* Lexington, MA: Lexington Books.
21. Kane, R.A., and Kane, R.L. (1981). *Assessing the elderly: A practical guide to measurement.* Lexington, MA: Lexington Books.
22. Kane, R.A. Assessing social function in the elderly. *Clin. Geriatr. Med., 3*, 87.
23. Katz, S., et al. (1963). Studies of illness in the aged. The index of ADL: A standardized measure of biological and psychosocial function. *JAMA, 185*, 914–919.

24. Kurianksy, J.B., and Gurland, B. (1976). Performance test of activities of daily living. *Int. J. Aging Hum. Dev., 7,* 343–352.
25. Kennie, D.C. (1986). Health maintenance in the elderly. *Clin. Geriatr. Med., 2,* 53–83.
26. Lawton, M.P., and Brody, E.M. (1969). Assessment of older people: Self-maintaining and instrumental activities of daily living. *Gerontologist, 9,* 179–186.
27. Lawton, M.P., (1972). Assessing the competence of older people. In D. Kent, R. Kastenbaum and S. Sherwood (Eds.), *Research planning and action of the elderly* (pp.   ). New York; Behavioral Publications.
27a. Linn, M.W. (1967). A rapid disability rating scale. *J. Am. Geriatr. Soc.* 15:211.
27b. Mahoney, F, and Barthel, D. (1965). Functional evaluation: The Barthel index. *Md. State Med. J.* 1.
28. Mangen, D., and Peterson W. (Eds.). (1982). *Research instruments in social gerontology.* Vol. 1: *Clinical and social psychology.* Minneapolis: University of Minnesota Press.
29. Mangen, D., and Peterson, W. (Eds.). (1982). *Research instruments in social gerontology.* Vol. 2: *Social roles and social participation.* Minneapolis: University of Minnesota Press.
30. Mangen, D., and Peterson, W. (Eds.). (1982). *Research instruments in social gerontology.* Vol. 3: *Health program evaluation, and demography.* Minneapolis: University of Minnesota Press.
31. Nagi, S. (1975). Disability concepts and prevalence. Presented at the First Mary Switzer Memorial Seminar, Cleveland, OH, May, 1975.
32. Ramsdell, J.W., Swart, J., Jackson, J.E., and Renvall, M. The yield of a home visit in the assessment of geriatric patients. *J. Am. Geriatr. Soc. 37,* 17, 1989.
33. Reifler, B.V., Larson, E., and Cox, G. (1981). Treatment results at a multi-specialty clinic for the impaired elderly and their families. *J. Am. Geriatr. Soc., 29,* 579.
33a. Sherwood, S.J., et al. (1977). *Compendium of measures for describing and assessing long-term care populations.* Boston: Hebrew Rehabilitation Center for the Aged.
34. Stewart, J.E. (1979). *Home health care* (pp. 58–66). St. Louis: Mosby.
35. Williams, M.E., and Williams, T.F. (1986). Evaluation of older persons in the ambulatory setting. *J. Am. Geriatr. Soc., 34,* 37.
36. Williams, M.E. (1986). Geriatric assessment. *Ann. Intern. MEd., 104,* 720.
37. Williamson, J., Stokoe, I.H., Gray, S., et al. (1964). Old people at home: Their unreported needs. *Lancet 1,* 1117.
38. Wylie, C.M. (1967). Gauging the response of stroke patients to rehabilitation. *J. Am. Geriatr. Soc. 15,* 797.

CHAPTER 3

The Psychosocial Context of Geriatric Rehabilitation

BRYAN KEMP

Contrary to popular belief, rehabilitation is not a medical specialty. Rehabilitation is a complex biopsychosocial process, which happens to occur within a medical context. Moreover, the features which distinguish rehabilitation care from other forms of health care are primarily psychologic and social in nature. The purposes of this chapter are to describe some of those psychologic features common to most older persons with a disability and to indicate how rehabilitation is unique from a psychosocial point of view. Of course, rehabilitation requires proper medical care to treat illnesses, reduce trauma, prevent secondary illnesses, and restore health. Naturally, during the early stages of rehabilitation, attention must be given first to lifesaving efforts and the restoration of biologic functioning. Talented physicians in the specialties of surgery, internal medicine, physical medicine, and family medicine make outstanding contributions to the patient's rehabilitation. And if it were not for early medical pioneers such as Howard Rusk, there probably wouldn't be as much rehabilitation in the United States. However, a disability causes life changes above and beyond any changes in health and it is these life changes that are of paramount importance to rehabilitation.

THE KEY OUTCOMES OF REHABILITATION: IMPROVING FUNCTION, PROMOTING LIFE SATISFACTION, AND PRESERVING SELF-ESTEEM

By definition, chronic diseases cannot be cured. Success of intervention, therefore, cannot be measured in terms of physical recovery. Chronic disease that results in disability must be viewed in terms of helping individuals adapt to a life that is permanently changed. The onset of a severe disability is possibly the most life-changing event that can happen to someone in terms of its impact on daily life, its future implications, and the need for ongoing adaptations. For older persons it appears to cause even more stress than the death of a spouse.[5]

The changes one encounters after a disabling condition are a major concern of rehabilitation. These changes include (1) a decrease in daily living skills and social independence, (2) an impact on sources of life satisfaction, and (3) the potential impact a disability has on self-esteem. Adaptation to these changes determines success in living with a disability. To the extent that rehabilitation programs help people deal with these changes they are successful. These issues may not always be the staff's greatest concern, but from the patient's point of view, these are usually the ones of greatest concern.

INDEPENDENCE

Two main goals of rehabilitation are improving function and promoting independence. These goals are not, however, simply a matter of increasing cardiovascular reserves, stabilizing gait, increasing muscular strength, improving activities of daily living (ADLs), or improving range of motion in a joint. Improving function means maximizing the person's ability to live in the least restrictive and most desirable environment. For older persons, living independently at home is often the most desired goal of rehabilitation. Living in a long-term care institution is often the most feared outcome of chronic illness.[7]

The ability to live independently after a disability is largely the result of two psychologic processes. The first is learning *skills* to compensate for the deficit the disability brought about. Physical therapy and occupational therapy are largely skill-learning procedures that are designed to help people learn or relearn how to perform a variety of tasks. The ability to learn and to retain what is learned is therefore of great importance to rehabilitation success. Older people frequently have different learning and memory processes. They often learn a task in a different manner than younger persons,[6] and usually take longer to learn to the same criterion.[6] For example, when compared with younger persons older persons benefit more from having complex tasks broken down into simpler ones, by providing more frequent feedback, by encouraging attempts even if they are wrong, by reducing fears of failure, by spacing out learning trials, and by allowing them to learn at a pace they prefer.[13]

In addition, older persons frequently have conditions that can interfere with learning or retention. Such conditions include adverse drug effects, undetected medical illness, or neurologic impairment. Geriatric rehabilitation requires careful assessment of learning and memory, screening for problems that may interfere with learning or memory, modification of teaching techniques, and tolerance for slower learning. Unfortunately, such screening and modification is often lacking. One study found that older persons in a hospital setting were not screened for cognitive problems[27] though as many as 50 percent of these patients were found on reexamination to have cognitive deficits. Cognitive assessment plays an important role in both rehabilitation evaluation and discharge planning.

Maximizing functional capabilities requires adopting the kind of *attitude* that will support independence at home. This attitude has variously been called "autonomy," "self-reliance," or "independence" (see, e.g., Cohen[10]). The passive, dependent, or unassuming patient in the hospital is often regarded as less trouble to staff. This type of patient, however, generally functions poorly in the community if a chronic illness is present. The risk becomes greater if the person also lives alone. Older persons who have a disability fare better with an attitude of assertiveness, self-responsibility, and realism. Such an attitude is needed in order to maintain health, secure assistance, defend one's rights, and direct the care of home aides. Cohen warns that the older person's independence is in great danger if he or she adopts the idea that the potential for growth, development, and continuing involvement in life disappears because of a disability.[10] The tendency to adopt a defeatist attitude may help to account for the high rate of depressive symptoms among older persons with disability.[4] If so, careful research needs to be directed toward ways to modify such negative viewpoints.

LIFE SATISFACTION

The second major impact a disability has is on life satisfaction. The sources of life satisfaction frequently are changed as a result of a severe disability. At least three factors usually contribute to life satisfaction. The first is sufficient pleasurable experiences to outweigh whatever painful ones may exist in daily life (physical *or* psychologic). Pleasurable experiences include those brought to us through our senses, including vision, touch, hearing, smell, taste, and through our own thought processes (fantasy). To the extent that these sources of pleasure are present, life has pleasure, and to the extent there is pleasure, there may be satisfaction. A good meal, a hug, the sight of a pleasant environment, the smell of flowers, the pleasure of sex, the sound of music all contribute to a pleasurable life.

A disability increases the sources of pain in life without equally corresponding increases in pleasure. When a disability is present in late life, it may be in addition to other painful losses such as decreased hearing, diminished vision, absence of spouse, and limited ability to get around in the community. For older persons, there may not be a high enough ratio of pleasure to pain to make life very satisfying. Rehabilitation programs should always consider the basic issue of pain versus pleasure and help people to increase their sources of pleasure and decrease their sources of pain. Often, the biggest pains are not physical, but psychologic. Unless care is available to help older persons deal with this kind of pain, life is not going to be as satisfying.

A second source of life satisfaction comes from the experience of success. The ability to control, improve, and influence everything from one's daily tasks to one's life circumstances leads to a sense of success. Older people frequently feel like they have little control or ability to influence their lives after a chronic illness. Many report problems doing daily activities. They are subject to the demands of their physicians, families, and routines. This lack of influence over their own lives may lead to feeling as though they are powerless and have lost their status as independent adults. When the balance of feelings is one of failure rather than success, demoralization or depression results. In support of this Murphy[29] found in a sample of severely disabled older persons that functional ability (as measured by the Barthel index) was an important predictor of overall life satisfaction. Kemp, Staples, and Lopez[23] found that decrements in daily living skills were among the highest correlates with depression scores among a large group of community-dwelling older persons. Stoedefalke[37] stresses that success in physical therapy increases dramatically for older persons if sufficient signs of success are provided to them. Improved ability in daily skills, therefore, may lead to overall improved life satisfaction through its impact on the older person's sense of success and control.

A third source of life satisfaction is having a sense of meaning or purpose in life. Victor Frankel[16] has stressed the importance of this issue. Eric Erikson[14] has described the conflict between meaning and despair which often occurs in late life as a normal developmental issue.

A chronic illness brings this issue to the forefront even sooner. Reestablishing a purpose and meaning in life after a major disability is difficult because what provided a sense of purpose may have been eliminated or greatly reduced by the disability. Determination of a sense of purpose is a new philosophic issue for most people. Life may have been rich with many pleasurable and successful experiences. One may have not worried about anything so ethereal as "purpose." Among older persons with a disability, however, issues surrounding the meaning of life are experienced by at least 75 percent of them.[38] People who suffer deep doubts about the purpose or value of their lives are at very high risk for depression and unhappiness.

The topic of life satisfaction after disability is crucial in rehabilitation. People with low satisfaction will not only lead unhappy lives, they will also develop more medical problems, more psychiatric disorders, and will probably need more health care and social support than others.[38] Examination of life satisfaction within a pleasure-plan, success-failure, meaning-despair context should be a part of any rehabilitation program.

SELF-ESTEEM

The third major impact of a disability is on self-esteem. Self-esteem means liking yourself exactly the way you are. People who can accept and appreciate themselves after a disability are minimally handicapped by it. People who cannot accept themselves (and therefore their lives) are more likely to experience unhappiness and are at risk for developing major mental health problems. Self-esteem is different from life satisfaction. Life satisfaction follows from an appraisal of one's life. Self-esteem follows from an appraisal of one's self. Typically, self-esteem arises from how one evaluates several parts of his or her life: what a person *does,* such as his or her occupation or role; what a person *has,* such as possessions; and what kind of person he or she *is,* such as honest or humorous. A disability usually affects self-esteem because it affects what a person can *do,* it affects what the person *has* (something undesirable, the disability), and it affects how the person is *seen* (disabled). To the extent that each of these are diminished, the person will suffer poor self-esteem. One of the major problems with poor self-esteem is that it often creates a self-perpetuating attitude that leads to a spiral of poor self-care ("I don't care"), little expectation of improvement ("what's the use"), and a tendency to assume that positive achievements are not the result of one's abilities ("I was just lucky"). Severely impaired self-esteem is believed by many psychiatrists and psychologists to be the root cause of most mental health problems; see Rogers,[33] for example).

Functional ability, life satisfaction, and self-esteem are therefore inter-related. Each can and does influence the other. Improvements in one area can cause improvements in others. Conversely, continuously low levels of life satisfaction or greatly impaired functional ability may eventually lead to low self-esteem. Continuous low levels of life satisfaction or impaired self-esteem are likely to lead to major mental health or physical health problems.

SOCIETY AS THE PRIMARY HANDICAP

It is customary to define impairment as a defect that exists at the organ level, a disability as a difficulty at the task level, and a handicap as a problem at the social level (e.g., Granger[18]). A person is handicapped to the extent that he or she is not integrated into society. In reality, it is usually not the person affected who does the handicapping. Society typically handicaps the person with a disability. Society does this by reducing the opportunities for open and free interaction with both the physical and social environments. As will be shown, handicapping of disabled persons happens in both subtle and not so subtle ways, but both are powerful forces with which to contend.

The design of the physical environment handicaps older persons with a disability because they cannot participate fully in it. Dykwald[12] has presented numerous examples of such practices: curbs that are too high, clothes with buttons instead of Velcro fasteners, traffic lights set at intervals too short to cross the street in time, glare in brightly lit rooms, stairs (only) leading into buildings, jars sealed too tightly to open, etc. The younger disabled population has expressed concern over these problems for years, and the lack of progress in this area was one of the primary factors that led to the development of the independent living movement in the 1960s and 1970s. Younger disabled persons began to take a more assertive role in determining the quality of their own lives and developed centers for independent living. Now that the older popula-tion is growing in numbers and becoming increasingly vocal about the same problems, additional positive action has begun. A growing number of programs promote technology to reduce barriers (e.g., the American Society on Aging's section on technology, the American Association of Retired Persons' focus on technology, the National Aeronautic and Space Administration (NASA) technology transfer program, and state architec-tural laws that are promoting greater accessibility). Other countries are also active in this area. Sweden has estimated that any given person will spend a significant amount of his or her life in a wheelchair. Therefore, *all* housing must be wheelchair-accessible.[32]

Older persons with a disability are probably handicapped even more than younger persons because of society's negative attitudes toward them. The general theme of the attitude toward disabled persons in general might be called *devaluation,* a term used by Vash.[39] Devaluation refers to the process of seeing someone as less valuable, less attractive, less desirable, and less acceptable than someone else. Older people in general have been and continue to be devalued in society because of the imputed negative qualities associated with aging.[9] Older persons with a disability have been more devalued because they suffer the "double jeopardy" of being both old and disabled.[34]

Devaluation attitudes are reflected in behavior, but only rarely are these behaviors open and direct. They are more apt to be manifested indirectly, in the form of exclusionary practices, styles of communication, and in setting expectations for improvement.

No profession seems to be free of such attitudes.[25] Health planners, administrators, and many health professionals also often demonstrate negative attitudes toward older people. Older patients are frequently seen as hopeless, uninteresting, somatisizing, complaining, and helpless by health providers. These attitudes translate into second-class treatment. For example, although the older population accounts for about 40 percent of all disabled persons,[3] fewer than 10 percent of older disabled persons are even referred for rehabilitation-type services to state agencies,[11] and perhaps only 10 to 15 percent of older persons who could use rehabilitation after acute care are referred for it. Fewer than 3 percent of hospital beds in the United States are for rehabilitation although it is clear that disability is becoming one of the biggest and costliest health problems. Older people are frequently not given the same range of health services given to others, especially rehabilitation services. Physicians are often overaggressive in providing diagnostic and procedural services but are underaggressive in providing function-improving services. Even staff on a rehabilitation team have been shown to be less aggressive in goal setting for older persons, even when there was no logical reason for it.[26] The bulk of evidence indicates that older persons do just as well as younger persons in rehabilitation if given the opportunity, although it may take 15 to 20 percent longer to achieve the same goals.[21,40]

Several authors have discussed why negative attitudes exist toward disabled and older persons.[9,28,40] Most negative attitudes are believed to develop because the qualities that are venerated by society as a whole are perceived to be lacking in these groups. In Western civilization, these venerated qualities include physical attractiveness, productiveness, physique, intellect, and wealth. Older and disabled persons are seen as not having these qualities. When a member of the target group senses the

negative attitude and feels the full impact of the rejection and devaluation, he or she may begin to lose self-esteem and may even begin to
accept the characteristics implied in the attitude as being true. Thus,
society creates the attitude and behaviors in the target group and then
blames them for having them!

Communication between staff and older patients can also reflect a
poor attitude and therefore create poor outcomes for the patient. For
example, older people with a disability are frequently described as
"frail." This is a terrible description. It creates an image of someone who
is virtually going to break apart and for whom any intervention is only
undertaken at great risk and with little expectation of benefit. This, in
turn, can create lower expectations of success, the withholding of
possible services, and the likelihood of neglect. Some older people have
been described as being "wheelchair-bound" or "confined" to a wheelchair. In fact, they are *liberated* by the wheelchair, because without it they
would not be able to get around at all. Such word choice may seem
innocuous, but subtle word choice actually creates powerful images that
subsequently serve to form the basis of action.

Even seemingly normal language can create a negative image of a
person and thus decrease his or her chances of receiving equal care and
opportunities. The designation "Older disabled person" creates a different image than does "older person with a disability" because the word
order emphasizes disability more than personhood. Negative attitudes
may also be communicated through subtle yet powerful actions. A
physician who hands a prescription to the daughter who accompanies
the older patient is implying dependency on the part of the older person.
A minister who asks the son a question about his mother even though
she is standing next to him reduces her stature. The older person may not
even consciously recognize what is going on yet over a series of such
communications he or she may begin to adopt the behavior implied in
the description.

Families can also be potent handicappers of older persons. It is true
that families care greatly about their older relatives and most families
have at least weekly contact with their older relatives. Family members
also provide over 80 percent of all daily care to older persons with health
problems.[8] Families, however, are not immune to negative attitudes,
poor communication, and faulty expectations concerning their older
relatives. As many as 60 percent of families may have faulty expectations
and negative attitudes toward older persons.[22] These families may foster
dependency through overprotection, create anxiety through inconsistent care, lower self-esteem by demoting the older person, or engender
guilt by being resentful about caregiving. Families are such a key
ingredient in the overall health and welfare of older persons that their

attitudes must be examined and aided with appropriate intervention. This topic is further examined in chapters that follow.

ADJUSTMENT TO DISABILITY AND PROBLEMS IN ADAPTATION

Rehabilitation cannot be successful without considering the person's psychologic reactions to his or her disability, because those reactions will determine how the person lives with the disability. In an era when the psychiatric syndrome approach to mental health problems is popular,[1] the adjustment model of the 1930s, 1940s, and 1950s, which stressed understanding the adjustment process, seems often to be minimized. A major emphasis is currently placed on diagnosing pathologic disorders and administering the proper medication to alleviate symptoms. Less emphasis is given to understanding the long, complex process of adjusting to something as life-changing as a major disability.

The shortsighted emphasis on pathology overlooks the fact that the person has had a permanent change in his or her life. The rehabilitation approach requires more than treating extreme (though common) reactions, such as depression. This approach helps the person adopt a new outlook, a new set of behaviors, and often a different attitude toward life.

To various degrees, a disability causes a crisis. The degree of the crisis is roughly equivalent to the person's loss of ability and what that loss means to him or her. Each person's experience of the crisis will be, to some degree, idiosyncratic. Everyone has a manner of responding to a perceived crisis, a "crisis style." After the crisis people ultimately develop some style of adaptation that "works" for them. But on the way to establishing a style of adaptation, and during the period of crisis (as long as that may last) some people may develop very disordered behaviors. Such disordered behavior must be viewed as an adaptive response, an attempt to come to grips with a crisis. If the person is labeled with a psychiatric diagnosis at that time they tend to be seen primarily that way rather than as a more or less normal person who is going through a very tough situation. Other chapters in this book will focus on the "mental health" problems of older persons with chronic illness. This section focuses on some of the issues involved in the usual process of adjusting to a disability.

Older persons have some unique characteristics which distinguish their adjustment to disability. First, a disability may be only one of a long series of losses in the later part of life. Prior to the disability the older person may have lost a spouse, may have changed residence, may have even lost a child. He or she may have had other physical health changes in the last years. By contrast, the younger person may have had "only" the onset of a disability (I am not trying to downplay the impact of disability on the younger person, but simply emphasizing age differences). Therefore, it is important to view the disability in the context of possible multiple losses.

Older persons in rehabilitation belong to a cohort of people who prided themselves on being independent and able to work through their own personal problems. They are often reticent to openly discuss personal matters or to rely on mental health help until after a close relationship is established. They may initially reveal less about what they are thinking and feeling. Practitioners must not overlook the fact, therefore, that increased complaints of pain may signify the equivalent of depressive or anxious feelings. Consequently, the rehabilitation professional usually has to try to establish a good working relationship first, then gently but thoroughly probe to determine the full extent of what is going on personally.

Older persons have a more foreshortened future than younger persons. In fact, the onset of a disability is how many people first define themselves as being old. A disability may herald a reduction in activities, a withdrawal from others — even thoughts of eventual death and finality. The older person's expectations about what is possible in late life after a disability, therefore, can be diminished. The general attitude of society further reinforces pessimism. Not realizing that physical recovery normally takes 20 to 25 percent longer in late life,[20] the older person may view his or her "slow" recovery as a failure. Some may even feel that their disability leaves little reason to live.

STAGES OF ADJUSTMENT

The process of adjustment to disability and crisis has several stages, each with critical issues and each with various possible outcomes. People do not necessarily go through all stages. They may go back and forth between various stages as additional problems and crises arise. For our purposes, however, we will divide the process into only two phases: an acute phase and a chronic phase.

It is not possible to discuss adjustment to crisis and change with reference to the patient only. Proper understanding requires that the person with a disability be seen in the context of at least two other influences: the family and the health care team. This group has been described as the "caregiving system."[32] The characteristics of each and how each relates to the other will determine success or failure. Thus the process and the outcomes of adjustment are a product of these three intersecting influences: the person, the family, and the team.

The acute phase of the adjustment process includes what others usually term the shock and denial phase.[2,36,39] During this phase the person may not be functioning very well intellectually or emotionally because the shock of the event and its potential implications may overwhelm his or her coping capacity. The nature of the onset and the perceived implications of the illness are two factors that will determine the response at this point. For older persons, approximately half of impairments are of sudden onset, such as a stroke, hip fracture, or heart attack. The other impairments are of gradual onset, such as pulmonary disease, diabetes, and Alzheimer's disease.

Shock is the most common response to problems of sudden onset. For a problem with a gradual onset, uncertainty regarding the future requires continuous adjustment. A common personal reaction to the onset of either is to deny the extent or the implications of the impairment. During this period there may even be an absence of psychologic problems. At this point, other people who try to "force" reality upon the patient may find themselves rejected or avoided.

While the patient's task during this period is to try to manage a crisis, the health care team's role during the acute phase is usually focused on analysis of the problem, life-preserving efforts, or minimizing further impairment. At this point, their *technical skills* are most important, but they also need to realize that what is communicated to the patient may not be well understood, appreciated, or remembered because of the patient's emotional shock. The family's chief task at this point is to be able to function as a unit and to help serve as a bridge between the patient and the physician. The ability of the family to mobilize itself, to reach decisions, and to tolerate ambiguity and uncertainty are the most important factors in determining the degree to which they can help. Cohesiveness, communication, and decision-making skills are the tools that are most important at this point.[32] Frequently, one person emerges to take on the "executive" role in directing activities. At this point any preexisting problems or conflicts the family had in acting as a unit usually become apparent to the health team. This is one of the main reasons for having a family conference after the patient's evaluation. Most families cope pretty well during this phase. Interestingly, the older person may even find enjoyment in some aspects of this stage because a great deal of attention and concern is centered upon him or her. This stage passes for the family when a diagnosis is made and a course of action is started. For the patient, this phase passes when reality sets in and the person begins to realize that what has happened is real and permanent.

The second phase of adjustment centers around the theme of acknowledgment. The most important tasks for the patient are to deal with the emotional problems, improve functioning as much as possible, find alternative ways of maintaining life satisfaction, and avoid equating self-worth with loss of functioning. Psychologic problems are very common at this point. The most common are depression, anxiety, somatization, substance abuse, and psychosis. Depression is particularly a problem in rehabilitation because it affects the very attributes needed to succeed: endurance, learning ability, optimism, good decision-making ability, reasonable interpersonal relations, and a desire to improve. During the first 5 years after onset, some form of severe emotional problem may occur in as many as 70 percent of older person with a major disability.[22]

This phase is marked medically by the establishment of a regular program of improvement and the routinization of care. The health care team's role at this point is to provide services which will help the older person achieve the goal of maximal functioning, including rehabilitation-oriented services, psychologic support, and education for the family. The health team members (especially the physician) must change modes from being primarily technical experts to being psychosocial advocates and "functional coaches." Some physicians (and other health professionals) may be unused to or uncomfortable with this change; however, the success of rehabilitation requires it. In this phase it is not a matter of the physician's specialty in making this transition, so much as it is a matter of his or her personality. Thus, any medical specialty can make an outstanding rehabilitation specialist. It is more a matter of temperament than training.

The family's task at this stage changes from arranging life-sustaining and acute care support to fostering increased independence. This stage can be very difficult for the families because they often do not know how to respond to the older person's emotional problems or how to determine what the older person really requires in care. There is also limited knowledge available to families about what older persons can accomplish after a disability. Finally, families often have their own issues which prevent optimal functioning. Therefore, families also need to be a focus of intervention at this point. During this phase the patient may receive less attention from the family. Some patients may view this as withdrawal of interest on the family's part. However, what needs to be worked out is a compromise between patient needs and family needs. Families who cannot reach a suitable compromise usually suffer from burnout or cycles of resentment, anger, and guilt.

The family members may feel that they don't need to do as much for the older person at this point but don't know how to withdraw from providing as much care without feeling guity or angry. The change from high involvement to low involvement may precipitate a minor crisis in either the family or the older person. In order to successfully navigate this phase, the family members must be accurately aware of the medical facts, must know how much support to give the older person without doing too much, and must clearly communicate with one another. They also must accept the fact that the older person is no longer a patient, but rather an older *person* who happens to have a disability.

PSYCHOSOCIAL FACTORS ASSOCIATED WITH REHABILITATION OUTCOMES

The factors that determine rehabilitation success or failure of an older person are frequently psychosocial. Rarely is success or failure due to a lack of technical skill on the part of the rehabilitation team. It is necessary to distinguish between those psychological factors likely to lead to failure in rehabilitation and those factors likely to lead to success because they are usually not the same.

At least four psychological variables are strong predictors of possible rehabilitation failure. The first is motivation that is counter to rehabilitation goals. Assessment and improvement of motivation has received little attention in the literature. Chapter 18 addresses this topic.

Sufficient cognitive ability is also important to rehabilitation success. Rehabilitation programs require learnhing new procedures, carryover of learning from one day to the next, and long-term retention for utilization of gains when the patient returns to the home environment. Obviously, persons with severe cognitive problems have a difficult time learning new material. However, *how much* cognitive ability is necessary for rehabilitation and *which* cognitive abilities are necessary? There are little data on either of these topics. It would be best if candidates for rehabilitation were given complete mental status examinations. In the absence of staff or expertise to do this, short versions of the mental status examination that focus on cognitive functioning have been developed, such as the mini-mental state examination.[15] Based on experiences at Rancho Los Amigos Medical Center in Downey, California, older persons with a reliable score of less than 22 (out of 30) on the Mini-Mental test have a difficult time with normal rehabilitation programs. (Care must be taken to establish that the low score is valid and not due to a reversible process, such as an infection.) It is equally important to determine which items present problems. Various items reflect different mental processes and functions, each with a different impact on rehabilitation. In other words, a person can get a score of 22 in many different ways. If the person got 22 because he or she missed all the memory items (-3), couldn't register three words (-3), was temporarily disoriented (-2), and if these were uncorrectable, there would probably be a great deal of trouble with a rehabilitation program. On the other hand, if the person missed copying a geometric figure (-1), couldn't write a sentence (-1), was not language-fluent (-1), was off a little on reversing the spelling of a word (-3), and missed the location of where they were (-2), but did well on everything else, a rehabilitation program may not be adversely affected.

Depression, if it goes unrecognized or is not properly treated, is also a predictor of possible rehabilitation failure. As long as depression is present, the person will be poorly motivated, pessimistic, easily fatigued, and show little retention because that is the nature of depression. It is equally true that where there is depression, there is reason for optimism. Most depressed older persons can be treated successfully and their rehabilitation can be positive. Unfortunately, many older depressed persons go untreated because their depression is poorly recognized, wrongly assessed, and undertreated.[3,19] Candidates for rehabilitation should be carefully evaluated and reevaluated for depression. Chapter 15 discusses depression fully.

A fourth factor predictive of poor rehabilitation outcome is longstanding personality traits that are counter to rehabilitation goals. The person with a high degree of passivity, dependency, antisocial, histrionic, or suspicious traits will not do well in a program that relies on initiative, independence, tolerance for frustration, endurance, and trust in others. Not only are these traits antithetical to rehabilitation, they usually drive the staff crazy. With the proper understanding and approaches, however, rehabilitation can be made more successful.[17]

A few psychologic variables are positive indicators of rehabilitation success. The first is the presence of assertiveness on the part of the older person. By assertiveness, we mean taking appropriate control and actions to influence one's own outcomes in life. Persons with this trait seek answers to questions, want things explained to them, stick up for their rights, don't always go along with what other suggest, and take responsibility for their decisions. Such persons are not always favored by all staff (who may prefer more passive patients), but experience indicates that these persons have better outcomes.

Another factor is close involvement with at least one other person on an intimate basis. This does not necessarily mean a sexual relationship. But people who have at least one "confidant" in life have been shown to cope better with adversity.[29] Perhaps they feel more supported or can more easily work through the emotional issues.

A third positive variable is the ability to focus on life goals. People do better in rehabilitation who can set goals to improve functioning so they can participate in other activities (like returning to work, participating in family activities, etc.). This has been established with younger persons,[28] and there is some evidence to support it with older persons. Quite naturally, in the early phases of disability most attention will be on physical functioning. But when rehabilitation begins, the person must want something more.

IMPLICATIONS FOR TREATMENT AND PROGRAMMING

Rehabilitation involves many psychosocial processes. As such, as much attention must be paid to the psychologic and social issues as is paid to the physical ones. On a social level, in order to achieve ultimate success in treating the chronic health problems of older persons, some factors will need to change. Attitudes toward the potential of older persons with chronic illness are generally negative. Older persons are frequently discriminated against in terms of access to rehabilitation services. Chronic illness must receive the attention the nation now shows for acute illness. Further, positive examples of rehabilitation programs for older persons need to be widely disseminated.

On a psychologic level, rehabilitation needs to be seen in the context of the health team, the patient, and the family. If any of these are functioning at a less than optimal level, then the outcomes of rehabilitation will be diminished. Attention to the psychologic process of older persons in rehabilitation is extremely important. Even though a high rate of mental health problems can impair success, treating these problems is not enough. Even without psychiatric syndromes, older persons with a disability, who must cope with the life-changing disability and who also are handicapped by society, need programs that will enhance their chances of achieving maximal functioning, life satisfaction, and self-esteem. Programs that focus on self-help, peer support, advocacy, education about disability, and other "strengthening" aspects are needed. If sufficient attention is paid to the psychosocial changes that occur as a result of a disability, older persons with a disability can lead satisfying lives.

REFERENCES

1. American Psychiatric Association (1980). *Diagnostic and statistical manual of mental diseases,* 3rd ed. Washington, DC: American Psychiatric Association.
2. Athelstan, G.T. (1981). Psychosocial adjustment to chronic disease and disability. In W.C. Stolov and M.C. Clowers (Eds), *Handbook of severe disability.* Washington, DC: U.S. Dept. of Education.

3. Blake, R. (1984). What disables America's elderly? *Generatios, 3,* 6.
4. Blazer, D. (1982). *Depression in late life.* St. Louis: Mosby.
5. Blazer, D., and Williams, C.D. (1980). Epidemiology of dysphoria and depression in an elderly population. *Am. Journal of Psychiatry, 137,* 439.
6. Botwinick, J. (1973). *Aging and behavior.* New York: Springer.
7. Brody, S.J., and Ruff, G.E. (1986). *Aging and rehabilitation: Advances in the state of the art.* New York: Springer.
8. Brody, F.M. (1986). Informal support systems in the rehabilitation of the disabled elderly. In S.J. Brody and G.E. Ruff (Eds.), *Aging and rehabilitation: Advances in the state of the art.* New York: Springer.
9. Butler, R.N. (1975). *Why survive? Being old in America.* New York: Harper & Row.
10. Cohen, E.S. (1988). The elderly mystique: Constraints on the autonomy of the elderly with disabilities. *Gerontologist, 28,* 24.
11. Dunn, D. (1981). Vocational rehabilitation of the older disabled worker. *J. Rehabil. 47,* 56–71.
12. Dychtwald, K. (1984). Aging and environments. Presented to the Gerontological Society of America, Boston.
13. Eisdorfer, C. (1965). Verbal learning and response time in the aged. *J. Gerontol. 107,* 15.
14. Erikson, E.R. (1959). *Psychological issues: Identity and life cycle.* New York: International Universities Press.
15. Folstein, M.F., Folstein, S.E., and McHugh, P.R. (1975). Mini-mental state: A practical method for grading the cognitive state of patients for the clinician. *J. Psychiatr. Res., 12,* 189.
16. Frankel, V. (1970). *The will to meaning: Foundations and applications of logotherapy.* New York: Plume Books.
17. Geringer, E.S., and Stern, T.A. (1986). Coping with medical illness. The impact of personality types. *Psychosomatics, 27,* 251.
18. Granger, C. (1986). Goals of rehabilitation of the disabled elderly: A conceptual approach. In S.J. Brody and G.E. Ruff (Eds.), *Aging and rehabilitation: Advances in the state of the art.* New York: Springer.
19. Jeneke, M.A. (1985). *Handbook of geriatric psychopharmacology.* Littleton, MA: PSG Publishing.
20. Jones, R. (1984). Physiological basis of rehabilitation therapy. In T.F. Williams (Ed), *Rehabilitation and the aging.* New York: Raven Press.
21. Katz, S., Jackson, B.A., and Jaffee, M.W. (1962). Multidisciplinary studies of illness in aged persons. VI: Comparison study of rehabilitated and non-rehabilitated patients with fracture of hip. *J. Chronic Dis., 15,* 979.
22. Kemp, B.J. (1985). Rehabilitation of the older adult. In J.E. Birren and K.W. Schaie (Eds.), *Handbook of the psychology of aging.* New York: Van Nostrand Reinhold.
23. Kemp, B.J., Staples, F., and Lopez, W. (1987). Epidemiology of depression and dysphoria in an elderly Hispanic population: Prevalence and correlates. *J. Am. Geriatr. Soc., 35,* 920.
24. Kemp, B.J., and Vash, C.L. (1971). Productivity after injury in a sample of spinal cord injured persons: A pilot study. *J. Chronic Dis., 24,* 51.
25. Kosberg, J.I., and Gorman, J.F. (1975). Perceptions toward the rehabilitation potential of institutionalized aged. *Gerontologist, 10,* 398.
26. Kvitek, S.D.B., et al. (1986). Age bias: Physical therapists and older patients. *J. Gerontol., 41,* 702.

27. McCartney, U.R., and Palmateer, L.M. (1985). Assessment of cognitive deficit in geriatric patients: A study of physician behavior. *J. Am. Geriatr. Soc., 33*, 467.
28. McTavish, C. (1971). Perceptions of old people: A review of research medhodologies and findings. *Gerontologist, 11,* 90.
29. Murphy, E. (1983). The prognosis of depression in old age. *Br. J. Psychiatry, 42,* 111.
30. Osberg, J.S., et al. (1987). Life satisfaction and quality of life among disabled elderly adults. *J. Gerontol., 42,* 228.
31. Reinius, K.L. (1984). The elderly and their environment. Research in Sweden. Stockholm: Swedish Council for Building Research.
32. Reiss, D., and Denour, A.K. (1987). The family and the medical team in chronic illness: A transactional and development perspective. Unpublished manuscript. Dept. of Psychiatry, George Washington University, Washington, DC.
33. Rogers, C. (1942). *Counseling and psychotherapy.* Boston: Houghton-Mifflin.
34. Rubenfeld, P. (1986). Ageism and disabilityism: Double jeopardy. In S.J. Brody and G.E. Ruff (Eds.), *Aging and rehabilitation: Advances in the state of the art.* New York: Springer.
35. Salthouse, T. (1985). Speed of behavior and its implications for cognition. In J.E. Birren and K.V. Schaie (Eds.), *Handbook of the psychology of aging, 2nd ed.* New York: Van Nostrand Reinhold.
36. Steger, R. (1976). Understanding the psychologic factors in rehabilitation. *Geriatrics, 27,* 68–73.
37. Stoedefalke, K.G. (1985). Motivating and sustaining the older adult in an exercise program. *Top. Geriatr. Rehabil., 11,* 78–83.
38. Trieschmann, R.B. (1987). *Aging with a disability.* New York: Demos Publications.
39. Vash, C. (1981). *The psychology of disability.* New York: Springer.
40. Wright, B. (1960). *Physical disability—A psychological approach.* New York: Harper & Row.
41. Yuker, H.E., Block, J.R., and Campbell, W.J. (1960). A scale to measure attitudes toward disabled persons. Human Resource Study No. 5. Albertson, NY: Human Resource Center.
42. Zuckerman, J.D., et al. (1988). Interdisciplinary care of geriatric hip fracture patients. Presented to American Geriatric Society, Anaheim, CA.

PART _____ II

Major Disabling Conditions

CHAPTER 4

Stroke Rehabilitation for Elderly Patients

JEREMIAH F. KELLY

Though major advances have been made in the prevention of stroke, it remains one of the most common causes of death, disability, and loss of independence for those over 65. Usually sudden in onset and always unexpected, it merits the designation "shock" commonly applied to it by patients. For the elderly person with multiple preexisting chronic illnesses and precarious functional reserve, a stroke may be devastating, causing paralysis and loss of ability to communicate and often meaning the difference between continuing to live at home and being institutionalized.

While there are promising treatments for stroke under investigation, none of these is yet accepted for use in routine clinical practice. The clinician must therefore focus on neurologic and medical diagnosis, a careful assessment of specific deficits, prevention and treatment of complicating problems, and appropriate formal rehabilitation. In the elderly stroke patient with multiple coexisting problems, rehabilitation requires a comprehensive approach that may extend over months and across a variety of different settings. Since the most important outcomes for those who survive a stroke are functional improvement and the capability to maintain independence, care must be based on periodic formal and informal assessments of function. The specifics of such an approach are rarely covered in traditional textbooks of internal medicine and neurology.

EPIDEMIOLOGY

Nearly 500,000 Americans have a first stroke each year.[1] The risk of stroke is strongly associated with advancing age. After age 55 the incidence doubles with each additional decade. Data from population surveys indicate that 75 percent of strokes are due to atherothrombotic brain infarction (ABI), 5 to 14 percent to emboli, and 14 to 20 percent to intraparenchymal and subarachnoid hemorrhages.[12] With increasing age the proportion due to atherothrombotic brain infarctions increases to nearly 90 percent.[78]

Stroke is the third most frequent cause of death for all ages in the United States. It is the second commonest cause of death for those over 85.[57] Mortality within the first 30 days of stroke is significant, averaging 20 to 30 percent for all causes. Age is associated with a higher early mortality.[57] Type of stroke is also an important predictor of early death. Data from the Framingham cohort indicate that early mortality differs markedly depending on stroke type; 15 percent of patients with atherothrombotic stroke and 16 percent with emboli died within 30 days compared to 46 percent of those with subarrachanoid hemorrhage and 82 percent with intracerebral hemorrhage.[63]

Although there has been a dramatic decline in the incidence of new stroke, 37 percent between 1968 and 1978,[18] improvements in survival and major increases in the population of elderly have resulted in a rise in the prevalence of stroke in the population.[57] Current estimates suggest that there are close to 2 million stroke survivors now living in the United States.[1] This has resulted in a large reservoir of people with stroke-related disability. Though 15 percent of patients with stroke are institutionalized, most continue to live in the community.[26]

Data from the Framingham study showed that 32 percent of stroke survivors were dependent in activities of daily living (ADLs), 22 percent in mobility, and 56 percent in instrumental ADLs (IADLs). Disability was not limited to physical functioning. Fifty-nine percent evidenced decreased socialization outside the home.[26] Even those individuals with no residual physical impairment had notable social disability.[38]

SPECIAL PROBLEMS OF THE ELDERLY STROKE PATIENT

The physiologic hallmark of advancing age is a decrease in homeostatic reserve capacity. This may result in atypical presentation of common illnesses and an enhanced vulnerability to complications associated with a host of physiologic and environmental stresses. Though there is substantial interindividual variability, advancing age brings with it decrements in the functioning of most organs. For example, such alterations in lung function as decreased forced expiratory volume in 1 second (FEV_1) and reduced ciliary clearance of secretions may predispose to pneumonia; alterations in baroreceptor sensitivity to postural hypotension and falls; and loss of subcutaneous tissue and skin vasculature to pressure sores. Age-associated loss of neurons may limit or slow recovery from brain injury felt to result from neuroplasticity.

Also characteristic of old age is an increasing burden of chronic disease. More than 80 percent of those over age 65 living in the community have at least one chronic condition and 22 percent have some degree of disability. Of those over 65, 41 percent have hypertension; 47 percent, arthritis; 16 percent, cataracts; 29 percent, hearing impairment; and 30 percent, heart disease.[54] In the stroke patient, the presence of significant comorbid cardiovascular disease correlates with increased early mortality, poorer functional outcome, and a higher risk of recurrent stroke.[62,63]

Social and economic problems are common in the elderly and may complicate the care of individual patients. Among these are widowhood, poverty or near poverty, the lower health status of minorities and those living alone,[54] and in some areas a lack of community alternatives to nursing homes.

THE FUNCTIONALLY ORIENTED HISTORY AND PHYSICAL EXAMINATION

Given the special health problems of the elderly patient, functional approach is an especially important element in care. This is particularly the case for the elderly stroke patient who may have multiple coexisting problems due to stroke, preexisting comorbid disease, and psychosocial difficulties. A functionally oriented history and physical examination permits the creation of a composite picture which may assist the physician, patient, and family in establishing a baseline, gauging process, planning for discharge, and speculating on prognosis for recovery. It may also provide an especially meaningful set of data on which to base key decisions about intensity of rehabilitation, discharge setting, amount and type of in-home services, and the need for aids, adaptive devices, and environmental modifications. This type of functionally oriented approach to patients with disability has been comprehensively described by Granger.[21]

For clinical purposes the functionally oriented examination into two types: informal and formal. The informal functional examination includes a functionally oriented history and physical examination. The history incorporates questions about the effect of chronic and acute illnesses on an individual's ability to perform particular ADLs, IADLs, and customary roles into the traditional medical history. It should provide information about prestroke function in at least five areas: physical, mental, social, economic, and environmental. In most cases patient interview data will need to be supplemented by discussions with family and friends.

Information gathered about physical functioning should include an account of the patient's previous level of activity and exercise tolerance, particularly exercise-related precipitation of such symptoms as dyspnea, arthritic pain, angina, or claudication. The ability to perform ADLs should be assessed using the Barthel index as a checklist. IADLs may be evaluated in a similar fashion by using the Lawton IADL scale.[39] Level of motivation and preferences for various activities should also be assessed. Specific inquiry should be made about adaptive equipment and walking aids, including their acceptability and usefulness. In addition, availability of assistance, including its current amount and type, should be noted.

Assessment of prestroke mental functioning should include questions about coping style and the existence of dementia or a history of depression. Since early dementia may often go unnoticed or be denied by family members, specific questions should be asked about memory, language, and behavior changes that may be an indicator of dementing illness. This is particularly relevant in the patient who is very old or who has had a previous stroke.

Social functioning should be assessed by asking about the nature of relationships with spouse or partner, siblings, children, friends, and neighbors. Included in this should be questions about whether the patient has a confidant and an inquiry about the frequency of social contacts inside and outside the home. Current or previous occupation, avocational activities, and hobbies should also be noted.

Economic circumstances should be investigated carefully as options for rehabilitation, in-home services, and community programs will be affected by level of income and insurance coverage.

Environmental assessment should include a description of the patient's dwelling including floor, number of steps inside and outside, the presence of an elevator, specific environmental barriers, and any previous modifications made to overcome them. Questions should also be asked about the layout of the household, particularly the distance from kitchen to living space and from bathroom to bedroom.

The functionally oriented physical examination incorporates bedside observation of actual or simulated functional activities like dressing and undressing, grooming, and eating into the traditional physical examination. Such observation provides preliminary information that is further objectified in the formal functional examination.

Formal functional examination of the stroke patient utilizes one or more formal scales designed for use in a rehabilitation setting. Multiple such instruments exist. Some, like the Long-Range Evaluation System (LRES),[21] are comprehensive, incorporating items that measure functioning in a variety of different domains: physical, cognitive, emotional, and social. These have the advantage of providing a complete assessment with one valid and reliable measure. However, such instruments are time-consuming to administer and therefore usually not practical for clinical purposes. More practical and efficient for clinical use are selected short scales in several domains. At a minimum, all stroke patients should be evaluated for physical functioning with a formal ADL scale. Among the most commonly used are the Katz index,[37] the Kenny self-care index,[68] and the Barthel index.[49] All of these have been found to be valid and reliable. In one study Gresham found a high degree of agreement among the three when used on patients with stroke.[26] Of the three, the Barthel index appears to possess several advantages, including completeness and sensitivity to change. For this reason, it is recommended for routine use by the primary care provider.

When using the Barthel index in clinical settings the same rater should be used for each measurement to maximize reliability. It is scored on a 100-point scale with the maximum score signifying independence in ADLs. Results on the Barthel index may be useful for planning service needs and judging rehabilitation potential. In planning in-home assistance, the score of 60 has been found to be a pivotal one. Individuals with scores less than this needed more than 4 hours a day of personal care assistance. Estimates of rehabilitation potential may also be made from Barthel index scores. In a study of 269 patients Granger found that individuals with scores between 41 and 60 were ideal candidates for an intensive rehabilitation program and that those with scores less than 20 had poor functional outcomes.[21]

THE PHASES OF STROKE CARE

Care of the stroke patient may be divided into three phases, each with unique goals. The acute phase extends from admission to 48 hours; the subacute phase encompasses the period from 48 hours to 3 months; and the chronic phase focuses on the continuing care of the stroke patient. The goals and areas of clinical focus differ importantly during each of these phases. These are listed in Table 4-1.

Table 4-1. *Care of the Elderly Stroke Patient*

Phase	Timing	Goals	Clinical Focus
Acute	Admission to 48 hr.	Diagnosis and stabilization	Traditional history, physical examination, diagnostic studies, treatment
		Creation of a functionally oriented database	Functionally oriented examination
			Functionally oriented history
			Cognitive status
			Affective status
			Communication
			Vision and hearing
			Swallowing
			Motor control
			Sensation
			Perception
			Postural control
			Caregivers' evaluation
			Initial assessment with Barthel index
Subacute	48 hr. to 3 mo.	Provision of rehabilitation to maximize functional status	Multidisciplinary rehabilation in acute, skilled nursing facility (SNF), home care, outpatient, and adult day health care settings
			Weekly assessment with Barthel index
		Prevention of complications	Complications (see Table 4-2)
Chronic	3 mo. and after	Maintenance of functional gains	Maintenance level rehabilitation; periodic assessment with Barthel index
		Prevention of recurrent stroke	Risk factor modification

There may be substantial overlap of tasks and concerns for individual patients within each phase. Although the phases are outlined sequentially, clinicians may in practice encounter an elderly stroke patient for the first time during any one of these periods. For example, patients with inadequately treated stroke-related disability may first be seen months or years after the event. In institutional long-term care settings, some elderly stroke patients may be treated nihilistically, neglecting potentially remediable problems like dysphasia, contractures, or spasticity. The clinician who takes a systematic approach to such patients may contribute substantially to their quality of life and level of independence.

ACUTE PHASE (ADMISSION TO 48 HOURS)

The traditional goals of care in the acute phase are anatomic and etiologic diagnoses and medical and neurologic stabilization. Diagnosis includes the task of differentiating between stroke and various stroke imitators. Some of the common causes of "pseudostroke" include seizure producing Todd's paralysis and hypoglycemia. In elderly persons with prior stroke, any acute medical illness can cause accentuation of the persisting neurologic deficit and the appearance of a new event.

Assessment of cause in the elderly patient should take into account the prestroke probability of specific stroke etiologies and relevant historical factors like mode of onset, associated symptoms like headache and seizure, and the presence of risk factors like hypertension and atrial fibrillation. Nonvalvular atrial fibrillation increases with advancing age. It is associated with a twofold increase in the risk of stroke; three-quarters of patients with this arrhythmia will have embolic stroke, though only 20 percent will have positive findings on echocardiograms.[12,79]

Initial treatment should be directed at stabilizing vital signs and treating coexisting medical illness. In patients with atherothrombotic stroke, elevated blood pressure should not be lowered to normal levels, as this has been associated with further neurologic deterioration. In the elderly patient particular attention needs to be directed to the treatment of coexisting acute medical problems that may be a cause of early mortality. Though recent advances have been made in understanding mechanisms of brain injury caused by stroke, most treatment remains experimental.[27] Therefore, after initial medical treatment has been instituted, the clinician must focus on creating a comprehensive picture of the patient's deficits and abilities that can be used to formulate a treatment plan and on counseling the patient and family.

The acute phase examination should therefore include a functionally oriented history and a physical examination that incorporates informal and formal functional assessment and a careful search for deficits commonly found in stroke.

Specific Stroke-Related Deficits

Cognitive Status. Confusion is a common and vexing problem in elderly stroke patients. Its origins may be multifactorial—related to stroke-preexisting cognitive impairment, acute medical illness, or medications. Its import for functional recovery and survival may be grave.

The prevalence of dementia rises steadily with advancing age. Twenty percent of community-dwelling elderly over 80 have significant cognitive impairment. Though there are exceptions to this, dementia is usually associated with poorer response to rehabilitation.[68]

Delirium may be present due to stroke, coexisting medical illness, or medication toxicity. Such life-threatening acute medical illnesses as myocardial infarction, pneumonia, or urosepsis may present atypically with delirium as the primary clinical manifestation. Medications may cause confusion by a variety of mechanisms including age-associated alterations in pharmacokinetics or pharmacodynamics and drug-drug interactions.[45]

Among the frail elderly it is common to encounter delirium superimposed on dementia. Delirium may be differentiated from dementia by its abrupt onset and fluctuating course, and by the presence of problems of attention, psychomotor retardation, or agitation or sleep disturbance.

All elderly stroke patients should be assessed with the standard mental status examination and a scored instrument like the Mini-Mental State Examination.[17] Because delirium may be a manifestation of a life threatening acute illness, it is essential to distinguish it from dementia so that proper diagnostic and therapeutic measures can be taken. Neuropsychologic evaluation of some demented patients may be helpful in designing a rehabilitation program as it may further characterize specific cognitive strengths and deficits.

Affective Status. Initial emotional reactions to stroke may include anxiety, frustration, anger, and grief. The individual elderly patient's reaction will depend on his or her life history and a variety of other factors. Goodstein[20] suggests several of these, including the general meaning of stroke as a disease, perceptions about the specific losses of function and their practical consequences, the reaction of significant others, the response of the patient's social network, the effect of the stroke on personal appearance and sexuality, any loss of status or finances, and the presence of preexisting medical problems that may interact with the stroke and its associated disability.

Specific affective problems may depend on the hemisphere affected.[6] Patients with nondominant hemispheric stroke may manifest a syndrome characterized by impaired initiative, lack of empathy, emotional lability, impulsivity, and poor judgment. This may produce misunderstanding and conflicts among staff and family members if it is not identified as a consequence of stroke. Though improvement may occur over time, this problem has major prognostic significance as it may interfere with rehabilitation efforts and complicate later attempts to care for the patient at home.

Another problem related to laterality is depression. It is most common in patients with lesions proximal to the left frontal pole of the brain and may manifest at any time following a stroke.[60] Depression is most important to identify and treat during the subacute phase when it may hamper efforts to provide rehabilitation. Diagnosis and treatment are discussed in detail subsequently.

Communication. Disorders of language and speech occur in nearly half of patients with stroke. If ineffectively addressed, they may isolate the patient from family and staff and reduce the chance of benefit from rehabilitation.

The two commonest communication problems encountered in stroke are dysphasia and dysarthria. Dysphasia may be classified into nonfluent and fluent forms.[2,21,29] The major nonfluent aphasias are Broca's and global aphasia; the major fluent aphasias are Wernicke's, anomic, and conduction aphasia. Broca's aphasia occurs when there is involvement of the third frontal gyrus proximal to the motor association area which coordinates the muscles used to create speech. Individuals with this disorder have a disturbance in ability to select, organize, and initiate muscle action. Severity may range from mild problems with articulation to complete inability to speak. Typically the speech of a Broca's aphasic is described as telegrammatic because of its paucity of syntax. Patients with Broca's aphasia generally have preserved comprehension.

Wernicke's aphasics have lesions that affect the posterior superior temporal gyrus of the dominant hemisphere. These patients have fluent, well-articulated speech that may contain verbal, literal, or neologistic paraphasias. Comprehension, naming, and repetition, however, are usually markedly impaired. Patients with Wernicke's aphasia only rarely have hemiplegia.

Conduction aphasics have lesions of the left angular and supramarginal gyrus regions and demonstrate major problems with repetition. Patients with anomic aphasia have injury of their second temporal gyrus and/or angular gyrus. These individuals' predominant communication problem is an inability to generate word names.

Global aphasics have massive injury of the dominant cortex that affects all aspects of speech and language. There is usually associated hemiplegia, hemisensory loss, and apraxia. Though these patients are severely impaired they commonly maintain the ability to understand gestures and communicate information through facial expression and intonation.

Dysarthria may occur in either hemispheric or brain stem infarction. It is commonly present in strokes that are bilateral or that affect the cerebellum or basal ganglia. Dysarthria may be associated with significant swallowing problems. Slurred speech due to absent dentures and medication should be differentiated from dysarthria.

Baseline assessment of communicative abilities should include an evaluation of language input and output components. Input components include the ability to comprehend spoken and written language. Output components include the ability to speak, to name, to write, and to repeat spoken language.

Several measures should be taken until a speech and language therapist can be consulted. First, the patient should always be addressed as an adult. Though this may seem to be a matter of common sense, it is often not practiced. In addition, a system of communication should be devised that makes optimal use of remaining abilities. In the aphasic patient this involves the combined use of spoken and gestural language and in the dysarthric a pad of paper and pencil or one of several commercially available communication boards.

Vision and Hearing. Impaired vision or hearing may also interfere with initial care and rehabilitation. It may, in addition, confound efforts to establish an adequate system of communication with the aphasic patient. Common stroke-related visual abnormalities include homonymous hemianopia or quadrantanopia. Less commonly found are cortical blindness or diplopia associated with posterior circulation strokes. Elderly patients frequently have cataracts, glaucoma, senile macular degeneration, or diabetic retinopathy that may add to visual loss associated with stroke. These may make new stroke-related deficits difficult to detect. In addition, hymonymous hemianopia may be hard to distinguish from unilateral neglect. These both may result in visual inattention on the affected side, though head turning may compensate in patients with hemianopia only. Any adverse affects of visual impairment can be minimized by good lighting and the regular use of eyeglasses.

Hearing loss due to stroke is rare. It is sometimes seen in brain stem infarction. Most commonly, impaired hearing is due to impacted cerumen or presbycusis. All patients should routinely have impacted cerumen cleared and have missing hearing aids brought to the hosital.

Swallowing. Swallowing disorders may be present in hemispheric or brain stem strokes. They may be a result of impairments in oromotor control, triggering of the swallowing reflex, pharyngeal peristalsis, or ability to protect the airway.[77] Often there are several coexisting abnormalities. Lack of careful assessment of swallowing disorders may result in fatal aspiration. Early detection will enable the clinician to provide a safe feeding program until a speech therapist can examine the patient and provide a more definitive diagnosis and therapeutic program.

Each patient should be carefully observed for swallowing dysfunction. Those with dysarthria, facial weakness, gurgling speech or respirations, poor cough, drooling, or altered level of consciousness are particularly likely to have a problem. Examination should include assessment of gag and observation of tongue control and attempts to swallow small sips of water. A trial of feeding with thick liquids (puddings and purees) closely supervised by nursing staff may be useful in evaluating patients with a questionable problem. Definitive evaluation of swallowing disorders requires videofluorography.

Motor Control. The most commonly noted initial finding in hemispheric stroke is hemiparesis. Infarction or hemorrhage in the territory of the middle cerebral artery (MCA) or its branches causes paresis of the contralateral side with facial and upper extremity involvement predominating over lower extremity. Hypotonia and decreased deep tendon reflexes are typical early findings. Complete flaccidity is relatively rare.

Following stroke, neurologic recovery proceeds from proximal to distal. In the typical MCA stroke, lower extremity improvement precedes that seen in the upper extremity and face. The pattern of motor recovery is one of initial hypotonia followed by spasticity, patterned synergistic movements, and then isolated motor control. In the individual patient, recovery may plateau at any of these stages or may consist of a combination of them. With the development of spasticity, synergy patterns predominate. These are mass contractions of synergistic muscles acting on different joints in an extremity. Flexor synergy patterns predominate in the upper extremity and extensor synergy patterns in the lower extremity.[74]

An accurate baseline assessment of motor deficits and remaining abilities is essential for treatment planning and for prognostic purposes. This should include an evaluation of strength, tone, reflexes, and range of motion. Muscle strength should be measured using the standard five-point grading system; fine motor control by observing the ability to rapidly appose the thumb to each finger; and hand function by having the patient attempt to pick up a quarter. It is important to recognize that the results obtained may be influenced by a variety of factors, including preexisting neurologic deficits from stroke or peripheral neuropathy, and changes in position. For example, in an apparently flaccid lower extremity the assumption of the upright position may result in increased extensor tone. In addition, cooperation with the examination may be influenced by such factors as aphasia, apraxia, and agnosia.

Sensation. Deficits in primary and cortical sensation often go unappreciated, but may contribute to functional impairment and pose safety hazards for walking and ADLs. Elderly persons with preexisting neuropathy due to diabetes or alcoholism may be particularly affected. The incidence of sensory deficits in stroke is not as well characterized as that of motor deficits. In one study by Van Buskirk and Webster, 80 percent of patients had sensory impairment.[76]

In general, the majority of patients with hemispheric stroke will have deficits in primary and cortical sensory modalities on the contralateral side. Individuals with brain stem lesions may have mixed findings. In patients with lacunar infarction there may be sensory impairment without coexisting motor loss — a pure motor stroke.

Assessment of sensation should include testing of primary sensory modalities — light touch, pain, temperature, vibration and proprioception, and cortical sensory modalities, — two-point discrimination, stereognosis, graphesthesia, baresthesia, and extinction. In the elderly stroke patient the presence of abnormal vibratory sensation may not be ascribed to stroke as it can be a normal accompaniment of aging.

Perceptual Function. Individuals with either left or right hemispheric stroke may display perceptual impairment. However, this problem is most commonly seen in nondominant or right brain injury where there may also be coexisting behavioral disturbances.[50] The most prevalent perceptual abnormalities are neglect for the affected side, distortion in body image, and impaired sense of true horizontal and vertical. The presence of any of these problems will complicate recovery. Significant hemineglect may make progress in rehabilitation difficult. Impaired sense of total body position in space may threaten safety and contribute to the tendency to fall.

A high likelihood of perceptual impairment may be assumed if the patient has a left hemiparesis. Gaze preference away from the affected side, inability to cross the midline, and lack of eyeblink response to visual threat strongly suggest hemineglect. In those patients able to draw, the presence of neglect and impaired spatial orientation may be unmasked by clock and figure drawing tasks. Omission of detail on the affected side and/or rotation from the normal axis suggest these problems. Subtle perceptual impairment may only be apparent later when ambulation and ADLs are attempted.

Patients found to have significant neglect should initially be approached on the unaffected side. During rehabilitation they should be actively encouraged to attend to the affected side.

Postural Control. Disturbances in postural control are often present in hemispheric stroke. Problems may be seen with head control, sitting balance, and standing balance and may impair performance of ADLs, transfers, wheelchair mobility, and walking. All patients should therefore be assessed for the ability to roll from side to side in bed, come to sitting, sit, come to standing, and stand.

Caregiver Support and Education

One of the most important factors determining functional recovery after stroke is the amount and quality of caregiver support. DeJong and Branch in a retrospective review of stroke patients showed that elderly men with spouses were less likely to be institutionalized.[8] Evans and colleagues have shown that good family function correlated with fewer days of rehospitalization and better adherence to treatment plans.[14,15]

It is therefore important during the acute phase to identify the family-caregiver group and evaluate its ability and willingness to participate in rehabilitation and assume responsibility for caregiving functions after discharge. Formal evaluation may be performed using the McMaster Family Assessment Device,[13] a scale that has been found to be useful in characterizing problems as well as strengths in particular families. It should be emphasized that "family" may include not only spouses and blood relatives, but same-sex lovers, common-law spouses, friends, and neighbors. These individuals may react to the stroke with shock, anger, frustration, disbelief, and denial and will require early support and education if they are to effectively assume ongoing care after the patient is discharged. Whenever available, social service personnel should be involved in assessment and counseling of the patient's family.

SUBACUTE PHASE (48 HOURS TO 3 MONTHS)

The subacute phase begins at 48 hours after admission or at the time of neurologic and medical stabilization. It extends over 3 months, the period during which most neurologic recovery has been found to occur.[36] The major goals of treatment in the subacute phase are to provide appropriate rehabilitation to maximize function and to prevent complications that may threaten life or limit recovery. Decisions about care provided during this phase depend importantly on the data obtained on specific deficits in the acute phase. Functional assessment, performed at weekly and later at monthly intervals, serves as a means of monitoring progress and detecting deterioration.

Estimating Prognosis for Recovery

The prognosis for most long-term stroke survivors is good: four out of five will achieve independent ambulation and two out of three will be independent in ADLs.[23] However, current data do not permit accurate functional prognostication for the individual patient. Multiple studies have sought to link particular patient characteristics with functional outcomes after stroke. Interpretation of most of these is complicated by flaws in design.[24] These include the presence of noncomparable study groups, incomplete classification of neurologic deficits, lack of investigation into the contribution of comorbid diseases, inconsistent outcome variables used from study to study, and lack of adequate documentation of time of entry into rehabilitation after stroke. In reviewing 33 such studies Jongbloed summarizes several variables that are consistently associated with negative functional outcomes.[32] These are listed in Table 4-2.

The question of whether advancing age per se exerts a negative influence on functional recovery is one that can be answered only with

Table 4-2. *Functional Outcome After Stroke: Negative Predictors*

Coma at outset
Incontinence 2 wk after stroke
Poor cognitive function
Severe hemiparesis or hemiplegia
No motor return after 1 mo.
Previous stroke
Perceptual-spatial deficit
Neglect or denial syndrome
Significant cardiovascular disease
Large or deep lesion on computed tomogram
Multiple neurologic deficits

Source: Adapted from Jongbloed, L. (1986). Prediction of function after stroke: A critical review. *Stroke, 17*, 765–776.

qualification.[10,32] Several studies that satisfy minimal design criteria suggest that old age is associated with poorer functional outcomes at discharge. Other studies that examine functional status at fixed intervals after stroke suggest that extent of functional recovery may not differ for the elderly, but that rate of recovery may be slower.[11] If proved to be correct in subsequent well-designed studies, this may provide a major justification for extended rehabilitation in a variety of settings.

Results of the acute phase assessment and subsequent bedside observation may be useful in estimating prognosis for recovery of particular functions.[41] For example, rate of motor recovery appears to correlate with extent of recovery. In general, recovery peaks at 2 to 3 months and is complete at 6 months. Prolonged hypotonia is a poor prognostic sign. Most patients will show an increase in deep tendon reflexes (DTRs) after 48 hours and development of clonus or clasp knife phenomena within 1 month. Bard and Hirschberg showed that in the typical MCA stroke, 40 percent of patients will regain full use of the upper extremity.[4] Most of these will have had return of voluntary movement in the first 2 weeks. However, full motor recovery may not imply normal function. Shah and Carones showed that at 12 weeks only 34 percent of 100 patients could grasp a coin and only 9 percent could pick up an object from the floor.[66] Function may also be affected adversely by apraxia, cognitive, sensory, or perceptual impairment.

The time course of sensory recovery has not been well studied. Van Buskirk and Webster found that it ranged from 1½ months for two-point discrimination to 4 months from vibratory sensation.[76] Persisting sensory deficits may have a major impact on function. For example, hand function may be impaired by the presence of sensory loss, and lower extremity sensory loss may pose safety problems and interfere with ambulation.

Recovery from aphasia has been shown to occur over a longer period of time than motor recovery. While motor recovery appears to plateau at 3 months, many individuals with aphasia show recovery for up to 2 years.[29] Evidence suggests that patients with Broca's aphasia have the best prognosis followed by Wernicke's aphasics and then global aphasics. From 20 to 30 percent of severe aphasics may show complete recovery over time.[29]

Rehabilitation Programs

Rehabilitation for the elderly stroke patient may be provided in a variety of different settings and at several different levels of intensity. Settings include acute rehabilitation units, chronic hospitals, skilled nursing facilities, adult day health centers, and the home. Many elderly patients will not be appropriate for intensive inpatient rehabilitation programs since these require participation in 3 hours of therapy each day.

Clinicians caring for the elderly stroke patient must be aware of treatment options and have an understanding of the goals and content of formal rehabilitation programs. This will enable them to plan and oversee treatment that will result in maximal functional gains and final discharge to a setting that allows the most independence. Data about specific deficits and comorbid conditions obtained during acute phase assessment will aid in decision making. In particular, it is essential for the clinician to characterize the nature of severity of limitations associated with such comorbid conditions as angina, chronic obstructive pulmonary disease, congestive heart failure, and intermittent claudication.

Most rehabilitation specialists advocate a 2-week trial of therapy for all patients. In order to benefit from this, patients should be medically stable and alert. Clinical experience suggests that the following factors are important in deciding whether formal rehabilitation should be continued: (1) the ability to comprehend verbal or nonverbal directions, (2) the ability to follow two- or three-step commands, and (3) the capacity to carry over or retain skills learned from one day to another.

Those patients found to be unsuitable for formal rehabilitation should be provided with a nursing care program that is functionally oriented. Physical and occupational therapists may be used as consultants. A basic program should consist of range-of-motion exercises, positioning to minimize spasticity, pressure relief to prevent pressure sores, a bowel and bladder regimen, mobilization to prevent deconditioning, and careful modulation of sensory stimulation. These are particularly crucial since resolution of acute medical illness or further neurologic recovery may permit a later response to formal rehabilitation.

The general goals of formal stroke rehabilitation include restoration of motor and sensory function in the affected limb; improvement and training in ADLs, transfers, and ambulation; and training and strengthening of the unaffected side.[41] In the acute rehabilitation settings these are most often pursued by a multidisciplinary team that consists of a physical therapist, occupational therapist, rehabilitation nurse, social worker, speech therapist, and physiatrist. In other settings personnel involved will be determined by the nature of the deficits and the regulations governing reimbursement.

Longstanding controversy exists about the relative benefits of different schools of therapy in achieving the gains in function seen after stroke. Two models of therapy are usually compared.[41] These are the traditional model and various neurophysiologic models. The traditional model emphasizes vigorous range-of-motion exercises to prevent contracture; early mobilization; training of unaffected limbs to compensate for lost function; and strengthening exercises. In a traditional program the patient quickly progresses from bed to chair to standing activities. The various neurophysiologic modes, whose major proponents are Rood, Bobath, Brunstrom, Kabat, Knott, and Voss, place much more emphasis on facilitation of movement in affected limbs. Features common to all of these include (1) use of sensory input to facilitate or inhibit motor function; (2) use of the sequence of normal human development in treatment; (3) an understanding of the central role of reflex activity in facilitation and inhibition of motor activity; (4) use of multiple motor repetitions; (5) integration of the body and its segments into a whole; and (6) stress on the importance of therapist and patient interaction. Comparisons between traditional and neurophysiologic approaches have not shown differences in functional outcome.[45] In practice, most therapists have been trained to incorporate elements of both schools into their treatment programs.

Preventing Complications

The hospital environment poses well-recognized risks for the elderly patient.[72] Stroke and related medical conditions may be associated with additional specific complications that increase mortality and morbidity.[53] During the subacute phase it is especially important for the clinician to focus attention on preventing complications. These may be divided into complications that may threaten life and complications that may limit functional recovery (Table 4-3).

Table 4-3. *Complication of Stroke*

LIFE-THREATENING COMPLICATIONS

Recurrent embolic stroke
Deep venous thrombosis, pulmonary embolism
Pneumonia (hypostatic or aspiration)
Seizures

COMPLICATIONS THAT MAY INTERFERE WITH FUNCTIONAL RECOVERY

Medication toxicity
Sensory deprivation syndrome
Depression
Spasticity
Contractures

(continued)

Table 4-3. *(continued)*

Shoulder problems
Pressure sores
Urinary incontinence
Constipation and fecal incontinence
Peripheral nerve palsies
Poor adjustment to disability
Caregiver withdrawal, burnout

Recurrent Embolic Stroke

For patients with embolic stroke, the risk of recurrent embolization is highest in the first 2 weeks after the event—1 percent per day or 14 to 16 percent in the first 2 weeks. Anticoagulation with heparin has been shown to reduce the risk of reembolization by 66 percent.[28] Care should be taken to establish an accurate diagnosis. A computer tomographic (CT) scan should therefore be performed on all patients to identify hemorrhage or cerebral edema. Once instituted, heparin should continue for 7 to 10 days with the activated partial thromboplastin time (APPT) maintained at 1½ to 2 times control. Chronic anticoagulation with warfarin should be provided for 6 months or longer unless the cause of embolization is eliminated or the patient is unsuitable.[28] Individuals with new onset atrial fibrillation should have a trial of pharmacologic cardioversion. Those with chronic nonvalvular atrial fibrillation may not respond to cardioversion and so may require continuing anticoagulation to reduce the significant risk of recurrent stroke.

Deep Venous Thrombosis, Pulmonary Embolism

Stroke has been found to be a major risk factor for the development of deep venous thrombosis (DVT). In a study conducted by Sioson, Crowe, and Dawson,[70] 105 consecutive stroke patients were examined with impedance plethysmography (IPG). Thirty-four percent of those with adequate studies had DVT,[47] all except two of these undetected on clinical examination. Logistic linear regression analysis indicated that profound weakness, male gender, interval between stroke and IPG, edema, and leg hyperpigmentation were independently associated with a positive study. The authors suggest routine screening with IPG for all stroke patients. An alternative is the use of subcutaneous heparin sodium 5000 units every 8 hours while the patient is immobile. This has been shown to be effective in prevention of DVT in stroke patients and is therefore recommended unless there is a specific contraindication.

Pneumonia

Pneumonia is one of the commonest non-stroke-related causes of death during the first month.[69] Hypostatic pneumonia may arise as a result of decreased ventilation of dependent lung segments, atelectasis, poor mucociliary function, and cough. In patients with significant swallowing dysfunction, aspiration of gastric contents may occur. This may develop silently in patients receiving nasogastric or gastrostomy tube feedings. In the elderly patient pneumonia may present atypically with absent fever and leukocytosis. All patients should be encouraged to cough and take deep breaths. Patients with preexisting lung disease may benefit from incentive spirometry and chest physiotherapy.

Poststroke Epilepsy

Seizures occur in up to 9 percent of patients who have had a stroke.[55] These may manifest as grand mal, partial, focal, or jacksonian seizures. In the elderly patient, other precipitants should be considered, particularly arrythmia, postural hypotension, and hypoxemia. Diagnostic evaluation should include an EEG. Depending on the type and severity of the seizure disorder, either intravenous or oral phenytoin sodium should be administered initially. Maintenance phenytoin therapy may be required. An alternative medication for patients who have unacceptable CNS effects from this agent is carbamazepine.

Medication Side Effects

The elderly stroke patient is likely to be receiving multiple medications that may potentially be detrimental to function. After stroke, careful attention should be paid to elimination of those drugs that may decrease alertness, cause postural hypotension, or contribute to weakness. Antihypertensive agents should, when possible, be restricted to classes of agents unlikely to cause CNS effects. Among these are the calcium channel blockers and angiotensin converting enzyme inhibitors. Though postural hypotension is a common effect of most agents, it can be minimized if small doses are used.

Sensory Deprivation Syndrome

The combination of stroke-related hemianopsia or neglect and preexisting deficits in cognition, vision, and hearing can lead to a sensory deprivation syndrome that may be difficult to distinguish from depression. Elderly stroke patients in a poorly lit single bedroom far removed from the nursing station may be especially prone to this complication. Exacerbating factors may include bed position resulting in the affected side facing a wall and the use of air flotation mattresses and waterbeds which may decrease kinesthetic sensory input. Prevention should consist of the provision of adequate sensory stimulation.

Depression

Depression is a frequent complication of stroke. It is present in over 50 percent of patients and its pathogenesis may be complex. Evidence from a series of studies performed by Robinson and Price has suggested that there may be a neurophysiologic basis for poststroke depression.[61] In a series of 103 patients they found a strong correlation between severity of depression and proximity of the lesion to the left frontal pole of the brain, an area that has a high concentration of catecholamine fibers.

The commonest time of onset of depression is early after stroke. However, it can occur anytime up to 2 years following the event.[56] Without treatment, the natural history of poststroke depression is persistence for 9 to 12 months.

All patients with strokes near the left frontal pole should be considered at high risk for depression. Diagnostic evaluation should include a review of current medications and efforts to identify problems that may masquerade as depression, particularly sensory deprivation due to lack of a hearing aid or eyeglasses.

Several studies have demonstrated that antidepressant medication is effective in poststroke depression.[58,60] Choice of a specific agent should be based on the potential to cause side effects that may complicate recovery or result in injury. Most tricyclic agents have anticholinergic, sedative, postural hypotensive, and cardiac conduction system side effects. Of the medications currently available, several have desirable side effect profiles. These include desipramine, nortriptyline, and trazadone. Among these agents, nortriptyline causes the least postural hypotension; desipramine has minimal sedative and anticholinergic activity; and trazadone, absent or minimal anticholinergic potency, though moderate sedative and postural hypotensive effects. In the elderly patient nortriptyline hydrochloride and desipramine hydrochloride should be started in a dose of 10 mg bid and then slowly titrated up to 50 to 75 mg daily over several weeks. Trazadone hydrochloride should be started at 25 mg bid and titrated on a total daily dose of 125 to 150 mg.

In patients for whom anticholinergic, sedative, and postural hypotensive effects are undesirable, methylphenidate is an alternative. Methylphenidate hydrochloride should be started in a dose of 2.5 mg bid, given at 8 A.M. and at 2 P.M. This may be titrated up to a total daily dose of 20 mg. Methylphenidate has been shown to be safe and effective in medically ill elderly patients and in individuals with poststroke depression.[35,42] There is also some evidence to suggest that stimulants may increase learning in individuals with brain injury.[3,16]

Spasticity

The onset of spasticity after stroke is a good prognostic sign. Depending on severity and location its persistence may be either beneficial or detrimental for function. Manifested clinically by the presence of clasp knife rigidity and clonus, spasticity is felt to be due to increased activity of alpha motor neurons. Patients with MCA stroke are likely to have prominent spasticity in shoulder adductors; elbow, wrist, and finger flexors; hip adductors; knee extensors; ankle inverters; and plantar flexors. Spasticity may be worsened by factors that increase nociceptive input, including constipation, urinary retention, and pain from arthritis or pressure sores.

Individuals with extensor spasticity in the lower extremity may begin to ambulate with the aid of a brace that maintains ankle stability and facilitates knee control.[40] Upper extremity spasticity, though, may interfere with volitional movement required for the performance of ADLs.[41] Persistent untreated spasticity in the upper or lower extremity may be associated with clonus that produces sudden movements, which may threaten safety. It may also contribute to the formation of contractures.

Mild to moderate spasticity can be minimized by the use of several measures.[34,44] These include bed positioning that utilizes antispasticity techniques, efforts to minimize factors that increase nociceptive input, and application of heat, cold, or vibratory stimulation. Physical modalities may be particularly useful in reducing spasticity prior to therapy. Severe, persisting spasticity may require the use of medication or neurolysis. A physiatrist should be consulted in such cases.

Contractures

Remolding of muscles and connective tissue surrounding an immobilized joint may occur in as little as 3 days. This occurs as a result of nonoptional positioning. Contractures can produce pain, contribute to skin breakdown and poor hygiene, and seriously retard functional gains.[28] They may be prevented by passive range-of-motion exercises of each joint performed 2 to 3 times a day or once each nursing shift. Patients who are able should be instructed in self-range activities and when this is not feasible family members should be taught to perform such exercises. In addition, wrist and hand contractures may be prevented by the use of orthotic devices fashioned from polyurethane by the occupational therapist.[48] Early contractures can be treated by a program of slow prolonged stretching preceded by superficial heat applied with hot packs or deep heat in the form of ultrasound. Severe contractures may need to be treated surgically.

Shoulder Problems

Shoulder problems are a serious but frequently unrecognized complication of stroke. A preventive approach and early recognition of specific disorders will minimize pain and contracture formation. The commonest shoulder problems are anteroinferior subluxation of the humeral head and reflex sympathetic dystrophy.[75] Other problems that may be seen include rotator cuff tears, tendonitis, bursitis, and heterotopic ossification. Spasticity is the most frequent contributing factor to shoulder pain.[75] To minimize shoulder problems patients with hemiparesis should never be lifted using the affected shoulder. In addition, the upper extremity should be positioned with the hand elevated on a pillow or foam wedge and the shoulder abducted, externally rotated, and forwardly flexed at 25 to 30 degrees from the body. Individuals with flaccidity should be provided with an arm trough when sitting and a sling for transfers and ambulation. Patients found to have reflex sympathetic dystrophy will require a vigorous program of occupational therapy that includes range-of-motion exercises and massage. Steroids or sympathetic blockade may be necessary for some patients.[65]

Pressure Sores

Pressure sores may develop insidiously in the skin overlying major bony prominences, particularly those over the sacrum, ischium, greater trochanter, and heels.[11] These may be a source of pain or infection and may prolong hospitalization. Inadequate relief of pressure is the primary factor responsible. Additional factors include friction from bed sheets, shearing forces produced from sliding down in bed, and moisture from urinary or fecal incontinence. Patients with poor nutrition, edema, vascular disease, or diabetes may be particularly prone to skin breakdown and delaying healing of established pressure sores. All patients should routinely be inspected for skin breakdown and turned at 2-hour intervals. Friction and shearing forces should be reduced by bed positioning and incontinence controlled by the use of a toileting program. Patients who are able should be taught to shift their weight in chair or wheelchair every 30 minutes for 15 seconds or every 60 minutes for 30 seconds.

Urinary Incontinence

Transient urinary incontinence may be present in stroke as a result of temporary loss of cortical inhibition on the sacral micturition center. Persisting urinary incontinence in the elderly patient may be due to a variety of factors including preexisting detrusor hyperreflexia with urge incontinence, prostatic hypertrophy with partial outlet obstruction and overflow incontinence or fecal impaction, delirium, urinary tract infection, or medications. Multiple coexisting factors may be involved. Therefore all patients require careful assessment. Each should have a rectal examination, straight catheterization to detect postvoid residual urine greater than 100 ml, and a urinalysis. Medications should be scrutinized carefully with particular attention paid to eliminating unnecessary sedative, diuretic, and anticholinergic drugs. Those patients without reversible causes of incontinence should be provided with an every-2-hour toileting program. Definitive evaluation of incontinence may require urologic consultation with cystoscopy and cystometrography.

Constipation and Fecal Incontinence

Fecal incontinence may be present early after stroke due to loss of normal inhibition of defecation. Persisting fecal incontinence is commonly a result of fecal impaction created by a combination of immobility, inadequate intake of fluid and fiber, and constipating medications. Fecal impaction may be of two types: colonic or dyschezic.[71] In the colonic type the impaction is high and is associated with a mucous diarrhea. In the dyschezic type soft stool overdistends the rectal vault causing defective emptying and continuous leakage of stool. In the former case a flat plate x-ray of the abdomen may be necessary to make the diagnosis. In the latter, rectal examination is sufficient. Patients with transient fecal incontinence due to stroke should be started on a bowel program that includes placement on the commode each morning after breakfast and efforts to prevent fecal impaction, including a high fiber diet with adequate fluids, early mobilization, and elimination of constipating medications.

Peripheral Nerve Palsies

Peripheral nerve palsies may be produced by improper positioning or lifting that creates pressure or traction on a peripheral nerve or nerve plexus.[52] Elderly thin patients who are wheelchair-bound may be particularly at risk.[31] Some common injuries include ulnar nerve palsy due to pressure over the ulnar groove from prolonged wheelchair sitting, peroneal nerve palsy from pressure over the fibular head, and long thoracic nerve or brachial plexus palsy associated with a flaccid arm dangling over the side of the wheelchair or between the bedrails. The presence of an atypical pattern of motor recovery should prompt a search for possible causes of this problem.

Poor Adjustment to Disability

Many patients will have difficulty adjusting to limitations imposed by the stroke. There may be major changes in physical abilities, ranging from slowed ambulation to need for a wheelchair. Self-care activities may require the assistance of a family member. Aphasia may interfere with the ability to communicate needs or discuss feelings. Hobbies or customary social activities may be less easy to accomplish due to the loss of ability to drive or use public transportation, decreased ability to read, or a lack of volitional control of hand muscles. Patients with right hemispheric syndrome may deny their disability, producing frustration in staff and caregivers. Changes in customary roles may be a cause of anger, frustration, and resentment. Sexual activity may decrease after stroke in both women and men. This may be due to the erroneous belief that it may precipitate another stroke.[51]

Acceptance of disability and future adaptation can be encouraged by emphasizing remaining abilities and the potential for further functional recovery with time. Short-term counseling with a social worker or mental health professional may be useful. A high index of suspicion should always be maintained for depression, particularly in those with left hemispheric involvement. Stroke clubs, present in many areas, may be an especially helpful means of providing needed support and information about practical ways of coping with particular disabilities.

Caregiver Withdrawal and Burnout

Some families may be overwhelmed by the prospect of caring for a multiply disabled elderly stroke patient at home. Results of the McMaster family assessment scale can be used to provide counseling for specific problems. All interested family members should be encouraged to learn how to assist with range-of-motion and self-care tasks. Materials from the American Heart Association can be used to supplement verbal information provided by nurses and therapists.

Plans for discharge should include a consideration of options for respite care in addition to extended therapy and in-home services. Many areas offer adult day health care programs which provide a combination of services well suited to the needs of elderly stroke patients and their families. These include continuing respite and nursing care, rehabilitation, and social activities.

CHRONIC PHASE (3 MONTHS AND AFTER)

Most patients will survive for years after their stroke. In the Framingham cohort, 50 percent of patients were alive at 5 years. Though neurologic recovery has been found to plateau at 3 months, functional recovery may continue for 2 years or longer.[9,36] The major goals of the chronic phase therefore are maintenance of functional gains and modification of risk factors that may increase the chance of recurrent stroke.

Maintaining Functional Gains

Functional gains achieved as a result of spontaneous neurologic recovery and rehabilitation may be preserved by a treatment plan that emphasizes continuing family education and support, prevention of complications, and intermittent short courses of formal rehabilitation. Results derived from periodic functional assessment with the Barthel index may be useful in encouraging compliance with treatment and detecting deterioration that warrants intervention.

Good medical care is a critical factor in the chronic care of elderly stroke patients. Particularly important is avoidance of medication toxicity and early diagnosis of acute medical illness. Repetitive hospitalizations are a common feature of the care of frail elderly patients. Patients with previous stroke may suffer additional declines in functional during stays for acute illness. This may be avoided by early mobilization and provision of appropriate therapies.

Risk Factor Modification

Nearly 30 percent of stroke patients will have another stroke within 10 years.[63] Efforts to prevent recurrent stroke should therefore be a priority in ongoing care.[19] While much evidence supports the benefit of risk factor modification in the prevention of first stroke, there are little data about the value of such intervention in decreasing recurrent stroke. Only hypertension and cardiac comorbidity have been associated with an increased risk of recurrent stroke in prospective studies. Until further evidence is available, clinicians should consider treating hypertension to reduce the blood pressure below 160/90 mm Hg and altering risk factors for atherosclerosis.

CONCLUSION

Effective rehabilitation of the elderly stroke patient demands an approach that is systematic and functionally oriented. It must take into account the special health and social problems of the elderly and the importance of caregiver education and support. The clinician who utilizes such an approach will maximize the chance of achieving meaningful functional improvement and independence, the outcomes most important to elderly stroke survivors and their families.

REFERENCES

1. American Heart Association. (1988). *Stroke facts.* Dallas, American Heart Association.
2. Albert, M.L., and Helm-Eastabrooks, N. (1988). Diagnosis and treatment of aphasia, parts I and II, *JAMA, 259,* 1043, 1205.
3. Back, Y., Rita, P., et al. (1988). Neural aspects of motor function as a basis of early and post-acute rehabilitation. In J.A. Delisa (Eds.), *Rehabilitation medicine: Principles and practice* (pp. 175–195). Philadelphia: Lippincott.
4. Bard, G., and Hirschberg, G.G. (1965). Recovery of voluntary motion in upper extremity following hemiplegia. *Arch. Phys. Rehabil., 46,* 567.
5. Bernspang, B., et al. (1987). Motor and perceptual impairments in acute stroke patients: Effects on self-care ability. *Stroke, 18,* 1081.
6. Binder, L. (1982). Emotional problems after stroke. *Curr. Concepts Cerebrovasc Dis. Stroke, 18,* 17.
7. Calliet, R. (1980). *The shoulder in hemiplegia.* Philadelphia: Davis.
8. Dejong, G., Branch, L.G. (1982). Predicting the stroke patient's ability to live independently. *Stroke, 13,* 648.
9. Dombovy, M.L., Bach, Y., Rita, P. (1988). Clinical observations on recovery from stroke. *Adv. Neurol., 47,* 265.
10. Dombovy, M.L., Sandok, B.A., and Basford, J.R. (1986). Rehabilitation for stroke: A review. *Stroke, 17,* 363.
11. Donovan, W.H., et al. (1988). Pressure ulcers. In J.A. Delisa, et al. (Eds.), *Rehabilitation medicine: Principles and practice* pp. 476–491). Philadelphia: Lippincott.
12. Dyken, M.L., et al. (1984). Risk factors in stroke. A statement for physicians by the subcommittee on risk factors in the stroke council. *Stroke, 15,* 1105.
13. Epstein, M.B., Baldwin, L.M., and Bishop, D.S. (1983). McMaster family assessment device. *J. Marital Fam. Ther., 8,* 71.
14. Evans, R.L., et al. (1987). Prestroke family interaction as a predictor of stroke outcome. *Arch. Phys. Med. Rehabil. 68,* 508.
15. Evans, R.L., et al. (1987). Family interaction and treatment adherence after stroke. *Arch. Phys. Med. Rehabil., 68,* 513.
16. Feeney, D.M., Gonzales, A., and Law, W.A. (1982). Amphetamine, haloperidol and experience interact to affect rate of recovery after motor cortex lesion. *Science, 217,* 855.

17. Folstein, M.F., Folstein, S., and McHugh, P.R. (1975). Mini-mental state: A practical method for grading the cognitive state of patients for the clinician. *J. Psychiatr. Res., 12,* 189.
18. Garraway, W.M., and Whisnat, J.P. (1987). The changing pattern of hypertension and the declining incidence of stroke, *JAMA, 258,* 214.
19. Goldberg, G., and Berger, G.G. (1988). Secondary prevention in stroke: A primary rehabilitation concern. *Arch. Phys. Med. Rehabil., 69,* 32.
20. Goodstein, R.K. (1983). Overview: Cerebrovascular accident and the hospitalized elderly — A multidimensional clinical problem. *Am. J. Psychiatry, 140,* 141.
21. Granger, C.V., Seltzer, G.B., and Fishbein, C.F. (Eds.) (1987). *Primary care of the functionally disabled: Assessment and management.* Philadelphia: Lippincott.
22. Greenblatt, D.J., Sellers, E.M., and Shader, R.I. (1982). Drug disposition in old age. *N. Engl. J. Med., 306,* 1081.
23. Gresham, G.E. (1986). The rehabilitation of the stroke survivor. In H.J.M. Barnet, B.M. Stein, J.P. Mohr, and F.M. Yatsu (Eds.), *Stroke: Pathophysiology, diagnosis and management* (pp. 1259–1274). New York: Churchill-Livingstone.
24. Gresham, G.E. (1986). Stroke outcome research. *Stroke, 17,* 358.
25. Gresham, G.E., Phillips, T.F. and Labi, M. (1980). ADL status in stroke: Relative merits of three standard indexes. *Arch. Phys. Med. Rehabil. 61,* 355.
26. Gresham, G.E., Therese, P.F., Wolf, P.H., McNamara, P.M. (1979). Epidemiologic profile of long term stroke disability: The Framingham study. *Arch. Phys. Med. Rehabil., 60,* 487.
27. Grotta, J.C. (1987). Current medical and surgical therapy for cerebrovascular disease. *New Engl. J. Med. 24,* 1505.
28. Halar, E.M. and Bell, K.R. (1988). Contracture and other deleterious effects of immobility. In J.A. Delisa, (Eds.) *Rehabilitation medicine: Principles and practice* (pp. 448–462). Philadelphia: Lippincott.
29. Halper, A.S., Mogil, S.I. (1986). Communication disorders: Diagnosis and treatment. In P.E. Kaplan and L.J. Cerulo (Eds.), *Stroke rehabilitation* (pp. 233–252). Boston: Butterworths.
30. Harper, C.M., and Lyles, Y.M. (1988). Physiology and complications of bed rest. *J. Am. Geriatr. Soc., 36,* 1047.
31. Hartig, D. (1982). The dangerous wheelchair. *J. Am. Geriatr. Soc. 30,* 572.
32. Jongbloed, L. (1986). Prediction of function after stroke: A critical review. *Stroke, 17,* 765.
33. Katz, R.T. (1988). Management of spasticity. *Am. J. Phys. Med. Rehabil.,* 108.
34. Katz, S., et al. (1970). Progress in development of the index of ADL. *Gerontologist, 10,* 20.
35. Kaufman, M.W., Cassen, N.H., Murray, G.B. et al. (1984). Use of psychostimulants in medically ill elderly patients with neurological disease and major depression. *Can. J. Psychiatry, 29,* 46.
36. Kelly-Hayes, M., and Wolf, P.A. (1988). Course of recovery following stroke: The Framingham study (abstract). Presented at Congress of Rehabilitation Medicine, Seattle.
37. Kelly-Hayes, M., et al. (1988). Factors influencing survival and need for institutionalization following stroke: The Framingham study. *Arch. Phys. Med. Rehabil., 69,* 415–418.

38. Labi, M.L., Phillips, T.F., and Gresham, G.E. (1980). Psychosocial disability in physically restored long term stroke survivors. *Arch. Phys. Med. Rehabil.*, 61, 561.
39. Lawton, M.P. (1971). The functional assessment of elderly people. *J. Am. Geriatr. Soc.*, 19, 465–481.
40. Lehmann, J.F. et al. (1987). Gait abnormalities in hemiplegia: Their correction by ankle-foot orthoses. *Arch. Phys. Med. Rehabil*, 68, 763–771.
41. Lieberman, J.S. (1986). Hemiplegia: Rehabilitation of the upper extremity. In P.E. Kaplan and L.J. Cerullo (Eds.), *Stroke rehabilitation* (pp. 95–117). Boston: Butterworth.
42. Lingham, V.R., et al. (1988). Methylphenidate in treating post stroke depression. *J. Clin. Psychiatry,* 49, 151–153.
43. Lipowski, A.J. (1983). Transient cognitive disorders (delirium, acute confusional states) in the elderly. *Am. J. Psychiatry,* 140, 1426.
44. Little, J.W., and Merritt, J.L. (1988). Spasticity and associated abnormalities of muscle tone. In J.A. Delisa (Eds.), *Rehabilitation medicine: Principles and practice* (pp. 430–447). Philadelphia: Lippincott.
45. Lord, J.P., and Hall, K. (1986). Neuromuscular reeducation versus traditional programs for stroke rehabilitation. *Arch. Phys. Med. Rehabil.,* 67, 88–91.
46. Mahony, F.I., and Barthel, D.W. (1965). Functional evaluation: The Barthel index. *Md. State Med. J.,* 14, 61.
47. McCarthy, S.T., et al. (1977). Low dose heparin as a prophylaxis against deep vein thrombosis after acute stroke. *Lancet, 2,* 800.
48. McCollough, N.C. (1978). Orthotic management in adult hemiplegia. *Clin. Orthop., 131,* 38.
49. Meissner, I. Whisnant, J.P., and Garraway, M.W. (1988). Hypertension management and stroke recurrence in a community (Rochester, Minnesota, 1950–1979). *Stroke, 19,* 459.
50. Mersulam, M.M. (1981). A cortical network for directed attention and unilateral neglect. *Neurology, 10,* 309.
51. Monga, T.N., Lawson, J.S., and Inglis, J. (1986). Sexual dysfunction in stroke patients. *Arch. Phys. Med. Rehabil.,* 67, 19.
52. Moskowitz, E., and Porter, J. (1963). Peripheral nerve lesions in the upper extremity in hemiplegic patients. *N. Engl. J. Med., 269,* 776.
53. Mulley, G. (1982). Avoidable complications of stroke. *J. Roy. Coll. Physicians Lond, 16,* 94.
54. *National health interview—Survey and supplement on aging.* National Center for Health Statistics, 1984.
55. Olsen, T.S., Hoogenhave, A., and Thage, O. (1987). Epilepsy after stroke. *Neurology, 37,* 1209.
56. Parikh, R.M., Lipsey, J.R., Robinson, R.G., and Price, T.R. (1987). Two year longitudinal study of post-stroke mood disorders: Dynamic changes in correlates of depression at one and two years. *Stroke, 18,* 579.
57. Posner, J.D., Gorman, K.M., and Woldow, A. (1984). Stroke in the elderly: I. Epidemiology. *J. Am. Geriatr. Soc., 32,* 95.
58. Reding, M.J., Orto, F.L.A., Winter, S.W., Fortuna, I.M., Di Ponte, P., and McDowell, F.H. (1986). Antidepressant therapy after stroke. *Arch. Neurol., 43,* 763.
59. *Rehabilitation nursing techniques. 1. Bed positioning and transfer techniques for the hemiplegic.* Minneapolis, Sister Kenney Rehabilitation Institute, 1962.

60. Robinson, R.G. (1986). Post-stroke mood disorders. *Hosp. Pract.,* 21 (April 15), 83.
61. Robinson, R.G., and Price, T.R. (1982). Post-stroke depressive disorders: A follow-up study of 103 patients. *Stroke, 13,* 635.
62. Roth, E.J., Mueller, K., and Green, D. (1988). Stroke rehabilitation outcome: Inpact of coronary artery disease. *Stroke, 19,* 42.
63. Sacco, R. L., et al. (1982). Survival and recurrence following stroke: The Framingham study. *Stroke, 13,* 290.
64. Schuman, J.E., et al. (1981). Geriatric patients with and without intellectual dysfunction: Effectiveness of a standard rehabilitation program. *Arch. Phys. Med. Rehabil., 62,* 612.
65. Schwartzman, R.J., and McLellan, T.L. (1987). Reflex sympathetic dystrophy: A review. *Arch. Neurol., 44,* 555.
66. Shah, S.K., and Corones, J. (1980). Volition following hemiplegia. *Arch. Phys. Med. Rehabil., 61,* 523.
67. Sharpless, J.W. (1982). *Mossman's a problem-oriented approach to stroke rehabilitation.* Springfield, IL: Thomas.
68. Shoening, H.A., and Iverson, I.A. (1968). Numerical scoring of self-care status: A study of Kenney self-care evaluation. *Arch. Phys. Med. Rehabil., 49,* 221.
69. Silver, F.L., et al. (1984). Early mortality following stroke: A prospective review. *Stroke, 15,* 492.
70. Sioson, E.R., Crowe, W.E., and Dawson, N.V. (1988). Occult proximal deep vein thrombosis. Its prevalence among patients admitted to a rehabilitation hospital. *Arch. Phys. Med. Rehabil., 69,* 183–185.
71. Smith, R.G. (1983). Fecal incontinence. *J. Am. Geriatr. Soc., 31,* 694.
72. Steel, K., et al. (1981). Iatrogenic illness on a general medical service at a university hospital. *N. Engl. J. Med., 304,* 638.
73. Turney, T.M., Garraway, W.M., and Sinake, M. (1984). Neurologic examination in stroke rehabilitation: Adequacy of its description in clinical textbooks. *Arch. Phys. Med. Rehabil., 66,* 92.
74. Twitchell, T.E. (1951). The restoration of motor function following hemiplegia in man. *Brain, 74,* 443.
75. Van Ouwenaller, C., Laplace, P.M., and Chantraine, A. (1986). Painful shoulder in hemiplegia. *Arch. Phys. Med. Rehabil., 67,* 23.
76. Van Buskirk, C., and Webster, D. (1955). Prognostic value of sensory defect in rehabilitation of hemiplegics. *Neurology, 5,* 407.
77. Veis, S.L., and Logemann, J.A. (1985). Swallowing disorders in persons with cerebrovascular accident. *Arch. Phys. Med. Rehabil. 66,* 372.
78. Weingard, F.D. (Ed.) (1981). The national survey of stroke. *Stroke, 12.* (Suppl 1, p 2), 1.
79. Wolf, P.A., Abbott, R.D., and Kannel, W.B. (1987). Atrial fibrillation, a major contributor to stroke in the elderly. The Framingham Study. *Arch. Intern. Med., 147,* 1561.

CHAPTER 5

Arthritis and Osteoporosis
EDWARD MONGAN

OSTEOARTHRITIS

Osteoarthritis is a noninflammatory disorder of movable joints characterized by deterioration and abrasion of articular cartilage and by the formation of new bone at the joint surfaces. It is by far the commonest type of arthritis. In a nationwide sample of 6,672 adults 18 to 79 years of age in the United States, 37 percent of subjects examined had radiographic evidence of osteoarthritis.[12]

All degrees of radiographic osteoarthritis increase steadily with age from 4 percent in persons 18 to 24 years of age to 85 percent of persons 75 to 79 years of age. Males are affected more commonly than females before age 45 but the sex ratio is reversed thereafter. Moderate or severe involvement, however, is twice as common in women (11%) as in males (6%).

Osteoarthritis is traditionally divided into two categories:

1. Primary osteoarthritis, which arises de novo
2. Secondary osteoarthritis, which results from the effects of an injury or mechanical derangement of the joint

The primary form is by far the commoner type of osteoarthritis and usually becomes symptomatic after age 50 years. While secondary osteoarthritis can occur in any joint, primary osteoarthritis favors certain target sites.

The pattern of distribution classically seen involves the following articulations[1]:

1. Distal interphalangeal joints of the hands
2. Joints around the base of the thumb
3. Lower cervical spine
4. Lumbosacral spine
5. Large weight-bearing joints (hips and knees)
6. Great toe joints
7. Temporomandibular joints

The cause of primary osteoarthritis is unknown so there is no way to prevent it.

Secondary osteoarthritis may arise as a direct consequence of trauma to a joint such as a fracture with subsequent malalignment. Other causes of secondary osteoarthritis are congenital anomalies such as congenital dislocation of the hip, local damage to a joint caused by bacterial infection or ischemic necrosis, metabolic diseases such as acromegaly or alcaptonuria, and neurologic abnormalities leading to neuropathic joints as in tabes dorsalis or syringomyelia. Even low-grade trauma over a number of years can lead to secondary osteoarthritis.[8].

DIAGNOSIS OF OSTEOARTHRITIS

The cardinal symptom of osteoarthritis is pain after joint use which is relieved by rest. Later the pain occurs with minimal motion or even at rest. Stiffness of short duration, aching at times of inclement weather, and crepitation on motion are other symptoms which are frequently found, but they are nonspecific because they are also found in many other types of arthritis. While the affected joints may be tender and enlarged, signs of inflammation are uncommon except for effusion. Range of motion may be limited and is particularly helpful in diagnosing osteoarthritis of the hips. Osteophytes can be palpated on the dorsal lateral aspect of the proximal and distal interphalangeal joints and malalignment of a extremity due to asymmetric involvement of joints is common.

Routine blood counts, sedimentation rate (ESR), urinaysis, electrolytes, serum calcium, phosphorus, alkaline phosphatase, serum proteins, and serologic tests for rheumatoid factor (RF) and antinuclear antibodies (ANA) are all normal in osteoarthritis. Synovial fluid from osteoarthritic joints is a type I or noninflammatory fluid (i.e., only a slight increase in the number of cells with most cells mononuclear in type). The one consistent abnormality in osteoarthritic joints is the x-ray finding. Indeed, osteoarthritis can probably not be diagnosed in a given joint unless characteristic radiographic findings are present. These findings include irregular joint space narrowing, subchondral bony sclerosis, marginal osteophyte formation, and, on occasion, bone cysts. It should be stressed, however, that only 30 percent of joints which show radiographic evidence of osteoarthritis are symptomatic (Table 5-1).

Table 5-1. *Osteoarthritis — Essentials of Diagnosis*

Pain relieved by rest
Lack of inflammatory signs
Normal laboratory findings
Type 1 synovial fluid
Characteristic x-ray findings

PREVALENCE OF OSTEOARTHRITIS

The prevalence of osteoarthritis is greater in men than in women up until age 45. This finding is felt to be due to more secondary osteoarthritis in younger men because of increased joint trauma, occupational stress, and mechanical factors. After age 45 osteoarthritis is more common in women. The pattern of joint involvement is similar in men and women up until age 55, but in older persons distal interphalangeal, proximal interphalangeal, and the first carpal metacarpal joints are more frequently involved in women and the hips more commonly affected in men. There is a well-known familial predominance of distal interphalangeal joint involvement (Heberden's nodes) and proximal interphalangeal joint involvement (Bouchard's nodes) in women.[13]

TREATMENT OF OSTEOARTHRITIS

Treatment in osteoarthritis must be individualized. Many patients require only reassurance that they do not have a severe form of arthritis. Rest of the involved joint and protection of joints from overuse is important, especially in weight-bearing joints. Forces on the lower extremity are increased threefold when weight is shifted to each leg in walking. For this reason weight reduction should be carried out in obese patients because, if successful, a significant reduction in pain can be achieved. Appliances such as canes or walkers are beneficial for joint protection when indicated. Physical therapy to relieve pain and associated muscle spasm and to maintain joint range of motion is important.

It has long been recognized by clinicians that obesity aggravates the pain in osteoarthritic weight-bearing joints. More controversial, however, is the question whether or not obesity predisposes to osteoarthritis. A recently published study[4] bears directly on this question. As part of a larger study of heart disease, a cohort in Framingham, Massachusetts was carefully examined in the period 1948 through 1951 and closely followed at 2-year intervals for the next 36 years. At entry to the study none of the group had known osteoarthritis. All individuals were placed in one of five groups depending on their body weight. Men in the highest weight group had significantly more osteoarthritis of their knees 36 years later, as did women in the two highest weight groups. The authors interpret these findings to mean that not only does obesity aggravate the symptoms of osteoarthritis, but it is probably a predisposing factor.

Pain relief in osteoarthritis can be obtained by two additional methods, the use of pharmacologic agents or elective joint surgery. In patients with mild osteoarthritis, analgesic drugs such as acetaminophen or propoxyphene hydrochloride may be effective when used on an as-needed basis. Narcotic preparations should be avoided. In moderate to severe cases of osteoarthritis, nonsteroidal antiinflammatory agents are often beneficial. Aspirin, which has both analgesic and antiinflammatory properties, is effective, often in moderate doses. Nonsteroidal agents such as indomethacin, ibuprofen, fenoprofen, naproxen, tolmetin, piroxicam, and sulindac are available for use. These agents have a number of side effects including rash, gastrointestinal (GI) upset, peptic ulceration, and, rarely, acute renal failure. There is evidence to suggest that there is an increased incidence of GI hemorrhage from peptic ulceration and acute renal failure in elderly patients on these medications.[5] These drugs, therefore, should be used carefully in the elderly and the smallest effective dose should be prescribed. Judicious intraarticular injections of corticosteroids may be beneficial in the management of acute joint flare-ups in osteoarthritis. Injections should be infrequent, especially into weight-bearing joints. The improvement is only temporary, rarely lasting more than 4 to 6 weeks. As a general rule, a given joint should not be injected with adrenocorticosteroids more than 3 times in 1 year.

In patients with advanced osteoarthritis of a weight-bearing joint with disabling pain, a number of orthopedic procedures are valuable. Osteotomy and joint fusion have been tried for many years with some success. In the past 20 years the judicious use of cemented hip and knee replacements has resulted in marked symptomatic improvement in most patients by providing striking pain relief and an improved range of motion. While total knee replacements are less consistently beneficial than are hip replacements, in patients able to cooperate in a vigorous physical therapy program postoperatively, significant pain relief and a gain in range of motion occurs. The benefits of artificial joint replacements must be weighed against the possible complications, which include thrombophlebitis, pulmonary emboli, nerve injury, and loosening of the prosthesis. While loosening of cemented prostheses has been a major problem in younger persons with knee or hip arthroplasties, it is much less common after age 60, presumably because the patients are less physically active. The most feared complication of total joint replacement is bacterial infection which often requires removal of the prosthesis to clear the infection (Table 5-2).

Table 5-2. *Osteoarthritis—Essentials of Treatment*

Weight loss
Rest
Joint protection techniques
Physical therapy
Medication
Joint replacement surgery

Overall, primary osteoarthritis is a disease of persons over age 50 and with current medications, physical therapy, and elective orthopedic procedures, the functional prognosis for such persons is quite good.

RHEUMATOID ARTHRITIS

Rheumatoid arthritis (RA) is a chronic inflammatory disease principally affecting the joints, resulting in swelling, pain, and deformity. While joint involvement is predominant, RA involves connective tissues throughout the body and may lead to severe disability and invalidism. The inflammation starts in the synovial membrane and progresses to involve the entire joint. Rheumatoid arthritis occurs in about 1 percent of the adult population and is 2 to 3 times more common in women than it is in men. About 750 new cases per million population occur annually. No racial predisposition has been noted.

Rheumatoid arthritis usually starts insidiously although, on occasion, there may be a sudden or episodic onset. Although RA can involve multiple joints or only a single joint, there is a predilection for symmetric involvement of small peripheral joints. The most frequent joints involved are (1) the proximal interphalangeal joints of the hands, (2) the metacarpophalangeal joints, (3) the metatarsophalangeal joints, (4) the small hinge joints (wrists, elbows, and ankles), (5) the hip and knees, (6) the temporomandibular joint, and (7) the upper cervical spine. While pain and joint swelling are the most common complaints, stiffness occurring after joint inactivity is also common. The stiffness which occurs when a patient arises is called morning stiffness. If it occurs after prolonged sitting (such as in a theater or after watching a television program), it is called gelling. Unlike osteoarthritis, which is solely a joint disease, RA is a connective tissue disease which involves many other organ systems. Systemic effects such as weight loss, muscle atrophy, and anemia are common in severe RA (Table 5-3).

Table 5-3. *Rheumatoid Arthritis—Essentials of Diagnosis*

Pain after inactivity
Symmetric involvement of small joints
Other organ systems involved
Anemia
Elevated sedimentation rate
Positive rheumatoid factor (usually)

EPIDEMIOLOGY OF RHEUMATOID ARTHRITIS

The peak age of onset of RA is 20 to 40 years of age. The onset of RA after age 60 is not uncommon and has been reported to represent 33 percent of all RA patients seen in some clinics.[7] The clinical picture in patients who present with RA after age 60 years is essentially the same as in younger persons although two studies report a more favorable course than that seen in younger persons.[3,14]

DIAGNOSIS OF RHEUMATOID ARTHRITIS

Although there are a number of characteristic clinical and laboratory finding in RA, there is no one clinical finding or laboratory test which establishes the diagnosis. Indeed, it is possible that more than one etiologic agent can result in the syndrome presently called rheumatoid arthritis. Common laboratory abnormalities include a normochromic normocytic anemia, an elevated ESR, a positive serologic test for RF and, on occasion, a positive test for ANA. It should be stressed that the absence of RF in a patient with joint symptoms does not rule out the diagnosis of RA. The presence of RF in a patient with joint symptoms, however, does not make the diagnosis of RA. A high serum titer of RF does have some prognostic value in RA because almost all of the extraarticular complications of RA occur in those patients who have high titers of circulating RF.[16]

TREATMENT OF RHEUMATOID ARTHRITIS

The first goal in treating patients with RA is to control the inflammatory synovitis, which is felt to be the initial site of the disease. Analgesic drugs are not useful here. One can either use antiinflammatory doses of salicylates (by achieving salicylate levels of from 15–30 mg/dl) or other nonsteroidal antiinflammatory drugs. When used at antiinflammatory levels salicylates have significant dose-related toxicity such as tinnitus, GI upset, and GI bleeding, which occur more often in elderly patients with RA.[6] Nonsteroidal antiinflammatory drugs are useful in mild cases of RA but with the same precautions noted in the elderly, as in patients with osteoarthritis. Moreover, since the dose of a nonsteroidal anti-inflammatory drug needed to successfully treat patients with RA is usually higher than in patients with osteoarthritis, side effects must be more carefully monitored. Adrenocorticosteroids should not be used to treat patients with uncomplicated RA because in time almost all treated RA patients develop serious untoward drug effect.

A number of "remittive" drugs are also widely used in the treatment of RA. These include hydroxychloroquine, parenteral or oral gold therapy, penicillamine, and immunosuppressive drugs such as cyclophospha-mide, azathioprine, and methotrexate. These drugs are used almost exclusively by rheumatologists, have significant untoward effects which must be carefully monitored, but have not been reported to have a greater risk in patients over age 50 than below that age.

A second goal in managing patients with RA is to prevent unnecess-ary joint contractures which interfere with function. For example, most patients with knee pain and swelling feel more comfortable when supine in bed if their knees are slightly flexed by having pillows behind them. If this is done routinely, however, the patient may develop a flexion contrac-ture that is, an inability to completely extend the knee. A flexion contracture of 20 degrees or more is a significant functional problem because such persons must use 3 times the total amount of muscle energy to walk as do persons without such flexion contractures.

A third goal in managing patients with RA is to maintain optimal function. A number of joint protection techniques are valuable and are usually taught by occupational therapists. A fourth goal in managing patients with RA is to correct deformities that already exist by elective joint surgery which has revolutionized the care of patients with severe RA in the last 20 years. Although a discussion of the role of surgery in RA patients is beyond the scope of this chapter, many patients with RA have operations prior to age 50 and, in general, the surgical results in RA patients are not as good as they are in patients with osteoarthritis. The major reason for this difference is that RA patients have multiple joint involvement which does not allow them to make the functional gains that most osteoarthritic patients achieve postoperatively. Moreover, since the RA patients are frequently younger at the time of surgery, the chance of prosthetic loosening is higher because the patients live longer.

In the last 3 to 4 years the widespread introduction of porous ingrowth prostheses for hip and knee replacement in rheumatoid patients under age 60 has become standard. While we will have to wait at least a decade from the introduction of porous ingrowth prostheses to be certain that their early promise is achieved, so far the record is good (Table 5-4).

Table 5-4. *Rheumatoid Arthritis—Essentials of Treatment*

Goal	Method
Control synovitis	Antiinflammatory drugs
Prevent contractures	Therapeutic exercises
Maintain optimal function	Therapy
Joint protection	Education and assistive aids
Correct deformities	Joint replacement surgery

GOUT

Gout is a group of disorders of purine metabolism that are characterized chemically by hyperuricemia. When clinically manifest they present with acute arthritis, tophaceous deposits of sodium urate, uric acid stones, and/or renal disease. It is estimated that 5 percent of all arthritis patients have gout yielding a total of over 1 million people in the United States with the disease. It affects primarily males (approximately 95%) and of these, 85 to 90 percent have an onset over age 40. A family history of the disease is found in approximately 25 percent of patients.

DIAGNOSIS OF GOUT

Gout has a very characteristic clinical picture. There is usually an acute dramatic onset involving one, two, or at most three joints simultaneously. The patient is usually a man over age 40 who cannot only tell the physician what day his joint symptoms started, but often the exact hour. The involved joint is red, hot, swollen, and exquisitely painful. Even without therapy the acute attack usually clears in 2 to 3 weeks. Although any joint can be involved, first metatarsophalangeal joint involvement occurs in 50 percent of initial attacks and in greater than 90 percent with subsequent attacks. At the time of the attack the serum uric acid level is usually elevated and synovial fluid examination reveals type II or inflammatory findings with an elevated white cell count (10,000–40,000), an increased percentage of polymorphonuclear leukocytes, and negatively birefringent uric acid crystals when examined under a polarized microscope. The diagnosis can only be unequivocally made by finding the characteristic crystals in the synovial fluid of an involved joint during an attack.

TREATMENT OF GOUT

Therapy is divided into two portions:

1. The treatment of the acute gouty attack is best done by rest of the affected joint, large doses of a nonsteroidal antiinflammatory drug, or, if the patient cannot take medication orally, by intravenous (IV) colchicine.
2. Treatment to lower serum uric acid levels to normal limits: This step is not done simultaneously with the treatment of the acute attack, because it may exacerbate the acute attack. Usually 7 to 10 days after the acute attack has subsided treatment is begun with either a uricosuric drug (such as probenecid or sulfinpyrazone), or a drug which interferes with uric acid production (allopurinol).

Allopurinol, an xanthine oxidase inhibitor, is a potent and useful drug in decreasing uric acid production and thereby reducing serum uric acid levels to normal. Allopurinol must be used carefully in elderly patients because almost all serious side effects of the drug occur in patients with decreased renal function who are taking multiple medications, conditions more likely to occur in the elderly.

The prognosis of gout has been completely altered by the discovery of drugs which effectively reduce serum uric acid levels to normal. Gout, which prior to 1950 was felt to be the most severe type of arthritis, is as common as ever, but is now usually well controlled by appropriate drug therapy. The dose of uricosuric drugs and allopurinol is monitored by serum uric acid levels. Once the desired uric acid level is reached, lifelong medication is indicated. In addition, there is good empiric data that small daily doses of oral colchicine markedly decrease the incidence of recurrent attacks.[17]

There are two instances where the age of the patient alters the way a patient with gout is treated:

1. While there is conclusive evidence that the use of a medication to reduce serum uric acid levels and a prophylactic medication to prevent acute attacks is worthwhile, patients who develop their first attack of acute gout over age 70 may be treated differently. Since the chances of recurrent gouty attacks leading to chronic tophaceous gout are so small in these elderly men, the treating

physician may elect just to treat acute attacks because the patients will probably not live long enough to develop chronic tophaceous gout. The average time from the first attack of acute gout to the onset of chronic tophaceous gout is over a decade.[9]

2. Now that there are a large number of people living into their 80s and 90s, most elderly women present with acute gout. Males develop gout approximately 20 to 30 years after the normal increase in serum uric acid levels occurs at puberty. This finding explains the peak incidence of gout in 40- to 60-year-old men. In women, serum uric acid levels do not rise until menopause. Now that many women are living 20 to 30 years after menopause, we are seeing acute gout in elderly women. Not only is gout usually not considered in elderly women, but the disease does not present as classically as it does in middle-aged men. If the disease is suspected, however, it can be as readily diagnosed with appropriate blood and synovial fluid studies as it can in men. Moreover, treatment is as successful as in men.

SYSTEMIC LUPUS ERYTHEMATOSUS (SLE)

Systemic lupus erythematosus (SLE) is a disease of unknown cause that affects many organ systems; it is characterized by the presence of multiple autoantibodies that participate in immunologically mediated tissue injury. SLE is approximately one-tenth as common as RA; 90 percent of cases occur in women, and blacks are 3 times as likely to have SLE as are whites. The peak age of onset of lupus is between ages 15 to 35 years but SLE occurs both in children and in the elderly. SLE is a connective tissue disease which usually presents with systemic symptoms such as fatigue, fever, and weight loss, all of these symptoms occurring in at least 90 percent of patients. The hallmark of SLE is that at least two different organ systems are involved before the diagnosis can be made. Frequently involved organ systems include the joints (90% of patients), skin (75%), renal involvement (50%), pulmonary involvement (45%), cardiac involvement (45%), GI involvement (40%), and CNS (30%). In addition to rather characteristic clinical systems, a number of laboratory abnormalities are usually found. Seventy percent of SLE patients are anemic, 55 percent are leukopenic, and 10 percent are thrombocytopenic. Ninety-six percent of patients have a positive test for ANA, 50 percent have antibodies to double-stranded DNA, and 15 percent have biologically false-positive tests for syphilis. While the cause of this disease remains unknown, the prognosis is considerably better today than it was 30 years ago (5-year survivals of over 90% are routinely reported from large centers).[15] It is, however, still a serious, potentially fatal disease.

SLE can have its onset in patients over 50 years of age. As in younger persons, SLE is really a syndrome rather than a disease and the diagnosis depends on a characteristic clinical presentation with compatible (but not pathognomonic) laboratory findings. When SLE has its onset after age 50, it is often more insidious than when it occurs in a young person. Nephritis, CNS dysfunction, and severe hematologic disorders are more frequent in SLE with onset under age 50. In contrast, pulmonary manifestations and a milder course are more typical when the diagnosis is made after age 50.[2]

The therapy of SLE in the elderly is essentially the same as it is in the young. In mild cases salicylates or nonsteroidal antiinflammatory drugs may suffice. Particularly in cases with dermatologic features, antimalarial drugs such as hydroxychloroquine are beneficial. Patients with moderate, severe, or life-threatening SLE are best treated with adrenocorticosteroids. There is good evidence that with renal or CNS involvement (the two organ systems most likely to cause death in SLE) large doses of steroids are beneficial.[10] Since SLE is more common in women and since postmenopausal women are most at risk for developing steroid-induced osteoporosis, the smallest daily dose of adrenocorticosteroid that suppresses symptoms is the desirable one. If SLE patients do not respond to steroid therapy, an immunosuppressive drug is usually added, although these drugs have low therapeutic indices and must be used with care.

While SLE is a life-threatening illness, it rarely causes joint deformities. The arthritis of SLE usually responds to modest doses (i.e., 10–20 mg prednisone daily) of adrenocorticosteroids so the patient's ability to care for himself at home depends more on the control of constitutional symptoms (such as fatigue, malaise, and weakness) than on control of joint pain per se. Elective joint surgery is rarely indicated in lupus patients unless prolonged high-dose steroids are needed to control renal or CNS findings. Such patients may develop ischemic necrosis of their femoral heads and, if severe, may need total hip replacement.

OSTEOPOROSIS

Osteoporosis is a generalized loss of bone density resulting in either spontaneous fractures or fractures caused by minimal trauma. Osteoporosis can occur by itself, can be a complication of any disease which markedly reduces physical activities (such as RA), or it can be a sequela of long-term high-dose adrenocorticosteroid therapy (such as that employed in SLE, severe asthma, ulcerative colitis, etc.). Disability from osteoporosis results from fractures, from increasing dorsal kyphosis, and from bone pain.[11] Because an increasing percentage of the population in the United States is elderly, the chief target group for osteoporosis, in the past decade there has been a tremendous amount of media attention concerning this disease. While there is considerable scientific knowledge about bone formation, predisposing factors for osteoporosis, and some data about treatment, many preventive, diagnostic, and therapeutic suggestions have been made which have not yet been validated scientifically.

Peak bone mass occurs between ages 20 and 30 with a gradual but progressive loss thereafter because bone formation does not keep up with bone reabsorption.[7] The loss of bone mass is approximately 0.5 to 1.0 percent per year. Since women initially have less bone mass than do men, by age 60 most women have lost approximately one-third of their peak bone mass, making them the most susceptible group to develop osteoporosis.

Bone is not a static structure but is continually being remodeled. Normally bone remodeling occurs in cellular units, first a rather rapid bone breakdown by osteoclasts, followed by a slower buildup by osteoblasts. These cells do not work simultaneously, for when osteoclasts are breaking down bone, osteoblasts are inactive and vice versa. Our knowledge of the bone growth factors which control this switching on and off of osteoblasts and osteoclasts is in its infant stage.

The risk factors for symptomatic osteoporisis are as follows:

1. Female gender
2. White or Oriental ancestry
3. Northern European background
4. Thinness
5. Positive family history of osteoporosis
6. Low sunlight exposure
7. Less than 3 hours per week of exercise against gravity
8. Smoking
9. Alcoholism
10. Low protein intake
11. Low calcium intake
12. Certain drugs, such as adrenocorticosteroids and anticonvulsants

All of these risk factors work over a period of years and are important in prevention but not in the treatment of osteoporosis. In addition, some of the factors cannot be altered by an individual patient.

It would be extremely useful if persons at risk for developing osteoporotic factors could be recognized early so that preventive measures could be started. To be effective in screening a general population, a measure of bone mass would have to be inexpensive, easily repeated, widely available, and the bone mass measured would have to be in a target fracture area. Unfortunately, at this time there are no screening procedures that meet all these criteria. Conventional x-rays are not sensitive enough. Single-photon absorptiometry is sensitive but cannot be used to measure axial sites directly. Dual-photon absorptiometry is predictable, relatively inexpensive, and generally available, but unfortunately it works best in the wrists, an area where fractures occur but are not especially disabling. The areas of the body where fractures lead to significant incapacity are the hip, femur, or vertebrae. A computed tomographic (CT) scan of vertebral bodies is accurate and easily repeatable, but is so expensive that its cost for screening purposes is prohibitive.

Even if we cannot accurately screen the general population in order to institute preventive therapy, is preventive therapy valuable to prevent further fractures in those who have had one fracture? The answer is probably yes. Although there is considerable difference of opinion among investigators and the data are conflicting, the following measures seem to help in preventing further osteoporotic fractures.

1. The more physically active a person is, the less likely he or she is to develop osteoporosis or to have it progress.
2. Since women are the major target for osteoporosis, premenopausal women should have at least 1,000 mg of calcium per day in their diet and postmenopausal women at least 1,500 mg. The calcium can be taken in the form of natural foods (the above dose would require about five glasses of milk daily) or as calcium supplements. Except for persons with renal stones or hypercalcemia of any cause, calcium supplementation is probably safe.
3. There is evidence that if estrogen is taken within 6 years of menopause, the incidence of osteoporotic fractures decreases. The estrogens can be given daily or can be cycled with a progesterone compound. Estrogens prevent bone loss by decreasing bone reabsorption and enhancing calcium absorption. In order to be effective the dose of estrogen has to be at least 0.625 mg daily. At this dose level, however, some side effects are noted. Fifty to 60 percent of women have some uterine bleeding. Moreover, there is a small but definite increase in the incidence of endometrial cancer in postmenopausal women who take estrogens. There is a suggestion that there may be an increase in breast cancer in these women, but the data are controversial. On the plus side, however, there are reports that the incidence of myocardial infarction in postmenopausal women is decreased if estrogen is taken regularly.

The most important problem for the patient who develops symptomatic osteoporosis with back pain and/or fractures is whether we now have successful treatment. The answer to this question is probably yes. Such persons will be helped with the following regimen.

1. Calcium supplementation, sometimes augmented by small weekly doses of vitamin D.
2. Sodium fluoride in relatively large doses, that is, 40 to 60 mg daily. It should be noted, however, that although fluoride is incorporated into bone, the bone that is formed is not normal bone. Moreover, approximately one-third of all patients cannot tolerate the dose of sodium fluoride necessary to achieve this beneficial effect.
3. Cyclic estrogens have been shown to reduce the incidence of further problems.

It would appear that many regimens for treating and/or preventing osteoporisis are currently being presented to the public with much greater enthusiasm than is warranted. More data are needed so that better preventive measures and treatments can be devised. Finally, there are several clinical points to be made about osteoporosis. First, even if a patient with osteoporosis suddenly has several spontaneous long bone fractures, the disease is not an inevitable progressive one with increasing fractures thereafter. For unknown reasons individuals will sometimes have to or three fractures in 1 month and then go for a decade without further fractures. Second, better screening methods are needed to identify persons at high risk for developing osteoporosis. Third, treatment for osteoporosis should probably be intermittent, not continuous, because osteoclasts and osteoblasts act at different times and at different rates. And last, the biggest hope for the future is that as our knowledge of bone growth factors (which switch osteoblasts and osteoclasts on and off) develops, an entire new area of treatment possibilities will arise.

REFERENCES

1. Bluestone, R. (1980). *Rheumatology* (p. 65). Boston: Houghton Mifflin.
2. Dimant, J., et al. (1979). SLE in the older age group: Computer analysis. *J. Am. Geriatr. Soc., 27*, 58.
3. Ehrlich, G. E., Katz, W. A., and Cohen, S. A. (1970). Rheumatoid arthritis in the aged. *Geriatrics, 25*, 103.
4. Felson, D. T., et al. (1988). Obesity and knee osteoarthritis. *Ann. Intern. Med., 109*, 18.

5. Griffin, M.R., Ray, W.A., and Schaffner, W. (1988). Nonsteroidal anti-inflammatory drug use and death from peptic ulcer in elderly persons.
6. Grigor, R.R., Spitz, P.W. and Furst, D.E. (1987). Salicylate toxicity in elderly patients with rheumatoid arthritis. *J. Rheumatol. 14*, 60.
7. Hahn, T.J., and Hahn, B.H. (1976). Osteopenia in patients with rheumatic diseases: Principles of diagnosis and therapy. *Semin. Arthritis Rheum., 6,* 230.
8. Handler, N.M., et al. (1978). Hand structure and function in an industrial setting: Influence of three patterns of sterotypes, repetitive usage. *Arthritis Rheuma., 21,* 210.
9. Hench, P.S. (1936). Diagnosis of gout and gouty arthritis. *J. Lab. Clin. Med., 22,* 48.
10. Kimberly, R.P., et al. (1981). High dose intravenous methylprednisolone pulse therapy in SLE. *Am. J. Med., 70,* 817.
11. McCarty, D.J. (1985). *Arthritis and allied conditions,* 10th ed (p. 1579). Tenth Edition, Philadelphia: Lea & Febiger.
12. National Center for Health Statistics (1966). Public Health Service publication No. 1000, Series II, No. 15, Washington, DC: Government Printing Office.
13. Stecher, R.M., et al. (1953). Herberden's nodes: Family history and radiographic appearance of a large family. *Am. J. Hum. Genet., 5,* 46.
14. Terkeltaub, R., et al. (1983). A clinical study of older age rheumatoid arthritis with comparison to a younger onset group. *J. Rheumatol., 10,* 418.
15. Urman, J.D., and Rothfield, N.F. (1977). Corticosteroid treatment in SLE: Survival studies. *JAMA, 238,* 2272.
16. Williams, R.C. (1974). *Rheumatoid arthritis as a systemic disease.* Philadelphia: Saunders.
17. Yu, T.F., and Gutman, A.B. (1961). Efficiency of colchicine prophylaxis in gout. *Ann. Intern. Med., 55,* 179.

CHAPTER 6

Pulmonary Rehabilitation

ANDREW L. RIES

The chronic obstructive pulmonary diseases (COPDs), including emphysema and chronic bronchitis, are major causes of death and disability.[7] In the United States, these diseases are recognized in approximately 10 percent of the adult population and rank as the fifth leading cause of death. Among causes of death for persons 55 to 74 years of age, COPD ranks third among men and fourth among women. In contrast to other major diseases, death rates from COPD have increased rapidly in recent years. For instance, from 1965 to 1985, death rates from heart disease, the number one cause of death, decreased 41 percent, while deaths from COPD increased 83 percent.

The natural history of COPD spans several decades associated primarily with cigarette smoking. These diseases typically develop insidiously and, because of the large reserve in lung function, do not produce significant symptoms or come to medical attention until at an advanced stage. Many patients with mild to moderate disease have few symptoms and are undiagnosed. On the other hand, when the disease is recognized later in life, lung function is often severely compromised and the disease process may be largely irreversible. In a classic study of 487 patients with a clinical and pulmonary function diagnosis of COPD, Renzetti, McClement, and Litt[16] reported that 59 percent of patients were in the seventh or eighth decade of life, whereas only 22 percent were below age 50. Similar data have been reported from Great Britain.[5]

Problems of morbidity and the resultant disability from these diseases are also significant.[7] In the United States, COPD is second only to coronary heart disease in the number of patients receiving social security disability payments for severe disease (estimated at more than 500,000 patients). Respiratory illnesses, often from acute respiratory infections, are the most common cause of lost time from work. In addition, the effects of respiratory infections are much more serious among patients with underlying chronic lung disease, many of whom are undiagnosed, unrecognized, and in the older age groups.

Standard medical therapy is important in alleviating symptoms of COPD, particularly the distressing symptom of breathlessness (dyspnea). However, many patients are left to cope with the problems of a chronic, largely irreversible disease process.

Comprehensive rehabilitation programs for patients with chronic pulmonary diseases are well established as a means to enhance standard medical therapy in order to control and alleviate symptoms and to optimize the patient's functional capacity.[1,2,11] The primary goal of these programs is to restore the patient to the highest possible level of independent function. This goal may be accomplished by helping patients to become more knowledgeable about their disease, more actively involved in their own health care, more independent in performing daily care activities, and, therefore, less dependent on family, friends, health professionals, and expensive medical resources. Rather than focusing solely on reversing a chronic, progressive disease process, rehabilitation programs attempt to reverse the patient's disability from disease.

In 1974, the American College of Chest Physicians' Committee on Pulmonary Rehabilitation adopted the following definition:

Pulmonary rehabilitation may be defined as an art of medical practice wherein an individually tailored, multidisciplinary program is formulated which through accurate diagnosis, therapy, emotional support, and education, stabilizes or reverses both the physio- and psychopathology of pulmonary diseases and attempts to return the patient to the highest possible functional capacity allowed by his pulmonary handicap and overall life situation.[1]

This definition focuses on three important features of successful rehabilitation programs:

1. Individual: Patients with disabling COPD require individual assessment of their needs, individual attention, and a program designed to meet realistic individual goals.
2. Multidisciplinary: Pulmonary rehabilitation programs provide access to information from a variety of health care disciplines which

is integrated by experienced staff into a comprehensive, cohesive program tailored to the needs of each patient.

3. Attention to physio- and psychopathology: To be successful, pulmonary rehabilitation programs must pay attention to psychologic and emotional problems as well as helping to optimize medical therapy to improve lung function.

Within this general framework, successful pulmonary rehabilitation programs have been established in various settings (i.e., inpatient or outpatient) and with different formats. The key to a successful program is often a dedicated and enthusiastic staff who are familiar with the problems of pulmonary patients and who can relate well to and motivate them. Since many of the patients are elderly, program staff should be particularly sensitive to the needs and problems of older persons.

Although pulmonary rehabilitation programs have been developed primarily for patients with COPD, these programs may also be useful for patients with other pulmonary diseases.

PATIENT SELECTION

Primary care practitioners play a key role in identifying potential patients and making referrals. It is important for patients to have an ongoing relationship with a primary care provider prior to entering a rehabilitation program. The role of the rehabilitation program is to provide support for the patient and his or her own physician and not, typically, to provide primary care. Therefore, the primary care physician is a vital link in maintaining continuity of care before, during, and after rehabilitation.

Any patient with symptomatic COPD is a candidate for a pulmonary rehabilitation program. Appropriate patients are those who recognize that they have symptoms due to lung disease, perceive some impairment or disability related to that disease, and are motivated to be active participants in their own care in order to improve their health status. Patients with mild disease may not recognize their disease or perceive their problem as severe enough to warrant a comprehensive care program. On the other hand, patients with severe disease without reserve in lung function may be too limited to benefit significantly.

Other factors are also important in evaluating patients as candidates for pulmonary rehabilitation. Pulmonary rehabilitation is not a primary mode of therapy for COPD. Therefore, patients should be stabilized on standard medical therapy before beginning a program. The assessment and treatment plan can then be based on the patient's optimal baseline level of function. Patients should not have other disabling or unstable conditions which would limit their ability to participate fully and to concentrate on rehabilitation activities. These include, but are not limited to, unstable heart disease, psychiatric illness, or concurrent evaluation for a potentially serious health problem.

The ideal patient for pulmonary rehabilitation, then, is one with moderate to moderately severe lung disease who is stable on standard medical therapy, not distracted or limited by other serious or unstable medical conditions, willing and able to learn about his or her disease, and motivated to devote the time and effort necessary to benefit from a comprehensive care program.

PATIENT EVALUATION

The initial step in evaluating patients for comprehensive pulmonary rehabilitation programs is a patient interview which thoroughly reviews the patient's medical history and attends to psychosocial problems and needs. Communication and cooperation with the primary care physician is important in this effort. This establishes the vital link with the rehabilitation program staff in clarifying questions or problems prior to the program and in facilitating communication during and after rehabilitation. Care and attention in this initial evaluation will result in setting appropriate individual goals compatible with both the patient's and physician's expectations and the program's objectives.

MEDICAL EVALUATION

Review of the patient's medical history from the primary care physician will allow characterization of the patient's lung disease and assessment of its severity. Other medical problems which might preclude or delay participation in the program should be identified. Pertinent laboratory data include available pulmonary function and exercise tests, rest and exercise arterial blood gases, chest radiographs, an electrocardiogram, and blood test results including blood cell counts, chemistries, and theophylline level monitoring. The program staff can then determine the need for additional information or action before the patient begins the rehabilitation program.

DIAGNOSTIC TESTING

To plan an appropriate program for each patient, it is important to have accurate, current information about the patient. The complexity of testing procedures performed depends on the individual patient and the facilities available.

Pulmonary function testing helps to characterize and quantify impairment resulting from the patient's lung disease. Spirometry and lung volume measurements are most useful and can be supplemented with other tests such as diffusing capacity, airway resistance, or other parameters as needed.

Exercise testing is necessary to assess the patient's exercise tolerance and to evaluate possible blood gas changes (hypoxemia or hypercapnia) with exercise. This may also help to uncover coexisting diseases which are common in elderly patients (e.g., heart disease). Other unstable or untreated diseases may contribute to the patient's symptoms or potentially interfere with the rehabilitation effort. The exercise test can also be used to establish a safe and appropriate prescription for subsequent training.

Maximal exercise tolerance of COPD patients is limited largely by their breathing capacity. Simple pulmonary function tests such as spirometry can be used to estimate a patient's capacity for sustained breathing (maximum ventilation) during physical activity or exercise. The forced expiratory volume in 1 second (FEV_1) is the most useful parameter in this regard. However, although the pulmonary function test measurements can be used to provide a rough estimate of a patient's maximum work capacity, the exercise tolerance of COPD patients will depend considerably on an individual's perception and tolerance of the subjective symptom of breathlessness (dyspnea).[17]

Many elderly patients are physically inactive and deconditioned due to their limited lung function and fear of dyspnea. Therefore, it is important to exercise patients to assess each patient's current level of function and tolerance for dyspnea. This assessment is best made utilizing the type of exercise which will be employed in training (e.g., treadmill testing for a walking exercise training program); however, test results from one type of exercise (e.g., cycle ergometer) can be translated to similar forms of exercise (e.g., walking).[22] Variables measured and/or monitored during testing should include workload, heart rate, ECG, and arterial oxygenation. Other measurements such as minute ventilation or expired gas analysis to calculate variables such as oxygen consumption (VO_2) may be performed, depending on the interest and expertise of referring physicians, program staff, and laboratory personnel.

Measurement of arterial blood gases at rest and during exercise is important because of the frequently unexpected and unpredictable occurrence of exercise-induced hypoxemia.[21] Blood gas sampling during exercise adds a significant degree of complexity to testing. Noninvasive techniques, such as cutaneous oximetry measurements of arterial oxygen saturation, are useful for continuous monitoring but should not be relied on for precise assessment of arterial oxygenation because of their limited accuracy (e.g., 95% confidence limits for measurement of arterial oxygen saturation by cutaneous oximetry = ± 4–5% saturation).[20]

PSYCHOSOCIAL ASSESSMENT

Successful rehabilitation requires attention not only to physical problems but also to psychologic, emotional, and social ones. Patients with chronic illnesses like COPD develop a number of psychosocial problems as they struggle to deal with symptoms that are often poorly understood. These problems are particularly difficult for older persons who must often cope with loss of loved ones, friends, self-esteem, and self-worth as well as the physical and physiologic changes of aging and disease. As mentioned previously, the majority of symptomatic COPD patients are in the older age groups beyond the sixth decade of life. Commonly, such patients become depressed, frightened, anxious, and more dependent on others to care for their needs. Progressive dyspnea is a frightening symptom and may lead to a vicious "fear-dyspnea" cycle: with progressive disease, less exertion results in more dyspnea which produces more fear and anxiety which, in turn, leads to more dyspnea. Ultimately, the patient avoids any physical activity associated with these unpleasant symptoms. In the extreme, patients may set up a stationary "command post" from which they rarely venture forth except to seek relief in physicians' offices and hospitals.

In order to overcome these problems, the initial evaluation should include an assessment of the patient's psychologic state (e.g., depression or other psychologic tests) and close attention to psychosocial clues during screening interviews (e.g., family and social support, living arrangement, activities of daily living, hobbies, employment potential). Cognitive impairment, which may limit the patient's ability to participate, must be recognized. Spouses, family members, and close friends may provide valuable insights and should be included in the screening process (and program).

SETTING GOALS

After evaluating a patient's medical, physiologic, and psychosocial state, it is important to set specific goals that are compatible with each individual patient's disease, needs, and expectations, and are realistic given the objectives of the rehabilitation program. Patients and family members should be included in this process so that everyone understands what can and cannot be expected. Communication with the primary care physician is also important in deciding what goals may be appropriate given the patient's medical condition and prognosis.

PROGRAM CONTENT

EDUCATION

It is important that patients and family members understand the patient's disease and learn specific means to deal with problems. Instruction can be given individually or in small groups, but must be adapted to the different learning abilities of individual patients. Particular attention should be given to the older patient in limiting the amount of material covered in each session and in providing ample opportunity to repeat and reinforce important subject matter. The educational program may consist of classroom, individual, and audiovisual formats. Classes may include topics such as: how normal lungs work, what is COPD, medications, nutrition, travel, stress reduction and relaxation, when to call your doctor, and planning a daily schedule. Individual instruction and coaching may be provided on the use of respiratory therapy equipment oxygen, breathing techniques, bronchial drainage, chest percussion, energy-saving techniques, and self-care tips. The general philosophy of the program should be to encourage patients to assume responsibility for and to become active participants and partners in providing their own care.[13]

RESPIRATORY AND CHEST PHYSIOTHERAPY

Many patients with COPD, especially older ones, use, abuse, and are confused about respiratory and chest physiotherapy techniques. Rehabilitation programs must assess each patient's needs and provide instruction in proper techniques. Good bronchial hygiene is important for all patients, especially those with excess mucus production. Patients should be taught appropriate coughing and postural drainage techniques. Instruction in pursed-lip and diaphragmatic breathing helps to improve the ventilatory pattern (e.g., slow respiratory rate) and gas exchange and assists patients in gaining control over symptoms of dyspnea. Relaxation training also helps with the latter. Patients with respiratory therapy equipment should be instructed in its proper use, care, and cleaning.

For patients who require supplemental oxygen therapy, available methods of oxygen delivery should be reviewed to help select the best system for their needs. The benefits of long-term, continuous oxygen therapy for COPD patients with significant resting hypoxemia are well established. Such therapy has been shown to improve survival and to reduce morbidity associated with these diseases.[12,14] However, maintaining patients on continuous oxygen therapy presents a number of problems for these patients who are often very physically limited. These problems are particularly difficult for older patients who may need assistance in handling, using, and caring safely for such equipment.

Several new developments in this area have improved the efficiency of gas delivery and patient compliance with continuous therapy.[23] Using liquid oxygen as a gas source provides more oxygen for less weight in portable systems. Also, the use of transtracheal oxygen increases the efficiency of gas delivery to the patient (reducing oxygen flow requirement and prolonging duration of portable sources), improves patient compliance, and avoids problems with nasal catheters.[4] However, patients need careful instruction in caring for and maintaining the catheter. The presence of another person (e.g., spouse) is particularly helpful in the daily care and replacement of the catheters. These problems are particularly important in older patients who should be screened carefully before implementing the procedure.

EXERCISE

Exercise reconditioning should be considered for all patients and is an important component of many rehabilitation programs. Benefits are both physiologic and psychologic. This is an ideal opportunity for patients to learn their capacity for physical work and to use and practice methods for controlling dyspnea (e.g., breathing and relaxation techniques).

The exercise program needs to be safe and appropriate for each patient's interest, environment, and level of function. It should be based on the results of initial exercise testing. Training should utilize methods easily adapted to the home setting. Walking programs are particularly useful for older and physically limited patients. They have the added benefit of encouraging patients to expand their social horizons. In inclement weather, patients can frequently walk indoors (e.g., shopping malls). Other types of exercise (e.g., cycling, swimming) are also effective. Patients should be encouraged to incorporate regular exercise into activities they enjoy (e.g., golf, gardening). Since many COPD patients have limited exercise tolerance, emphasis during training should be placed on increasing endurance. This will allow patients to become more functional within their physical limits. Increase in exercise level is also frequently possible as patients gain experience and confidence with their exercise program.

Exercise Prescription

After the initial exercise test to assess a patient's maximal exercise tolerance, training should begin at a level that the patient can sustain with reasonable comfort for several minutes. This is an adequate starting point for training which emphasizes increasing endurance as well as the level of tolerance.

It must be remembered that principles of exercise testing and training derived from normal populations are often not applicable to pulmonary patients who are limited by ventilation and dyspnea. For instance, most patients with significant chronic lung disease can be trained at higher percentages of maximum exercise tolerance than normals because they can often sustain ventilation at high percentages of their maximum ventilatory capacity. Therefore, training levels may often approach (or even exceed) the maximal level demonstrated on the initial exercise tolerance test.[18] Patients with more mild disease can be trained at submaximal levels which are higher than the usual 60 to 70 percent of maximum expected in normals. In addition, many patients will not reach maximum predicted heart rates, and exercise capacity may vary significantly from day to day depending on changes in lung function. Therefore, it is often not necessary (or helpful) to set standard heart rate targets. Exercise should be "titrated" to a level that pushes a patient toward his or her maximum and is adjusted according to the patient's perception and tolerance for dyspnea which, after all, is the symptom limiting exercise performance. Ratings of perceived symptoms (e.g., breathlessness) help in teaching patients to exercise "target" levels of breathing discomfort.[7]

A major problem in planning a safe exercise program for COPD patients is the potential occurrence of exercise-induced hypoxemia.[21] Patients who may or may not be hypoxemic at rest develop changes in arterial oxygenation which cannot be predicted reliably from resting measurements of pulmonary function or gas exchange. Normal persons do not develop hypoxemia with exercise. Patients with mild COPD may demonstrate no change, or an improvement in PaO_2 with exercise. In patients with moderate to severe COPD, PaO_2 may increase, decrease or, not change. Therefore, it is important to measure arterial blood gases at rest and during exercise to detect significant exercise-induced hypoxemia and to decide how much oxygen is necessary for safe training. With the availability of convenient, portable systems for ambulatory oxygen delivery, hypoxemia is not a contraindication to exercise training.

Other Forms of Exercise

Exercise programs for COPD patients have emphasized lower extremity training (e.g., walking). Other types of exercise may also be beneficial for the many physically limited patients who have difficulty performing even simple activities of daily living (ADLs).

Older patients with COPD frequently report disabling dyspnea for daily activities involving the upper extremities (e.g., lifting, grooming) at work levels much lower than for the lower extremities. Upper extremity exercise is accompanied by a higher ventilatory demand (for a given level of oxygen consumption) than for lower extremity exercise. Also, exercise training is generally specific to the muscles and tasks involved in training. Therefore, exercise training of the upper extremities may also be beneficial for these patients.[19]

The potential role of respiratory muscle fatigue as a cause of respiratory failure and ventilatory limitation in COPD patients has stimulated attempts to train the ventilatory muscles. Both isocapnic hyperventilation and inspiratory resistive loading have been shown to improve function of these muscles. However, improvement in exercise performance in COPD patients from ventilatory muscle training alone has not been demonstrated consistently. Pardy and coworkers reported that the benefits of ventilatory muscle training are most evident in the subset of COPD patients who demonstrate electromyographic evidence of diaphragmatic fatigue during exercise.[15] However, at present, there is no simple method to select patients most likely to benefit from this type of exercise training.

PSYCHOSOCIAL SUPPORT

The final important component of a comprehensive pulmonary rehabilitation program is psychosocial support. From the realization that their disease is chronic and incurable, COPD patients develop a variety of psychosocial symptoms reflecting their progressive feelings of hopelessness and inability to cope with their disease.[6] Depression and anxiety (particularly fear of dyspnea) are common. Patients show symptoms of denial, anger, and isolation and become sedentary and dependent upon family members, friends, and medical services to provide for their needs. They become overly concerned with other physical problems and psychosomatic symptoms. Sexual dysfunction and fear of sexual activities is a common, often unspoken, consequence contributing to personal and family difficulties. COPD patients have evidence of cognitive and neuropsychologic dysfunction, possibly related to or exacerbated by the effects of hypoxemia on the brain. All of these problems, which develop commonly in older people, are even more difficult for patients with significant chronic lung disease.

Successful pulmonary rehabilitation programs must attend not only to physical problems but also to psychosocial ones. This is provided best by enthusiastic and supportive staff who are able to communicate effectively with patients and devote the time and effort necessary to understand and motivate them. Important family members and friends should be included in program activities so that they can understand and cope better with the patient's disease. Support groups and group therapy sessions are very effective. Patients with severe psychologic disorders may benefit from individual counseling and psychotherapy. Psychotropic drugs should generally be reserved for patients with severe levels of psychologic dysfunction. Their use should be coordinated by the primary care physician.

RESULTS OF PULMONARY REHABILITATION

Comprehensive pulmonary rehabilitation programs have been shown to a cost-effective means of producing significant benefits for COPD patients. Several studies have demonstrated the cost-benefit of pulmonary rehabilitation which results in a decrease in hospitalization days and in the use of medical resources.[8,9] After rehabilitation, patients have an improved quality of life with a reduction in respiratory symptoms, increase in exercise tolerance and level of physical activity, more independence and ability to perform ADLs, and improvement in psychologic function with less anxiety and depression and increased feelings of hope, control, and self-esteem. Studies which have examined the effects of the individual program components have shown that even patients with severe disease can learn to understand their disease better, increase their activity level, and improve their exercise tolerance from training.

Pulmonary rehabilitation programs have not resulted in a significant improvement in pulmonary function in patients with COPD. Studies which have examined the survival of COPD patients after pulmonary rehabilitation have shown variable results. Vocational benefits may be difficult to achieve in the presence of severe, disabling disease. However, patients with less severe disease may be able to return to work and increase their performance of vocational and recreational activities. The success of vocational rehabilitation will also depend on factors other than the degree of respiratory impairment including the patient's age, motivation, level of education, capability for retraining, physical demands of a particular job, and support and understanding from an employer.

FUTURE OF PULMONARY REHABILITATION

Despite the demonstrated benefits of comprehensive pulmonary rehabilitation programs, there remain unanswered questions and fruitful areas for further investigation. COPD is a chronic, progressive, and largely irreversible disease which develops insidiously over many years and is generally moderate to severe when recognized. The goals of medical therapy are, first, to slow the decline in lung function and, second, if possible, to improve lung function. After stabilizing patients on standard medical therapy, it is unlikely that significant improvement in pulmonary function will result. The benefits of any treatment for COPD, therefore, would be evaluated best in a prospective, randomly controlled clinical trial comparing the effects of experimental intervention to a control group of COPD patients whose function would be expected to decline over time. Such a study has not yet been done.

In addition, the benefits of pulmonary rehabilitation are most evident in quality-of-life changes which are difficult to measure but which may be critical in understanding the benefits and cost-effectiveness of these programs. Recently, quality-of-life measurement instruments have been developed and used to assess the cost-benefit of clinical interventions.[10] Clinical trials which critically examine and characterize the benefits of pulmonary rehabilitation are needed.

In addition to assessing the overall benefits of comprehensive pulmonary rehabilitation programs, it is important to gain a better understanding of specific components. Much needs to be learned about the optimal methods for performing exercise testing and training in pulmonary patients. Guidelines for assessing and treating exercise-induced hypoxemia, an unpredictable threat in these patients, are needed. Exercise training is the most difficult component to provide in pulmonary rehabilitation programs and more knowledge is needed about the best methods of exercise training for these patients. Providing a multidisciplinary, individualized program requires a significant effort from both patients and staff and better means are needed for selecting appropriate patients who are motivated to complete a program and likely to benefit. The effects of age as an independent variable in assessing rehabilitation potential and in planning individual components such as exercise have not been studied.

THE PRIMARY CARE PHYSICIAN IN PULMONARY REHABILITATION

The primary care physician plays an important and integral role in the ultimate success of pulmonary rehabilitation for the individual patient. This is the key person in identifying the patient's lung disease, initiating primary therapy, and considering a referral for rehabilitation for patients who note significant symptomatology or disability from lung disease and are motivated to learn about and be active participants in their own treatment program. The primary care physician is the most appropriate person to make the suggestion and initiate this action. In choosing a program for referral, the physician should look for one that provides comprehensive evaluation and treatment including the components noted (e.g., education, exercise, psychosocial support). Communicating with the program staff will enable the physician to assess the program structure and content, initiate the referral process, if appropriate, and also open the essential lines of communication for continued support and follow-up during and after the program. At the end of the program, the physician should also expect a summary of the patient's progress and recommendations for continued maintenance.

REFERENCES

1. American Thoracic Society (1981). Pulmonary rehabilitation. *Am. Rev. Respir. Dis., 124,* 663.
2. American Thoracic Society (1987). Standards for the diagnosis and care of patients with chronic obstructive pulmonary disease (COPD) and asthma. *Am. Rev. Respir. Dis., 136,* 225.
3. Borg, G.A.V. (1982). Psychophysical bases of perceived exertion. *Med. Sci. Sports Exerc., 14,* 377.
4. Christopher, K.L., et al. (1987). A program for transtracheal oxygen delivery: Assessment of safety and efficacy. *Ann. Intern. Med., 107,* 802.
5. Cotes, J.E., et al. (1981). Disabling chest disease: Prevention and care. A report of the Royal College of Physicians by the College Committee on Thoracic Medicine. *J. R. Coll. Physicians Lond., 15,* 69.
6. Dudley, D.L., et al. (1980). Psychosocial concomitants to rehabilitation in chronic obstructive pulmonary disease: Part 1. Psychosocial and psychological considerations; Part 2. Psychosocial treatment; Part 3. Dealing with psychiatric disease (as distinguished from psychosocial or psychophysiologic problems). *Chest, 77,* 413, 544, 677.
7. Higgins, I.T.T. (1988). Epidemiology of bronchitis and emphysema. In A.P. Fishman (ed), *Pulmonary diseases and disorders,* 2nd edi. (pp. 1237–1246). New York: McGraw-Hill.
8. Hodgkin, J.E., Zorn, E.G., and Connors, G.L. (Eds.) (1984). *Pulmonary rehabilitation—Guidelines to success.* Boston: Butterworth.
9. Hudson, L.D., Tyler, M.L., and Petty, T.L. (1976). Hospitalization needs during an outpatient rehabilitation program for severe chronic airway obstruction. *Chest, 70,* 606.
10. Kaplan, R.M., Atkins, C.J., and Timms, R. (1984). Validity of a quality of well-being scale as an outcome measure in chronic obstructive pulmonary disease. *J. Chronic. Dis., 37,* 85.
11. Lertzman, M.M., Chyerniack, R.M. (1976). Rehabilitation of patients with chronic obstructive pulmonary disease. *Am. Rev. Respir. Dis., 114,* 1145.

12. Medical Research Council Working Party. (1981). Long-term domiciliary oxygen therapy in chronic hypoxic cor pulmonale complicating chronic bronchitis and emphysema. *Lancet, 1,* 681.
13. Moser, K.M., et al. (1983). *Shortness of breath*—A guide to better living and breathing, 3d ed. St. Louis: Mosby.
14. Nocturnal Oxygen Therapy Trial Group (1980). Continuous or nocturnal oxygen therapy in hypoxemic chronic obstructive lung disease: A clinical trial. *Ann. Intern. Med., 93,* 391.
15. Pardy, R.L., et al. (1981). The effects of inspiratory muscle training on exercise performance in chronic airflow limitation. *Am. Rev. Respir. Dis., 123,* 426.
16. Renzetti, A.D. Jr., McClement, H.Y., and Litt, B.D. (1966). The Veterans Administration cooperative study of pulmonary function: III. Mortality in relation to respiratory function in chronic obstructive pulmonary disease. *Am. J. Med., 41,* 115.
17. Ries, A.L. (1987). The role of exercise testing in pulmonary diagnosis. *Clin. Chest Med., 8,* 81.
18. Ries, A.L., and Archibald, C.J. (1987). Endurance exercise training at maximal targets in patients with chronic obstructive pulmonary disease. *J. Cardiopulmonary Rehabil., 7,* 594.
19. Ries, A.L., Ellis, B., and Hawkins, R.W. (1988). Upper extremity exercise training in chronic obstructive pulmonary disease. *Chest, 93,* 688.
20. Ries, A.L., Farrow, J.T., and Clausen, J.L. (1985). Accuracy of two ear oximeters at rest and during exercise in pulmonary patients. *Am. Rev. Respir. Dis., 132,* 685.
21. Ries, A.L., Farrow, J.T., and Clausen, J.L. (1988). Pulmonary function tests cannot predict exercise-induced hypoxemia in chronic obstructive pulmonary disease. *Chest, 93,* 454.
22. Ries, A.L., and Moser, K.M. (1982). Predicting treadmill/walking speed from cycle ergometry exercise in chronic obstructive pulmonary disease. *Am. Rev. Respir. Dis., 126,* 924.
23. Tiep, B.L., and Lewis, M.I. (1987). Oxygen conservation and oxygen-conserving devices in chronic lung disease. *Chest, 92,* 263.

CHAPTER 7

Parkinson's Disease: New Developments in Understanding and Treatment

CLIFFORD W. SHULTS

In 1817 James Parkinson gave the first concise description of the disease which now bears his name. He wrote that the malady is characterized by "involuntary tremulous motion, with lessened muscular power, in parts not in action and even when supported; with a propensity to bend the trunk forward, and to pass from a walking to a running pace, the senses and intellect being uninjured."[21]

Parkinson's disease is the most common and most thoroughly understood degenerative neurologic disease that results in progressive impairment of mobility in the elderly (Table 7-1). Cerebrovascular disease, which also often results in impairment in movement, is discussed in Chapter 4. Because Parkinson's disease is commonly encountered by those providing care to the elderly, a basic understanding of the disorder is critical to geriatric primary care and geriatric rehabilitation. In addition, less common movement disorders, such as progressive supranuclear palsy, share certain pathologic and clinical features with Parkinson's disease and understanding of Parkinson's disease aids in understanding and management of other movement disorders.

Table 7-1. *Other Diseases Sharing Symptoms of Idiopathic Parkinson's Disease*

Postencephalitic parkinsonism

Drug-induced parkinsonism—neuroleptics, reserpine, tetrabenazine, methyldopa, lithium, MPTP, carbon monoxide, manganese

Hereditary neurologic diseases—Wilson's disease, Huntington's disease, Hallervorden-Spatz disease

Multiple system atrophies—Striatonigral degeneration, Shy-Drager syndrome, progressive supranuclear palsy, olivopontocerebellar degeneration

Other CNS disorders—Normal pressure hydrocephalus, stroke, tumor, subdural hematoma, essential tremor

MPTP = methyl-4-phenyl-1,2,3,6-tetrahydropyridine.

This chapter reviews the clinical features of Parkinson's disease, the pathologic changes in the brain, recent discoveries pertinent to possible causes, current and experimental treatments, and rehabilitative therapy. It also discusses the role of the primary care physician in working with the neurologist and the rehabilitation team in managing these patients.

MOVEMENT DISORDERS IN THE ELDERLY

Idiopathic Parkinson's disease occurs commonly in elderly patients. The prevalence in the United States is 90 to 165 in 100,000 population, and the incidence increases into the eighth decade. Schoenberg has provided an excellent review of the epidemiology of movement disorders.[25] Essential tremor, which typically causes tremor of the arms and/or head, does not usually impair mobility, and is the only movement disorder that occurs more frequently than Parkinson's disease; the prevalence is approximately 306 in 100,000 in the United States. Other movement disorders occur rarely. Postencephalitic Parkinson's disease, which occurred only in patients who had suffered von Economo's encephalitis after World War I, is rarely seen today. Huntington's disease has an average prevalence of 4.8 in 100,000 in Western populations.[15] Wilson's disease occurs with a prevalence of only 1.6 in 100,000.[25] Golbe and colleagues have estimated the prevalence of progressive supranuclear palsy to be 1.39 in 100,000.[9] Multiple system atrophy and olivopontocerebellar degeneration are actually heterogeneous disorders so estimation of prevalence is difficult and would be misleading. Clearly, idiopathic Parkinson's disease is the most common degenerative disease resulting in impaired mobility in the elderly. However, when considering the diagnosis of idiopathic Parkinson's disease, the clinician should carefully consider other diseases which may mimic it.

CARDINAL FEATURES OF PARKINSON'S DISEASE

Parkinson painted a clear picture of the patient with his stooped posture, festinating gait, and resting tremor. Interestingly he described the intellect as being uninjured. During the last decade neurologists have recognized that a certain percentage of Parkinsonian patients will eventually develop dementia. The cardinal features of the illness are bradykinesia, rigidity, tremor, postural instability, and in some but not all patients, a cognitive decline. The principal functional impairment associated with Parkinson's disease is the compromise of mobility which results from the first four of these features.

Bradykinesia describes the paucity and slowness of movement. This may be one of the earliest and most subtle signs of the illness. The patient usually exhibits an expressionless face, for which we have coined the term "masked facies." The patient sits with an unblinking, exaggerated poker face. In fact, Karson and colleagues found that the rate of blinking is reduced from the normal rate of 24 blinks per minute to 12 blinks per minute in parkinsonian patients.[13]

Patients with Parkinson's disease exhibit a tremor, which is often the most conspicuous manifestation of the illness. The tremor is frequently described as a pill-rolling tremor. This term depicts the flexion-extension of the fingers combined with the abduction-adduction of the thumb. The tremor has a frequency of 4 to 6 Hz and its amplitude may fluctuate with the level of anxiety of the patient. The arm is often involved with pronation-supination movements. The legs, jaw, lips, and tongue can be involved. The parkinsonian tremor is characterized as a resting tremor because it is most conspicuous when the patient is at rest. When the patient performs a volitional action, the tremor usually diminishes and the act is performed relatively unimpeded by the tremor. However, the term "resting tremor" is somewhat misleading because when the patient is fully resting, asleep, the tremor disappears. Electromyographic studies of parkinsonian tremor reveal alternating bursts of activity in agonist and antagonist muscles. A second type of tremor is also common in patients with Parkinson's disease. This is a fine 8- to 10-Hz tremor which is brought out by asking the patient to reach for an object or to hold his or her hands outstretched.

When one examines a patient with Parkinson's disease, the examiner finds that the muscles are more rigid than usual. This increase in tone, which predominates in the flexors of the limbs and trunk, causes the characteristic posture of parkinsonian patients: the arms flexed at the elbows, the trunk moderately stooped, and the legs bent at the hips and knees. As the examiner passively flexes and extends the elbow or rotates the wrist, he notices that the movement has a rachetlike feel to it, which we term *cogwheel rigidity*. In a very early case of Parkinson's disease the rigidity may only be appreciated in a limb if the patient performs a volitional movement of the contralateral limb. For example, it may be necessary for the examiner to ask the patient to open and close the left hand as the examiner passively rotates the right wrist, to elicit rigidity in the right wrist.

Parkinsonian patients also have a tendency toward postural instability. A patient pushed slightly off balance will often fall whereas persons without neurologic impairment are able to catch themselves and keep from toppling over. This explains the frequency of falling in patients with Parkinson's disease. David Marsden's group in London studied the anticipatory postural responses in the calf muscles in response to a small pull to the arm in standing subjects.[28] The pull normally elicits a brisk automatic compensatory contraction of the calf muscles. This response was found in 50 normal subjects but was absent or greatly reduced in many parkinsonian patients.

In addition to the movement disorder, neurologists have recently noted that certain parkinsonian patients suffer progressive intellectual decline. One must be careful, however, in ascribing cognitive deficits in patients with Parkinson's disease to the disease for a number of reasons. First, certain illnesses, which have cognitive impairment as one of their features, may superficially resemble Parkinson's disease but are clinically and pathologically distinct from Parkinson's disease. Progressive supranuclear palsy, a disease characterized by axial rigidity, abnormalities of eye movement, and impaired cognition, is such a disease. Second, due to the disease the parkinsonian patient is at risk for certain misfortunes which can impair the intellect. These include subdural hematoma, due to the patient's tendency to fall, and drug-induced delirium. Finally, the parkinsonian patient is not immune to the more common causes of dementia such as Alzheimer's disease and multiple strokes. However, if one factors out these other causes, a minimum of 20 percent of parkinsonian patients appear to develop a dementia which cannot be explained on other grounds,[22] and the percentage may be higher.[1]

When examining a patient who demonstrates some of the features of idiopathic Parkinson's disease, the clinician must consider other diseases that may share certain manifestations similar to idiopathic Parkinson's disease (Table 7-1). A discussion of the differential diagnosis of parkinsonism is beyond the scope of this chapter. The reader is referred to the recent volume by Kollar for an excellent review of Parkinson's disease.[14]

NEUROPATHOLOGIC CHANGES IN PARKINSON'S DISEASE

It was not until 100 years after Parkinson described the clinical features of this disease that the salient pathologic features of the illness, the presence of abnormal intracytoplasmic inclusions—Lewy bodies—and the loss of cells in the substantia nigra, were noted. In 1912 Lewy described the pathognomonic abnormality which now bears his name. The Lewy body is a concentric hyaline cytoplasmic inclusion that has a characteristic eosinophilic appearance when the tissue is stained with hematoxylin and eosin. There may be a single Lewy body in a neuron or up to six or seven in large neurons. They are most commonly found in the pigmented nuclei of the brain stem: the substantia nigra, locus ceruleus, and dorsal motor nucleus of the vagus. However, Lewy bodies are also found in the lateral horns of the thoracic cord, facial nucleus, oculomotor nuclei, sympathetic ganglia, and even in the adrenal medulla. It is very unusual to find Lewy bodies in the striatum and globus pallidus. Lewy bodies are found in approximately 4 to 5 percent of control brains, but perhaps these persons would have developed Parkinson's disease if they had lived longer. Lewy bodies are not characteristically found in patients with postencephalitic parkinsonism.

Electron microscopy has demonstrated that Lewy bodies consist of filaments which are loosely packed in the outer portions and densely packed and mixed with granular material in the central core. The filaments in Lewy bodies are not helical as are those in the paired helical filaments of neurofibrillary tangles.

In 1919 the loss of cells in the substantia nigra was noted by Tretiakoff. In the 1960s cells of the pars compacta division of the substantia nigra were found to produce the neurotransmitter dopamine. Cell loss also occurs in the locus ceruleus in parkinsonian patients.

The loss of cells in the substantia nigra stimulated investigators in the early 1960s to measure levels of dopamine and its metabolites in brains of patients with Parkinson's disease. Hornykiewicz found striking reductions of dopamine, its metabolites, and synthetic enzymes in the basal ganglia of parkinsonian brains and noted that the degree of decrease appeared to reflect the severity of bradykinesia.[11] This discovery led to the introduction of levodopa as a very successful treatment for Parkinson's disease.

Not only is dopamine reduced in parkinsonian brains, as one might expect from the loss of the dopaminergic cells in the pars compacta of the substantia nigra, but other biogenic amines are also reduced as a result of the cell loss in other pigmented nuclei of the brain stem. For example norepinephrine, produced by cells of the locus ceruleus, and serotonin, produced by cells in the dorsal raphe, are also reduced. However, these reductions are not of the magnitude of that of dopamine.

A major advance in the study of Parkinson's disease occurred in 1982 when Langston and colleagues at Santa Clara Medical Center uncovered four young persons who had acutely developed parkinsonian symptoms after intravenously injecting a synthetic opiate. These patients were described as follows:

Examination in each revealed near total immobility, marked generalized increase in tone, a complete inability to speak intelligibly, a fixed stare, marked diminution of blinking, facial seborrhea, constant drooling, a positive glabellar tap test, and cogwheel rigidity in the upper extremities. One patient exhibited a "pill rolling" tremor (5–6 cycles per second) at rest in the right hand. All patients exhibited a flexed posture typical of fully developed Parkinson's disease.[16]

This report clearly describes the findings typical of idiopathic Parkinson's disease. All four patients responded to treatment with levodopa. Langston and his coworkers analyzed the synthetic heroin and tentatively identified the toxin as methyl-4-phenyl-1,2,3,6-tetrahydropyridine (MPTP).

Soon after identification of MPTP as a potential neurotoxin a number of groups were able to show that administration of MPTP to various primates would induce a parkinsonian syndrome complete with loss of dopaminergic cells and depletion of dopamine.

The current proposed mechanism of toxicity is that MPTP is taken up by astrocytes and oxidized by monoamine oxidase B to -1-methyl-4-phenylpyridiniumion (MPP+), which is the actual toxic compound. MPP+ is transported into dopaminergic cells by the dopamine uptake system. In the dopaminergic cell neuromelanin may bind the MPP+ and act as a reservoir for the toxin. MPP+ is next taken up into the mitochondria by a second carrier system. In the mitochondria, MPP+ inhibits NADH dehydrogenase. For a brief review of the toxicity of MPTP the reader is referred to the article of Singer, Trevor, and Castagnoli.[27]

Where does this serendipity followed by good scientific research take us? One obvious direction is an attempt to identify certain environmental toxins that resemble MPTO or MPP+. MPP+ has been used as a herbicide, and both MPTP and MPP+ resemble the herbicide paraquat. Andre Barbeau compared the use of herbicides in the rural regions of his native province of Quebec to the prevalence of Parkinson's disease and found a strong correlation.[2]

MANAGEMENT OF PARKINSON'S DISEASE AND RELATED MOVEMENT DISORDERS

The management of patients with Parkinson's disease and other neurogenic movement disorders begins with a careful effort to correctly diagnose the disorder. This is best done by a neurologist. The neurologist should then work with the primary care physician and rehabilitation specialists to provide optimal care for the patient. Because the neurologist has the greatest experience in treating Parkinson's disease and knowledge of new developments in management, he should assume responsibility for care of this disorder. A number of medications are available for treatment of Parkinson's disease and other movement disorders. Patients can also benefit from programs and devices provided by physical and occupational therapists. However, the patient may see his primary care physician more often than he sees his neurologist, and the primary care physician should adjust the parkinsonian medications in consultation with the neurologist. Because Parkinson's disease is a progressive disease, optimal management will require more frequent evaluation by the neurologist as the disease progresses. When appropriate, the neurologist should refer the patient to occupational therapists and physical therapists.

CURRENT AND EXPERIMENTAL DRUG THERAPIES OF PARKINSON'S DISEASE

Once the clinician is certain of the diagnosis of Parkinson's disease, then the questions are when to start therapy and what drug or drugs to begin with. There are a number of medications useful in treating Parkinson's disease (Table 7-2). Their correct use requires a clear understanding of their therapeutic effects, side effects, and limitations.

Levodopa, the precursor of dopamine, remains the most effective therapy for Parkinson's disease. Levodopa is used rather than dopamine

Table 7-2. *Antiparkinsonian Medications*

Anticholinergic drugs
Dopamine releasing agents
Levodopa
Dopaminergic agonists
Monoamine oxidase B inhibitors

because, unlike dopamine, it can be transported across the blood-brain barrier. Levodopa is usually administered with an inhibitor of dopa decarboxylase to prevent the peripheral conversion of it to dopamine. The addition of the decarboxylase inhibitor allows reduction in the amount of levodopa that is required and also reduces the incidence of side effects, particularly nausea. In the United States levodopa is combined with carbidopa (Sinemet) which is formulated in three combinations: 10 mg carbidopa per 100 mg levodopa, and 25/100 and 25/250.

Levodopa ameliorates bradykinesia, tremor, and rigidity. Side effects noted with levodopa therapy include nausea and hypotension. Like the other drugs used in the treatment of Parkinson's disease levodopa can cause confusion and hallucinations. The psychiatric side effects are seen more commonly in patients who are older, demented, on other psychoactive drugs, or have an intercurrent infection.

A major issue in the use of levodopa has been the timing of the initiation of this therapy. The question arose when the first investigators using levodopa noted that after a few years on the medication patients often developed new phenomena, such as dramatic fluctuations in the ability to move and dyskinesia. The dosages employed at that time were generally higher than those used now. This observation led some neurologists to hypothesize that duration of therapy might contribute to emergence of side effects. Rajput, Stern, and Laverty in Canada[23] and recently de Jong, Meerwaldt, and Schmitz in Holland[5] retrospectively reviewed their experience and noted that patients who had been on therapy with levodopa for longer periods were more likely to develop motor fluctuations. However, Rajput et al were not able to control for duration of disease in their study. de Jong and colleagues noted that although patients who had symptoms for over 5 years before beginning levodopa had a somewhat lower incidence of fluctuations, the duration of disease before levodopa therapy was started did not significantly influence the occurrence of response variations. Markham and Diamond reviewed their considerable experience and found that it was duration of disease rather than duration of therapy which correlated best with a patient's response to medication.[18]

Recently four centers in this country reviewed their experience and noted that patients who were begun on therapy with levodopa earlier had a lower mortality rate than those patients in whom treatment had been delayed.[6] Although there are some difficulties in comparing the studies of the three groups, Markham and Diamond's work appears to be the most convincing.

It is reasonable to begin therapy when the patient's disease begins to impair his function in his personal life or job. Often a patient with a slight tremor will be seen and medication will not be prescribed until the tremor has become a significant impediment or movements have become uncomfortably slow. The patient's function guides decisions of when to begin therapy. The timing of antiparkinsonian drug therapy is not standard and some would begin treatment with other medications such as an anticholinergic drug or amantadine (Symmetrel) in an attempt to delay use of levodopa.

When the decision has been made to begin a patient on therapy with levodopa, the patient can start with ½ tablet of carbidopa-levodopa 25/100 tid. Because certain amino acids contained in protein can interfere with the absorption of levodopa and its transport into the brain, it is best if patients take their medication 1 hour before or after a meal. However, some patients experience nausea after taking the medication, and those patients need to take medication with a small amount of carbohydrate such as fruit. The dose of carbidopa-levodopa is gradually increased until the patient's symptoms are satisfactorily, but not necessarily entirely, relieved.

As noted before, patients often become less responsive to levodopa and develop side effects within a few years of developing symptoms and institution of treatment. The most common problems are development of dyskinesias, "wearing off" of the benefit of a dose of medication, and emergency of sudden "on/off" fluctuations in response. The etiologies of these problems have not been fully elucidated but clearly further loss of the nigrostriatal fibers contributes to deterioration. Dyskinesias correlate with peak serum levels of levodopa. Fluctuations in mobility also appear to correlate with fluctuation in serum levels of levodopa. Fluctuations are often managed by prescribing smaller, more frequent doses of carbidopa-levodopa. However, the work of Nutt suggests that this may contribute to fluctuations by maintaining the patient's serum level of levodopa just above, or often below, the threshold for a clinical response.[19] Anticholinergic drugs were the first drugs found to be useful in the treatment of Parkinson's disease. Charcot recommended use of scopolamine in the nineteenth century, and anticholinergics remained the mainstay of parkinsonian therapy until the introduction of levodopa. The anticholinergic drugs commonly used include trihexyphenidyl (Artane), benztropine (Cogentin), procyclidine (Kemadrin), and ethopropazine (Parsidol). These drugs generally result in a modest improvement in a patient's symptoms. Rigidity and tremor respond to some extent and bradykinesia is less responsive. Use of the anticholinergics is greatly limited by their side effects. Peripheral side effects commonly noted are dryness of the mouth, constipation, urinary retention, and difficulty with near vision. The most troublesome side effects are impairment in memory and confusion. Memory impairment is seen even in younger patients. Older patients often become confused on anticholinergics, and delirium can occur. Because of the limitations of the anticholinergics, they should be avoided in patients in whom there is any sign of intellectual impairment and in elderly patients.

Amantadine is another drug which by serendipity was found to be useful for treatment of Parkinson's disease. The mechanism of action appears to be through stimulation of release of dopamine from remaining terminals. It appears to benefit tremor, rigidity, and bradykinesia equally and it can be useful as a single therapy or as an adjunct to levodopa. Common side effects include ankle edema and livedo reticularis, which subside with discontinuation of the drug. Amantadine is often used as an initial therapy in Parkinson's disease or as an adjunct to levodopa therapy. Unfortunately the benefit may wane after a few months.

Drugs which act directly on the dopamine receptor, such as the ergots, are often of benefit to patients with advanced disease. Bromocriptine is the only direct dopamine receptor agonist currently available in the United States, but pergolide may be marketed soon. When bromocriptine is used as an adjunct with levodopa, the sode of levodopa can usually be reduced and fluctuations dampened. The use of bromocriptine is limited by side effects. These include nausea, hypotension, confusion, and rarely pleural thickening. Treatment with bromocriptine is begun with a low dose, 1.25 to 2.5 mg per day, and increased gradually by 2.5 mg per day at 2-week intervals. Patients usually require 10 mg per day before improvement is noted.[10] It is seldom necessary to prescribe more than 30 mg per day. Rinne reported that initiation of therapy with a combination of levodopa and bromocriptine reduced the incidence of complications seen later in patients.[24] This claim will hopefully be replicated by other investigators.

The therapies described above treat only the symptoms of Parkinson's disease and do nothing to slow or reverse the progression of the illness. Recently attention has begun to be directed to possible pathogenic mechanisms in Parkinson's disease and remedies for these processes. The Parkinson's study group in 1987 began a 5-year study of 800 patients to determine whether certain antioxidative agents, high-dose vitamin E and deprenyl, could slow the progression of the illness. Deprenyl, which is a specific inhibitor of monoamine oxidase B (see above section on MPTP toxicity), has been claimed to slow the progression of Parkinson's disease.[4]

SURGICAL TREATMENT

Prior to development of levodopa therapy thalamotomy was sometimes employed to treat Parkinson's disease. Dopaminergic therapy has largely made thalamotomy unnecessary. However, some patients will have a disabling tremor that is not responsive to dopaminergic or anti-cholinergic agents. In these few patients unilateral lesions of subregions of the ventral lateral nucleus of the thalamus may abolish the tremor and reduce the rigidity in the contralateral limb. However, the tremor may return. Bilateral surgery often results in apathy and severe dysarthria, and should be avoided. Thalamotomy should be undertaken only at centers experienced in this stereotaxic technique.

In 1987 groups in Mexico[17] and China[12] reported that autologous transplantation of adrenal medulla to the caudate of parkinsonian patients caused dramatic improvement in their patients. Swedish physicians had earlier been unable to produce sustained benefit using a somewhat different transplant technique. A number of medical centers in North America have undertaken studies to try to replicate these claims. To date no American group has replicated the claims of dramatic improvement made by Madrazo and his colleagues, but some American investigators feel that certain of their patients are mildly to moderately improved. A number of groups, including Madrazo and his colleagues, have encountered serious morbidity and mortality from this operation.

REHABILITATION IN THE TREATMENT OF PARKINSON'S DISEASE

There is little in the literature regarding approaches to or the effectiveness of rehabilitation in movement disorders other than Parkinson's disease. However, it is reasonable to assume that inasmuch as rehabilitation deals more with impairments and disability than disease per se, and other movement disorders share certain features with Parkinson's disease, the experience with parkinsonian patients may apply also to movement disorders other than Parkinson's disease. Specialists in rehabilitation medicine can provide valuable assistance to parkinsonian patients by helping them to maximize their motor function and to make adjustments to accommodate their limitations. Occupational, physical, and speech therapists provide special expertise to such patients.

Beattie and Caird found that visits to the homes of parkinsonian patients by occupational therapists were considered to be very useful by the patients.[3] The occupational therapists provided devices to assist in toileting, bathing, and eating, which most of the patients found helpful. Because Parkinson's disease is a progressive illness, these investigators suggested that the occupational therapists should periodically visit the patients to identify and deal with new problems that may arise.

The long-term benefit of physical therapy has been controversial since the report by Gibberd and coworkers that a short course of physical therapy did not improve the function of parkinsonian patients whose disease and medical regimen were stable.[8] However, this study was limited because the therapy was carried out within a hospital apparently without exercise by the patients at home. Subsequent studies have documented functional improvement due to physical therapy.[7,20,26] These investigators all employed group therapy for a number of reasons. First, other parkinsonian patients are able to provide suggestions and encouragement to the parkinsonian patient, who tends to become isolated because of the disease. Second, a social setting, unlike individual therapy sessions, reflects the world the patient will have to interact in. Finally, group therapy can be carried out much more inexpensively than individual therapy. The studies also encouraged the patients to practice their exercises at home. The study by Palmer and coworkers was the most quantitative in its assessment of rigidity, tremor, and bradykinesia.[20] They did not document changes in rigidity or maximum speed of movement. They did demonstrate improvement in gait, tremor, grip strength, and motor coordination on tasks requiring fine control. Other studies have also demonstrated improvement in tremor and gait.[7,26]

The goals of physical therapy are to counteract the effects of rigidity, which may reduce the range of motion of the joints and result in contractures of the limbs, and to increase motor function. A therapy session usually begins with warm-up exercises in which the patients carry out exercises to attain full range of motion at various joints. A therapist may assist the patient with passive stretching. Exercises which may be employed include trunk rotation, side leg raises, and knee bends. Patients may use an exercise bicycle and pulleys to achieve reciprocal motion and maintain mobility of the legs and arms. Exercises to increase motor function include deep breaths, smiling, standing on one leg, rocking on toes, hopping on one leg, and doing dance steps. Games which can be employed include shuffleboard and ball tossing. Of course, the therapist must determine the capabilities of each patient and may assist patients with some activities.

Speech therapists are able to provide patients with a number of exercises to improve their speech. These include drills to increase the depth of breath between phrases, modulation of tone, and clarity of articulation.

Information regarding exercise programs and equipment which may be helpful to patients can be obtained from the United Parkinson Foundation, 360 West Superior St., Chicago, IL 60610, and the American Parkinson Disease Association, 116 John St., New York, NY 10038.

We currently understand some of the pathology of Parkinson's disease and are beginning to study the pathogenesis. We have therapies which will greatly improve the symptoms in the early stages of the disease but do not yet have remedies to slow or reverse the progression of the disease. Patients with advanced Parkinson's disease remain a challenge. The challenge for the neurologist, primary care physician, and rehabilitation specialist is to work together to determine when the patient's impairment necessitates treatment, to devise the optimal regimen of antiparkinsonian medications during the early and later stages of the illness, and to utilize the expertise of occupational, physical, and speech therapists to help the patient to maximize his or her capabilities.

REFERENCES

1. Agid, Y., et al. (1986). Parkinson's disease and dementia. *Clin. Neuropharmacol., 9,* 22.
2. Barbeau, A., et al. (1987). Ecogenetics of Parkinson's disease: Prevalence and environmental aspects in rural areas. *Can. J. Neurol. Sci., 14,* 36.
3. Beattie, A., and Caird, F.I. (1980). The occupational therapist and the patient with Parkinson's disease. *Br. Med. J., 280,* 1354.
4. Birkmayer, W., et al. (1983). (-)-Deprenyl leads to prolongation of L-dopa efficacy in Parkinson's disease. *Mod. Probl. Pharmacopsychiatry, 19,* 170.
5. de Jong, G.J., Meerwaldt, M.D., and Schmitz, P.I.M. (1987). Factors that influence the occurrence of response variations in Parkinson's disease. *Ann. Neurol, 22,* 4.
6. Diamond, S.G., et al. (1987). Multi-center study of Parkinson mortality with early versus later dopa therapy. *Ann. Neurol, 22,* 8.
7. Gauthier, L., Dalziel, S., and Gauthier, S. (1987). The benefits of group occupational therapy for patients with Parkinson's disease. *Am. J. Occup. Ther., 41,* 360.
8. Gibberd, F.B., et al. (1981). Controlled trial of physiotherapy and occupational therapy for Parkinson's disease. *Br. Med. J., 282,* 1196.
9. Golbe, L.I., et al. (1988). Prevalence and natural history of progressive supranuclear palsy. *Neurology, 38,* 1031.
10. Hoehn, M.M.M., and Elton, R.L. (1985). Low dosages of bromocriptine added to levodopa in Parkinson's disease. *Neurology, 35,* 199.
11. Hornykiewicz, O. (1982). Brain neurotransmitter changes in Parkinson's disease. In C.D. Marsden and S. Fahn (Eds.), *Movement disorders* (pp. 41–58). London: Butterworth.
12. Jiao, S., et al. The clinical study of adrenal medullary tissue transplantation to striatum in Parkinsonism. Presented at Schmitt Neurological Sciences Symposium, Rochester, NY, 1987.
13. Karson, C.N., et al. (1984). Blink rates and disorders of movement. *Neurology, 34,* 677.
14. Koller, W.C. (1987). *Handbook of Parkinson's disease.* New York: Marcel Dekker.
15. Kurtzke, J.F., and Kurland, L.T. (1987). The epidemiology of neurologic disease. In A.B. Baker and R.J. Joynt (Eds.), *Clinical neurology,* chap. 66. Philadelphia: Harper & Row.
16. Langston, J.W., et al. (1983). Chronic parkinsonism in humans due to a product of meperidine analog synthesis. *Science, 219,* 979.

17. Madroza, I. et al. (1987). Open microsurgical autograft of adrenal medulla to the right caudate nucleus in two patients with intractable Parkinson's disease. *N. Eng. J. Med., 316,* 831.
18. Markham, C.H., and Diamond, S.G. (1981). Evidence to support early levodopa therapy in Parkinson disease. *Neurology, 31,* 125.
19. Nutt, J.G. (1987). On-off phenomenon: Relation to levodopa pharmacokinetics and pharmacodynamics. *Ann. Neurol., 22,* 535.
20. Palmer, S.S., et al. (1986). Exercise therapy for Parkinson's disease. *Arch. Phys. Med. Rehabil, 67,* 741.
21. Parkinson, J. (1817). *An essay on the shaking palsy.* London: Sherwood, Neely, & Jones.
22. Quinn, N.P., Rossor, M.N., and Marsden, C.D. (1986). Dementia and Parkinson's disease—Pathological and neurochemical considerations. *Br. Med. Bull., 42,* 86.
23. Rajput, A.H., Stern, W., and Laverty, W.H. (1984). Chronic low dose levodopa therapy in Parkinson's disease: An argument for delaying levodopa therapy. *Neurology, 34,* 991.
24. Rinne, U.K. (1987). Early combination of bromocriptine and levodopa in the treatment of Parkinson's disease: A 5 year follow-up. *Neurology, 37,* 826.
25. Schoenberg, B.S. (1987). Epidemiology of movement disorders. In C.D. Marsden and S. Fahn (Eds.), *Movement disorders* (pp. 17–32). London: Butterworth.
26. Szekely, B.C., Kosanovich, N.N., and Sheppard, W. (1982). Adjunctive treatment in Parkinson's disease: Physical therapy and comprehensive group therapy. *Rehabil. Lit., 43,* 72.
27. Singer, T.P., Trevor, A.J., and Castagnoli, N. (1987). Biochemistry of the neurotoxic action of MPTP: or how a faulty batch of "designer drug" led to Parkinsonism in drug abusers. *Trends Biochem. Sci., 12,* 266.
28. Traub, M.M., Rothwell, J.C., and Marsden, C.D. (1980). Anticipatory postural reflexes in Parkinson's disease and other akinetic-rigid syndromes and in cerebellar ataxia. *Brain, 103,* 393.

PART   III

Improving Functional Abilities

CHAPTER 8

Improving the Ability to Perform Daily Tasks

JOAN C. ROGERS

Every day, we get out of bed, wash, dress, eat breakfast, and go off to work or play. Many of these activities are done quite automatically. However, if we were to experience macular degeneration, or fall and fracture a hip, or incur a stroke, or become clinically depressed, these same taken-for-granted, habitual tasks would become difficult to perform and complete. The term *activities of daily living (ADLs)* refers to those routine tasks which are essential to a person's day-to-day living.

ADLs often become problematic for older adults due to impairments which are of sufficient magnitude to cause ADL disabilities. An *impairment* is a loss or abnormality of psychologic, physiologic, or anatomic structure or function. A *disability*, the residual consequences of an impairment, represents any restriction or inability to perform an activity in the manner considered normal for a person of the same age, culture, or education.[30]

In the elderly, ADL disabilities are precipitated by impairments of several origins. The most familiar source is a medical or psychiatric disorder, with diagnoses such as stroke, arthritis, cancer, depression, and dementia accounting for a substantive proportion of the referrals for rehabilitation. Another less well-recognized source of ADL disability are age-related changes. Decreased stamina, for instance, which accompanies physiologic changes in the heart, lungs, and muscles, can result in decreases in ADL performance that mimic those found with chronic cardiac, pulmonary, and neuromuscular diseases. Other, and even lesser acknowledged sources of ADL disability, are physical incapacity and environmental deprivation.[3,17,26] As disease-associated and age-related impairments accumulate, older adults become less mobile and less active. Hence, they are more susceptible to the deleterious effects of inactivity, such as muscular weakness, cardiovascular deconditioning, decreased mental acuity, and reduced motivation. In turn, these symptoms of disuse may be intensified by living environments that lack opportunity for adequate sensory and social stimulation.

Impairments disrupt ADL performance in multiple ways. To understand the nature of this disruption and its meaning to the patient, the clinician obtains relevant data about the patient through assessment. These data are integrated into an explanation of the patient's ADL function and dysfunction and are used to generate therapeutic options. From the available options, a course of treatment is selected that is best suited for the patient. Linking patient status to therapeutic action involves professional judgment. This chapter provides a conceptual basis for guiding the clinical decisions involved in ADL programming and discusses these in relation to those aspects of rehabilitation that are unique to geriatric practice. ADL programming addresses the continuum from screening for ADL disabilities to assessing more specifically the extent and nature of performance dysfunctions through intervention and the reestablishment of optimal ADL function.

ADL ASSESSMENT

ADL performance involves an interaction among the functional capability of the patient, the demands of the specific task, and the qualities of the task environment. Thus, the parameters of ADL assessment are both intrinsic and extrinsic to the patient. For the purposes of ADL programming, the patient's functional capability is viewed as a composite of preskills, skills, habits, and perceived self-competence. Task demands are conceptualized in terms of specific ADLs, subtasks composing each ADL, and task components. The physical and social conditions under which task performance occurs constitute the task environment. A model depicting the salient elements of the ADL assessment is given in Figure 8-1.

In assessing ADL performance, there is a tendency to ignore the extrinsic parameters, reflected in the task demands and task environment, and concentrate on the internal parameters represented by func-

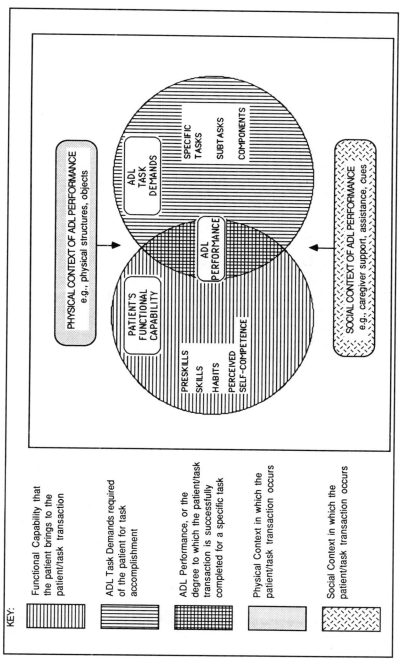

Fig. 8-1. The ADL assessment.

tional capability.[19,20] Thus, it is important to underscore that the ADL performance is as dependent on task and environmental factors as it is on the patient's functional capacity, and hence an appraisal of the extrinsic parameters is a necessary complement to the patient assessment.

NATURE OF ADL TASKS: TASK DEMANDS

When the requirements of a task exceed the functional capabilities of the patient to perform them, ADL disabilities emerge. A general understanding of task requirements is obtained through task analysis. However, the demand quality of a task, or the challenge that it presents, can be assessed only in relation to a particular patient.

ADL Tasks

The fabric of daily life is pieced together by three broad categories of ADL, namely, self-care, work, and leisure. These categories demarcate the daily living activities that are relevant for programming.[4,15,21] *Self-care* refers to bodily oriented tasks like eating, bathing, brushing teeth, combing hair, shaving, trimming toenails, toileting, and sleeping. *Work* considers tasks done in and around the home, as well as salaried and volunteer positions. Home management includes an array of tasks such as housecleaning, laundering, shopping, preparing food, managing finances, managing medications, mending clothing, using transportation, using the telephone, repairing equipment, doing yardwork, and caring for others. *Leisure* takes into account activities done primarily for pleasure and enjoyment. It encompasses arts and crafts, sports, games, intellectual and educational pursuits, and socialization. Each ADL category takes place within a sociocultural context. Except for tasks catalogued as self-care, which are generally viewed as normative for adults, routine tasks in the work and leisure categories are individually defined.

ADL programming is often restricted to self-care and home management due to its prevalent application with severely involved clinical populations and the critical role that these tasks play in maintaining independent living. However, a more adequate measure of ADL disability in the older population requires the inclusion of valued activities involving paid and volunteer work and leisure. These tasks are essential to the productive and meaningful use of time in later maturity and for maintaining physical, mental, and social abilities. Furthermore, they often provide the incentive for performing more basic ADLs, for if there is nothing to do and no place to go, why should one bother to eat or get dressed?

Subtasks and Components

Regardless of ADL category, the nature of the task is ascertained through task analysis.[5,7,9] Task analysis is a process of breaking the task down into logical steps or functional units. Eating, for example, might be broken down into the following six subtasks: (1) selecting food, (2) bringing food to the mouth, (3) chewing or drinking, (4) swallowing, (5) maintaining table manners, and (6) engaging in appropriate conversation. These subtasks are further analyzed in terms of their sensory, perceptual, cognitive, affective, motoric, and social components. Taken as a whole, the subtasks and components define the skill requirements needed by the patient for task accomplishment. Task analysis is a critical part of the ADL assessment, because it serves as a basis for determining if the patient currently has the functional capability needed to do the task; if the patient has the potential to develop this functional capability; or if the task needs to be adapted to match the patient's functional capability and how this adaptation might be accomplished.

TASK ENVIRONMENT

Tasks are carried out within a physical and social context which has the potential for facilitating or hindering the use of functional capabilities. Push-button controls placed at the front of a range assist patients with low vision, whereas dial controls situated at the back of the range handicap them. Similarly, caregivers can enhance functional independence by providing patients with needed adaptive equipment, such as plate guards, bath brushes with elongated handles, and sock aids, or they can promote dependence by feeding, bathing, and dressing the patient. Evaluation of the task environment is more difficult than task analysis because the environment of concern is the one in which the patient actually lives, works, and plays rather than the hospital or assessment setting. Evaluation of physical space aims at ascertaining architectural barriers, safety and functional features, and the extent to which available equipment can be operated by and/or assist the patient. Evaluation of the social context probes the availability of caregivers, their skills in rendering care and their need for training, their attitudes toward functional independence, and their experience of caregiver burden.

NATURE OF THE PATIENT: FUNCTIONAL CAPABILITY

A major purpose of functional capability assessment is the identification of deficits in ADL preskills, skills, habits, and perceived self-competence. These deficits serve as focal points for ADL intervention and provide insight into the nature of ADL performance dysfunction. Equally important, however, is the delineation of functional strengths, since these can be used to compensate for deficiencies.

Preskills

ADL performance involves preskills that are generic to many tasks as well as specific skills unique to each task.[25] Thus, even though manipulative ability is needed for both typing and piano playing, the skilled typist cannot necessarily play the piano. Preskills, such as attention, memory, eye-hand coordination, problem solving, balance, mobility, and communication of needs and feelings, are integrated in various combinations and permeate a number of tasks. Preskills are evaluated through standardized tests as well as clinical observations and procedures. Examples of evaluations tapping the biologic preskills are tests of joint range of motion, muscular strength, manual dexterity, and balance. Appraisals of mental status, affect, and perceptual abilities probe psychologic preskills. Trait rating scales are often used for evaluating psychosocial preskills, such as assertiveness and empathy.

Skills

The parameter of skill appraises a patient's ability to do a particular task.[22] Skill evaluation addresses the basic question: What can the older adult do now despite impairment? Skill is measured along a continuum ranging from independence to dependence. Skill ratings may be further graded in terms of the efficiency and safety of task performance, the amount and kind of help needed from another person, and the use of specialized aids or equipment. ADLs graded as dependent become potential targets for intervention. Those graded as independent are earmarked for safeguarding.

Skill is assessed by observing the patient's performance in the actual or simulated living, working, or playing environment. When evaluation takes place in the situation where the individual actually performs the task, as occurs in home health or industrial settings, testing takes advantage of the patient's *familiarity* with the task environment. In preparing a meal in one's kitchen, for example, experience enables one to find the ingredients and cookware, operate the range and stove, and solicit assistance from reluctant helpers. Testing in the actual task setting also allows the clinician to take into account the manner in which the patient uses the environment. A home appraisal, for example, might document the presence of bathtub safety rails, while observation of bathing might suggest that the rails are not used.

Although evaluation in the actual task environment is generally preferable, testing in simulated settings is more common and is not devoid of advantages. Simulations of ADL environments, like those found in occupational therapy clinics, generally include more ideal task conditions, since they are designed to accommodate a variety of impairments. Furniture is arranged for wheelchairs. Control panels on equipment are selected to reduce confusion and accommodate low vision. Caregivers are supportive of functional independence. Environmental assists such as these facilitate the assessment of optimal performance capability, that is, of what the patient is capable of doing in an adapted environment.

Habits

In contrast to the skill parameter, which accents capability, the habit parameter ascertains what the patient actually *does routinely* and the context in which it is done.[22] The evaluation of habits provides a portrait of what daily life is like for the patient and how time is allocated for self-care, leisure, and work. Habit evaluation extends beyond an investigation of current status to the premorbid pattern of functioning, the emergence of ADL disabilities, and reasons for task discontinuation. Projections into the future probe habits that need to be developed due to changing desires or capabilities and the activity pattern that appears feasible in the discharge setting.

A primary yield of habit evaluation is the detection of disabilities situated in habit structures rather than skills. In the healthy person, activities are organized to provide a dynamic balance of self-care, work, and leisure. The time devoted to each area is adequate for accomplishing responsibilities and achieving goals. Habit dysfunction is manifested when there is an absence or severe constriction of activity in one or more of the ADL categories. A second manifestation of habit dysfunction is a disorganized and ineffective lifestyle. At the other extreme is the rigid activity pattern that rapidly deteriorates when flexibility is needed. Activity patterns are rated on a continuum of effective to ineffective ADL routines.

For the patient with skill dysfunction, habit evaluation yields an indication of the patient's ADL priorities, because time is usually spent in valued activities when capability is unrestrained. It also provides a background for interpreting whether skill dysfunctions are attributable to disuse or a failure to learn a skill that is now needed, rather than skill breakdown. Lastly, discrepancies between what a person can do and does do suggest possible areas for ADL intervention.

Direct observation of daily living habits is usually impractical since it requires 24-hour observation over an extended time period. While behavioral cues, like unkept appearance, are used, the primary data-gathering methodology is questioning via interviews or questionnaires. Habit information is usually obtained from the patient and knowledgeable proxies to obtain as accurate information as possible.

Perceived Self-Competence

Perceived self-competence refers to patients' beliefs about their ability to do certain ADL tasks.[22] Normally, people do not attempt to do things unless they feel that they can, or at least have a chance of being successful. Self-perceptions of the capacity to meet task demands may range from accurate to inaccurate.

Self-perceptions are predictive of what a patient does or will do. By comparing the patient's perceptions of ADL competence with objective measures of ADL competence, the extent of agreement can be ascertained. When subjective and objective data closely correspond, patients are said to possess insight into their ADL functioning.

Information about perceived self-competence is obtained through self-report. Beliefs about task abilities and inabilities, degree of skill, ease of performance, and satisfaction with performance are queried. When incapacity is stated or implied, questioning centers on the perceived reasons for dysfunction.

ADL ASSESSMENT DECISION MAKING

Functional capability, task demands, and the physical and social environment provide a framework for the assessment of ADL performance. However, for each patient, the scope of the assessment must be narrowed to manageable limits. Several principles operate to focus the assessment. One principle is based on the patient's or caregiver's chief complaints. Many patients are able to indicate the tasks that they are unable to do or have difficulty doing. A second principle is based on common patterns of ADL disability emerging from a medical or a psychiatric diagnosis.[18] For example, a patient with a stroke, which leads to a one-handed impairment, could be predicted to have difficulty putting on panty hose and opening a milk carton. A patient with a hip fracture, however, would be expected to have the former problem but not the latter. Similarly, depression generally results in a deterioration of habits rather than skills. Diagnostically oriented ADL assessment works best when impairments are highly specific. When conditions are more generalized, or when there are multiple impairments, the approach works less well. A third principle emerges from the notion of task hierarchy.[24] Tasks whose demands closely match the strengths of the patient are tried before those where this fit is more incongruent. Chief complaint, diagnostic category, and task hierarchy strategies are often used in combination to identify a starting point for ADL assessment.

Measurement of ADL status itself usually begins with an evaluation of skill in the selected tasks. Skill serves as a pivotal point for in-depth evaluation of preskills, habits, and perceived competence. The identification of skill dysfunction leads to an examination of its causes in terms of deficits in preskills. Failure to find skill dysfunction leads to evaluations of ADL habits and beliefs. Each aspect of functional capability is considered in relation to task demands and the ambient physical and social environment.

In rehabilitation, the overall goal of the ADL assessment is to improve ADL status. This goal places requirements on the assessment process beyond those needed when functional assessment is done for purposes such as determining needed supportive services. The clinician is challenged to respond to the question: To what extent will the patient's ADL status be improved through rehabilitation? Or, in other words, what *could* the patient do as a result of intervention? Thus, the evaluation of ADL status incorporates an evaluation of rehabilitation potential.

To determine ADL potential, the clinician seeks evidence of the patient's adaptability.[12–14] Once an ADL disability has been detected, such as a failure to pass the dressing test, testing is modified to make success more feasible. In other words, an intervention, such as the demonstration of a new dressing procedure or the provision of a piece of adaptive clothing, is introduced. If the patient's performance improves, the patient is seen as having ADL potential.

Although the "test-intervene-retest" assessment methodology is highly individualized, it is also systematic.[13] It is a dynamic process which is guided by the successive generation and testing of clinical hypotheses about the causes of ADL disability in a particular patient and how it can be remedied. When several treatment options are available, the least intrusive solution is generally tried first. Accordingly, if a patient were unable to get out of bed independently, a new procedure would be tried before a self-help aid was used and an aid would be tried before a mechanical lift. In the course of these trials, task instructions are varied to include verbal (oral and written), visual (demonstration and pictorial), and physical (guidance and passive motion) modes to determine learning requirements. Thus in addition to a judgment about ADL potential, the intervention phase also provides cues about the means through which functional change can be promoted.

In practice, ADL assessment and treatment are intermingled and interant processes. As some ADLs are mastered, other, more complex, ones are brought into focus until optimal performance capability is achieved.

ADL INTERVENTION

The ADL assessment thus yields a description of patient performance that not only gives a picture of capability and incapability in terms of preskills, skills, habits, and perceived self-competence, but also yields data about the patient's adaptive potential and the types of interventions that can facilitate change. The underlying premise of all ADL intervention approaches is to strengthen abilities and alleviate deficits. This premise is particularly obvious in regard to interventions targeted for ADL preskills or environmental qualities; however it pervades all intervention approaches. The distinguishing features of the six intervention approaches to be discussed are outlined in Table 8-1.

DEFICIT

ADL interventions are either deficit- or ability-oriented.[1,8,10] The *deficit* approach is centered on restoring a dysfunctional structure or function to its normal or characteristic condition. Treatment involves a deficit-alleviating action that is appropriate for the specific type of impairment or environmental aberration. For example, a joint contracture might be reduced through splinting, passive stretching of tissue, and active motion applied to the joint of concern. The deficit approach is most suited to discrete problems where some improvement can reasonably be expected. Examples of deficits that are often amenable to remediation are joint contractures, muscular weakness, incoordination, visual-perceptual dysfunction, attention deficit, incorrect positioning, and improper caregiver technique. Once the deficit is removed, ADL function can presumably be resumed.

The deficit approach is applicable as a preventive as well as remedial strategy. As a preventive action, treatment might include activities to avoid as well as those to do. Thus, patients with rheumatoid arthritis might be advised to stop knitting because the hand positions and contractions required for holding the needles promote ulnar-deviating hand impairment. A woman having a recent mastectomy, on the other hand, might be encouraged to comb her hair because the repetitive contraction and relaxation of upper extremity musculature assists in preventing edema.

Table 8-1. *ADL Interventional Approaches*

Rehabilitation approaches for ADL programming	Rehabilitation outcomes	ADL parameters	Method
Deficit	Absence of impairment or environmental constraints	Patient's preskills Task environment	Deficit-alleviating action Removal of attitudinal & physical barriers
Ability	Strengthened intact preskills	Patient's preskills	Graduated, therapeutic exercise
Skills	Integration of preskills into specific ADL skills	Patient's ADL skills Task demands	Graduated, therapeutic activity Task adaptations
Habits	Habits and routines to support ADL efficiency and effectiveness	Patient's ADL habits	Habit training Context specific learning
Environment	Maintenance of ADL skills and habits	Task demands Task environment	Passive and active environmental assistance
Perceived self-competence	Realistic self-perception of competence in ADL skills and habits	Patient's perceived self-competence	Guided self-evaluation in conjunction with skill development and habit training

ABILITY

In contrast to the deficit approach, in the *ability* approach intervention is focused on strengthening an asset rather than eliminating a deficit. Whereas the impairment approach focuses on the paralyzed upper extremity of the hemiplegic patient, the ability approach focuses on the unaffected limb. Treatment aims at developing sufficient skill in the unaffected hand so that it can eventually replace the affected hand in skilled tasks. Compensation for lack of function is the goal, not restoration of function. Impairments are acknowledged as placing limitations on activity. However, treatment concentrates on the development of the remaining abilities.

Ability interventions are designed to develop preskills. As such, they aim at improving performance so that more effective action is possible. Facility in moving from place to place, using one's hands to manipulate objects, communicating ADL needs, solving problems, and making decisions are among the target behaviors of concern. The underlying rationale is that as preskills improve so will the specific ADL skills requiring them. The transfer of preskills to activities is assumed to occur automatically.

Preskills programming requires appropriate exercise selection, instruction in technique, and supervised practice. An exercise is therapeutic if it places a feasible demand on the preskill that is being developed and has no untoward negative effects. Initially, exercises are used that match the patient's present level of competence. Once an exercise is completed and success is experienced, progressively harder exercises are introduced to challenge and extend the patient's capabilities. The exercises themselves provide a medium for skill development and hence are less important than the competence that is being developed. Thus, recognizing that weaving is a good activity for relearning fine motor skill, patients may agree to weave, even though they have no particular interest in weaving.

SKILL

The *skill* approach is similar to the ability approach in its focus on skill development.[16,28,29] However, skill is developed in relevant ADLs, not preskills. Competence in specific tasks, like shopping by mail or repairing a hem, is the goal. The rationale underlying this approach is that the preskills constituting a task need to be practiced together rather than in isolation to link them into an integrated whole. Consequently, the training modality shifts from therapeutic exercise to therapeutic activity.

As in the ability approach, treatment revolves around a graded activity program. However, implicit in the transition from isolated to integrated preskills is the pursuit of activity for its own sake as opposed to a means to an end. To be therapeutic, the progressive program activities must be meaningful to the patient. Activity selection is a collaborative process between the patient and the clinician, with the patient sharing activity values, goals, and needs and the clinician matching these to patient capabilities and task demands. Task difficulty is dependent on the match between patient capabilities and task demands. If the capabilities-demand agreement is close, the task represents an acceptable level of difficulty.

Following task selection, attention is directed toward accomplishing it. Techniques that minimize the effects of impairment or circumvent them may be taught so that a routine task can be done in a new way. For example, if inflamed finger joints prevent lifting cups by the handle, a two-handed grasp may be used. If a patient is unable to use standard objects, self-help aids or adaptive equipment are introduced, and the patient is trained in their use. For instance, a raised toilet seat may be introduced to the patient who has difficulty rising from a regular commode. Skill in the activity is developed through practice under supervised, controlled conditions. Task demands are varied to enhance generalization. Dressing training, for example, might cover slipover and front-buttoning shirts as well as sweaters.

Since impairment often precludes continued participation in some activities, the skill approach allows for the learning of new activities. Patients are encouraged to try out tasks and discover latent abilities and interests. In the process of self-discovery, one can comfortably fail. Competence emerges as the activity process is repeatedly mastered.

HABIT

Relearned, newly learned, and previously learned skills are combined into an effective activity pattern in the *habit* approach.[11,23] ADLs are not just done, they are organized into routines like undressing, taking a bath, putting on nightclothes, taking medication, and going to bed. These routines provide economy and efficiency of action and reduce the need for planning. The goal of habit training is to provide the endurance, consistency, initiative, and autonomy needed to develop and sustain an ordered yet flexible pattern of ADL routines.

The habit approach involves context-specific learning. At issue is the generalization of ADLs from the structured, treatment situation to the less structured home and community setting at the appropriate time. Habit training aims at stabilizing ADLs in time and space. Initially, values are clarified to create an awareness of activity priorities. Then, formal training is given in time management, energy conservation, good body mechanics, stress management, and task delegation to preserve energy for valued goals. Finally, ADL routines are practiced in the context in which they are to be done. A cooperative environment for habit usage is achieved by working with patients, family members, employers, and others to remove attitudinal and architectural barriers and to put into place needed caregiving skills, adaptive equipment, and self-help aids.

ENVIRONMENT

The habit approach assumes that the patient can exercise control over day-to-day activities. In the absence of this capacity, ADL skills and habits may be maintained through *environmental* intervention.[2,27] The environment may be structured to interact both passively and actively with the patient. Passive assistance uses environmental design, such as color, furniture type and arrangement, and directional signs. Active assistance uses caregiver resources to schedule ADLs, provide needed materials, and give the level and type of help appropriate for managing the disability. Environmental mediations are intended to elicit behavioral routines that would otherwise not occur or would be incomplete or inadequate.

PERCEIVED SELF-COMPETENCE

A realistic self-assessment of one's skills and habits is the basis of the self-competence approach. Perceived self-competence is generally a natural outcome of skill and habit training. Competence emerges as the activity process is mastered in progressively harder tasks and more extensive behavioral routines. The results of action are concretely displayed in task accomplishments and successes are appropriately acclaimed. The experience of controlling personally valued ADLs rekindles a sense of competence. Sometimes this naturally emergent process requires supplementation with interventions specifically designed to increase self-awareness of abilities. This is done by eliciting self-evaluations of performance and guiding them with tangible examples of ADL improvements, using verbal feedback, graphs, and videotapes, so that positive gains are accentuated.

ADL INTERVENTION DECISION MAKING

In planning treatment, the patient's ability to learn must be considered first. If this is severely compromised, the environmental approach, in conjunction with passively instituted deficit-alleviating actions in which the patient is the recipient of care, is the primary option. To the extent that learning capacity is intact, approaches requiring active learning are available.

Although the six approaches differ in their target behaviors and intended goals, they are not incompatible and are often used simultaneously or sequentially. For example, recognizing that full recovery of a paralyzed arm is unlikely, exercises to improve motor control of the impaired limb (an impairment-alleviating action) and exercises to increase coordination in the noninjured limb (an ability approach) may be combined. Functional gains in preskills made possible through therapeutic exercise are subsequently integrated into specific ADL skills, and ADL skills subsequently into habits. Achievement of preskills, skills, and routines, along with accurate beliefs about one's capabilities, fosters competence and motivates the patient for continued achievement.

UNIQUENESS OF GERIATRIC REHABILITATION

There are some aspects of the interactions between the aging experience and the rehabilitation process that merit attention in both practice and research.

One of the most salient hallmarks of geriatric medicine is the simultaneous management of multiple conditions. For the rehabilitation specialist, these multiple diagnoses translate into multiple, and often multidimensional impairments which complicate ADL recovery. While an over-the-head activity might be recommended for a patient with upper extremity hemiparesis and contraindicated for one with cardiac insufficiency, the ADL prescription is confused when the two conditions coexist. Similarly, the older patient with a hip fracture and dementia must be taught to use the walker to prevent joint stress despite his or her memory loss and decreased learning capacity. It is imperative that there be clear communication between the primary care physician and the medical consultants, such as the physiatrist and psychiatrist, and the therapist when dealing with such patients.

The presence of multiple impairments has implications for assessment as well as treatment. Testing dressing skill by handing a patient a shirt and slacks to don would be an appropriate test for physical disabilities. It is less likely to elicit cognitive disabilities, however, because it eliminates the decision making needed for clothing selection and sequencing, which are the subtasks where cognitive problems are apt to be exhibited. When the patient population is likely to have multiple impairments, ADL testing must be carried out in a manner that has the possibility of eliciting a variety of impairments.

Research indicates that with advancing age the capacity to learn is retained but that learning takes longer. The older, impaired adult is thus doubly handicapped in the skill-learning essential to ADL training. The longer time required to learn implies an extended time to make an accurate determination of rehabilitation potential and to ascertain treatment gains.

When considering rehabilitation approaches for older adults, the direct learning of ADLs in the skill approach appears to have an advantage over the indirect learning of the ability approach. The relevance of ADL skills is more readily perceived than that of preskills. Because the environment plays an increasingly important role in regulating behavior as competence decreases, the contextually based interventions and those designed to increase the older adult's control over ADLs in time and space warrant more consideration. A greater extension of ADL training from the confines of the bathroom and bedroom to the total life space of the older adult is needed to meet emergent goals for independent living and continued work.

In assessing rehabilitation outcomes, functional interdependence becomes as important a therapeutic end point as functional independence. When complete independence is not feasible or desired, patient and caregiver need to learn to work in a synergistic manner to improve therapeutic outcomes for both. Teaching caregivers ADL techniques so that they can better manage the patient and themselves contributes to quality care and the relief of caregiver burden.

IMPLICATIONS FOR PRIMARY CARE PHYSICIANS

The source of impairment has implications for access to ADL rehabilitation. Presently, referrals for rehabilitation come largely through the medical system and provide for ADL disabilities due to impairments from medical conditions. There is no effective referral mechanism for ADL disabilities attributable to age-related changes or the disuse syndrome unless these coexist with medical disorders or until the changes become severe enough to cause a medically discernible problem. Furthermore, even in the medical system, older adults tend to frequent primary care physicians, such as geriatricians, internists, and family practitioners, whose medical education provided little exposure to rehabilitation concepts. Thus, it is likely that a substantive proportion of the elderly suffer needlessly from the accumulation of ADL disabilities that shred the fabric of daily life for themselves and those who care for and about them. These persons could be helped by a more adequate referral mechanism which channels them to practitioners skilled in managing ADL performance problems.

Primary care physicians can play a vital role in screening for ADL disability and initiating referrals to occupational and physical therapy. To assist in systematically collecting data about functional capability, screening tools such as the Activities of Daily Living section of the OARS Multidimensional Assessment Questionnaire,[6] which covers personal self-care and home management tasks, may be administered. This is an interview measure which can be completed in about 10 minutes. It can readily be supplemented with leading questions about the productive use of time such as: If you weren't at the doctor's now, how would you be spending your time? Do you have enough to do or are you bored most of the time? What do you do for fun?

During the office visit, the physician or an assistant can also take the opportunity to observe the patient performing ADLs such as rising from the chair, getting onto the examination table, undressing and dressing, and interpreting medication instructions. Performance observations like these provide valuable data about the patient's neuromuscular and cognitive capabilities as well as about the accuracy of information obtained through self- or caregiver reports. When referring patients for ADL assessment and treatment, physicians should alert therapists to any activity restrictions or precautions. Because the ADL parameters are broad, personal communication with therapists about the screening results is particularly advantageous in focusing rehabilitation efforts.

ADL disability in older adults is a multifactorial problem which has the potential to be prevented as well as remedied. A conceptual framework has been presented to promote examination and dialogue regarding those factors which guide professional decision making about ADL programming in geriatric rehabilitation.

REFERENCES

1. Allen, C.K. (1985). *Occupational therapy for psychiatric diseases: Measurement and management of cognitive disabilities.* Boston: Little, Brown.
2. Barris, R., et al. (1985). Occupation as interaction with the environment. In G. Kielhofner (Ed.), *A model of human occupation: Theory and application,* (pp. 42–62). Baltimore: Williams & Wilkins.
3. Bortz, W.M. (1982). Disuse and aging. *JAMA, 248,* 1203.
4. Clark, P.N. (1979). Human development through occupation: Theoretic frameworks in contemporary occupational therapy practice, part 1. *Am. J. Occup. Ther., 33,* 505.

5. Dicmonas, E. (1981). A psychoneuropsychologically based activity analysis. In B.C. Abreu (Ed.), *Physical disabilities manual,* (pp. 201–223). New York: Raven Press.

6. Duke University Center for the Study of Aging and Human Development. (1978). *Multidimensional functional assessment: The OARS methodology,* 2nd ed. Durham, NC: Duke University.

7. Faletti, M.V. (1984). Human factors research and functional environments for the aged. In I. Altman, J. Wohlwill, and M.P. Lawton (Eds.), *Human behavior and environment: Advances in theory and research,* (pp. 191–237), Vol. 7. New York: Plenum Press.

8. Farber, S.D. (1982). *Neurorehabilitation: A multisensory approach.* Philadelphia: Saunders.

9. Hopkins, H.L., Smith, H.D., and Tiffany, E.G. (1983). The therapeutic application of activity. In H.L. Hopkins and H.D. Smith (Eds.), *Willard and Spackman's occupational therapy,* (pp. 223–229). 6th ed. Philadelphia: Lippincott.

10. Hopkins, H.L., and Smith, H.D. (Eds.) (1983). *Willard and Spackman's occupational therapy,* 6th ed. Philadelphia: Lippincott.

11. Kielhofner, G., and Burke, J.P. (1985). Components and determinants of human occupation. In G. Kielhofner (Ed.): *A model of human occupation: Theory and application,* (pp. 12–36). Baltimore: Williams & Wilkins.

12. Lidz, C.S. (1983). Dynamic assessment and the preschool child. *J. Psychoeduc. Assess., 1,* 59.

13. Meyers, J., Pfeffer, J., and Erlbaum, V. (1985). Process assessment: A model for broadening assessment. *J. Special Educ., 19,* 73.

14. Missiuna, C. (1987). Dynamic assessment: A model for broadening assessment in occupational therapy. *Can. J. Occup. Ther., 54,* 7.

15. National Center for Health Statistics, Dawson, D., Hendershot, G., and Fulton, J. (1987). *Aging in the eighties, functional limitations of individuals 65 years and over. Advance data from vital and health statistics,* No. 133. U.S. Dept. of Health and Human Services publication No. (PHS) 87-1250. Hyattsville, MD; Public Health Service.

16. Palmer, M.L., and Toms, J.E. (1986). *Manual for functional training,* 2nd ed. Philadelphia: Davis.

17. Roberts, A.H. (1986). Excess disability in the elderly: exercise management. In L. Teri and P.M. Lewinsohn (Eds.), *Geropsychological assessment and treatment* (pp. 87–119). New York: Springer.

18. Rogers, J.C., and Masagatani, G. (1982). Clinical reasoning of occupational therapists during the initial assessment of physically disabled patients. *Occup. Ther. J. Res., 2,* 195.

19. Rogers, J.C. (1982). The spirit of independence: The evolution of a philosophy. *Am. J. Occup. Ther., 36,* 709.

20. Rogers, J.C. (1983). Clinical reasoning: The ethics, science and art. *Am. J. Occup. Ther., 37,* 601.

21. Rogers, J.C. (1984). I can: Restoring courage through occupational therapy. *Generations,* Summer, 20.

22. Rogers, J.C. (1987). Occupational therapy assessment for older adults with depression. *J. Phys. Occup. Ther., 5,* 13.

23. Snow, T.L., and Rogers, J.C. (1985). Dysfunctional older adults. In G. Kielhofner (Ed.), *A model of human occupation: Theory and application,* (pp. 352–370). Baltimore: Williams & Wilkins.

24. Spector, W.D., et al. (1987). The hierarchical relationship between activities of daily living and instrumental activities of daily living. *J. Chronic Dis., 40,* 481.
25. Stallings, L.M. (1982). Motor learning: From theory to practice. St. Louis, Mosby.
26. Suedfeld, P. (1980). *Restricted environmental stimulation.* New York: Wiley.
27. Trombly, C.A. (1983). Environmental evaluation and community reintegration. In C.A. Trombly (Ed.), *Occupational therapy for physical dysfunction,* (pp. 493–503). Baltimore: Williams & Wilkins.
28. Trombly, C.A. (1983). Activities of daily living. In C.A. Trombly (Ed.), *Occupational therapy for physical dysfunction,* (pp. 458–479). Baltimore: Williams & Wilkins.
29. Wehman, P., Renzaglish, A., and Bates, P. (1985). *Functional living skills for moderately and severely handicapped individuals.* Austin, TX: Pro-Ed.
30. World Health Organization. (1980). *International classification of impairments, disabilities, and handicaps.* Geneva, World Health Organization.

CHAPTER 9

Physical Therapy

LOIS A. AXTELL
MARION B. SCHONEBERGER

As the elderly population increases, physical therapists will be increasingly called upon to address the unique needs of older persons many of whom suffer from a primary disease or disability such as arthritis, stroke, or diabetes which result in pain, decreased motor control and loss of strength, and limitations of motion.[37] The uniqueness of these patients comes from the combined and interacting effects of the aging process, a deconditioned state associated with a sedentary lifestyle, and at least one disease process. One must understand how aging and deconditioning may alter the evaluation, goals, and treatment of the elderly. Payton and Poland suggest that physical therapy for the elderly falls into three categories: (1) prevention of disuse or restoration of function in the healthy elderly; (2) prevention or restoration in the acute or chronically ill; and (3) rehabilitation of functional losses secondary to trauma or disease.[42] Because of wide variation from individual to individual in the effects of both aging and disease processes, physical therapists need to be prepared to address a myriad of problems with the geriatric patient.

The purpose of this chapter is to provide the reader with an appreciation of the physical changes seen with aging and disuse and their impact on the evaluation and treatment of this population. The unique needs of the elderly population can then be met with an effect and well-designed program.

THE EFFECTS OF AGING

Many physical and functional problems associated with aging are related to changes in the neuromuscular, skeletal, and cardiovascular systems. Loss of muscular strength is a frequently cited change that can cause decline in motor or functional performance.[11,14,28] There is a decrease in both the size and the number of muscle fibers. Significant differences in muscular strength have been identified between younger and older persons, with age inversely related to strength.[23,27] Loss of strength results from impairment of contractile properties of the muscle, alterations in biochemical functions,[20,40] and a slowing in the speed of conduction at the myoneural junction.[46]

Declines in neuromuscular performance also can be attributed to a reduction in nerve conduction velocity, the speed and magnitude of reflex response, as well as a general loss of sensation. Changes in the vestibular system can affect balance and perception of body position in space, which then can contribute to problems with sitting, standing, and walking, resulting in falls.

Several skeletal changes are seen with aging. Declines in joint function are due to loss of elasticity in ligaments and cartilage and degeneration and calcification of articular joint surfaces. Demineralization of bones results in a propensity for fractures. Osteoporosis is 4 times more common in elderly women than men, affecting 30 percent of women over 65 years of age.[7] Functionally, the older person may have weaker muscles, stiffer joints, and move more slowly.

The cardiopulmonary changes related to aging include increased blood pressure and decreased maximum cardiac output.[54] Maximal heart rate and maximal oxygen consumption also decline.[55]

Lung changes are characterized by an increase in residual volume accompanied by a decrease in vital capacity. Declines are seen in maximal voluntary ventilation, the surface area for gas exchange as well as the rate of diffusion.[47] Both the lung tissue and chest wall lose elasticity. Cardiopulmonary demands usually can be met, but when disease or deconditioning are present the demands may exceed the available reserve. All of these changes result in a reduced tolerance for physical activity and are important to consider with regard to rate and intensity of activities for the older person. Declines occur gradually. Due to the wide variability in lifestyles, the rate and magnitude of changes cannot be predicted and may not be apparent until they impact on day-to-day functioning.

Declines in hearing, vision, and cutaneous sensation affect functional abilities and have implications for both evaluation and treatment. Perceptual, social, and psychologic changes further impact on the aging process and affect daily functioning. Keeping these in mind should enable physical therapists to more effectively treat the elderly.

EFFECTS OF DISUSE

Changes associated with normal aging are similar to those changes associated with lessened activity, inactivity, or bed rest.[9] Some of the common changes associated with bed rest include loss in muscle strength and range of joint motion, demineralization of bones, orthostatic hypotension, decreased coordination, and declines in vital capacity, maximum stroke volume, and oxygen consumption and endurance.[21,51] Immobilization or bed rest can have a potentially devastating effect on the functional capacity of the elderly, particularly on mobility. At this time it is difficult to define which changes are attributable to aging and which are caused by disuse. Much of the research on aging has been cross-sectional, comparing age differences between groups.[11] More longitudinal studies in large well-defined populations are needed. Age-induced changes may in fact be the result of disuse associated with a sedentary lifestyle. Fortunately, the effects of habitual exercise and endurance training with the elderly have been shown to be beneficial in maintaining optimal function of the human body.[4]

RESPONSE TO EXERCISE

Available data do not yet tell us the extent to which the aging process can be modified by activity. However, physical conditioning is possible for the older adult although improvement occurs at a slower rate than for a younger person. Multiple studies, which include persons over the age of 55, show improvement in muscle strength[24,29,36] and muscle morphology[29,36] as a result of resistive exercises. The benefits of physical activity on coordination and reaction time have been documented.[48,56,57] Total body calcium increases with exercise in both young and aged adults. Longitudinal studies are necessary to determine the intensity, frequency, and duration of exercise required to maintain bone density.[45] Endurance training, even when begun in old age, can significantly improve maximal oxygen consumption, ventilatory function, and maximum work output.[1,15,44,53,62]

These benefits of exercise for the older adult are important because some elderly function dangerously close to the point where further decline in strength or aerobic power may make them incapable of caring for themselves or being independently mobile. Maximum exercise capacity progressively declines with advancing age. Daily activities, such as walking, require a greater percentage of maximum exercise capacity for older persons.[61] If deconditioning is superimposed on age-related decline, the margin between maximum capacity and functional demands narrows.[63] Getting out of bed may require maximal effort. Therefore, exercise programs which produce even small gains in strength and endurance may render the person capable of regaining a higher level of function.

Research is showing that even low-level exercise programs such as calisthenics, walking, or biking produce a training effect in the elderly.[6,15] Therefore, intensity and duration of activity can be regulated according to the physical ability of each individual to enhance his or her well-being.

EFFECTS OF DISABILITY

Many elderly persons also suffer the effects of a specific disabling disease or disability such as arthritis or a stroke. Weakness, joint limitations, neurologic impairment, and pain are common problems associated with many disabilities. Musculoskeletal problems and arthritis often result in the elderly being homebound. The combined effects of aging, disuse, and disease place the individual at high risk for loss of functional independence and mobility.

EVALUATION

Several different approaches have been used for evaluation of the elderly. Some settings use standard physical therapy tests to evaluate musculoskeletal, neurologic, and cardiopulmonary status as well as functional abilities. In addition, several assessment tools are available specifically for the geriatric patient such as Lawton's Activities of Daily Living Scale, the OARS Multidimensional Functional Assessment Questionnaire, the Functional Life Scale, and the Philadelphia Geriatric Center Multilevel Assessment instrument.[22] Regardless of the specific evaluation tools or process used, the focus is on evaluation of functional abilities including basic activities of daily living (ADLs) such as hygiene, dressing, transfers, mobility, and home and community skills (cooking, housekeeping, shopping, etc.). Results or scores from such assessments provide information for goal setting and treatment planning. In an interdisciplinary setting occupational therapists and physical therapists work together in collecting evaluation information in order to minimize duplication.

Evaluation begins with a chart review noting medical history and the results and interpretations of laboratory and diagnostic tests to help determine rehabilitation potential. Special attention is given to medications, since action alone or interaction with other medications can affect the patient's response to treatment.

Finally, information about the patient's family and living situation, education, lifestyle, and economic situation is important and can be obtained from several sources—the patient, family members, and psychologists or social workers when available. Psychosocial information is critical to setting realistic goals and obtaining compliance with treatment programs. If transportation is a problem, perhaps home treatment is better than outpatient treatment. The patient may need a family member to follow through with and reinforce new skills learned in therapy. If money is a concern, it is helpful to discuss costs and insurance coverage before beginning treatment. The elderly person often has multiple and compounding medical problems as well as a complicated and difficult psychosocial and economic situation. These patients present a great challenge to all members of a multidisciplinary team.

Evaluation includes range of motion, muscle strength and control, sensation, gait, physiologic response to exercise, and functional skills. Normal age-related declines in range of motion seem to be more statistically significant than clinically significant.[8] The important range-of-motion limitations are those that interfere with function. Shoulder and elbow joint range-of-motion restrictions are significant for those who need to use their arms for transfers and manual wheelchair mobility.

A number of studies have documented the penalties of joint restrictions on gait. The important of reducing or preventing knee flexion deformity was illustrated in a group of normal subjects who walked with one knee in 15 degrees, 30 degrees, and 45 degrees of flexion. Walking efficiency was reduced by 12 percent, 21 percent, and 32 percent, respectively. Walking velocity declined with increasing amounts of joint restriction.[61] Another study demonstrated the effects of immobilization with unilateral lower extremity casts. Walking efficiency was reduced by 21 percent with a short leg cast, by 25 percent with a cylinder cast, and by 38 percent with a long leg cast.[60] Walking efficiency for persons with unilateral arthrodesis of the hip and ankle has been measured. A 12 percent reduction in walking efficiency was found in subjects with ankle fusion and a 32 percent reduction in those with hip fusion.[59] These studies illustrate the relative importance of specific joint movements in the gait cycle.

Clinically, the elderly patient often shows disproportionately weaker hip extensors, abductors, and plantar flexors than other lower extremity musculature, which can contribute to decreased walking velocity and

efficiency. The patient with lower extremity weakness may need orthoses and upper extremity assistive devices, or even a wheelchair, in order
to maintain mobility. It is therefore important to evaluate upper extremity strength for these activities.

Several studies indicate that the greater the reliance on upper extremities for walking, the greater the energy cost. Normal subjects forced to
walk with crutches significantly decrease their velocity and efficiency.[58]
Reliance on the arms presents two problems. First, the greater the
muscle mass involved, the greater the oxygen demand for the activity.
Therefore the older person may place a greater demand on the cardiopulmonary system. Secondly, upper extremity work requires higher
arterial blood pressure and heart rate for a given oxygen consumption
than leg work.[5] This may pose a problem for the elderly diabetic
amputee with underlying heart disease who must use crutches to walk.

Particular attention should be given to cutaneous sensory changes,
especially over bony prominence where skin problems may develop.

Assessment of sitting and standing balance is important when evaluating independence in transfers and walking. Evaluation of lower
extremity motor control in the standing position is important for patients with neurologic disorders. This helps determine the influence of
spasticity on stance stability and limb advancement in walking.[35]

Pain impacts on function and mobility since it can limit joint movement and muscular effort. Brown, Batten, and Porell studied 30 osteoarthritis patients pre- and postunilateral total hip replacement.[10] They
demonstrated a 17 percent increase in walking velocity and a 20 percent
improvement in walking efficiency with their new hips, which was
attributed partly to improved joint motion but mostly to pain relief.[10]

Observational gait analysis provides a systematic way to identify
swing and stance deviations and to determine the appropriate treatment
intervention such as stretching, strengthing, lower extremity orthoses,
and upper extremity aids.[38] Determination of walking velocity and
ability to negotiate architectural barriers provides information that
relates directly to functional goals.

In order for walking to be functional a person needs to be able to walk
certain distances to perform specific activities in a reasonable period of
time. Several studies have looked at the requirements for independent
ambulation in the community.[13,18,49] Distance requirements were variable ranging from 37 m for a beauty parlor or barbershop to 360 m for a
department store. In general, distances were shorter in rural and small
towns than in cities. Velocity requirements for safe street crossing at a
controlled signal was also variable, ranging from 30 to 82.5 m per
minute. Walking velocity is important when considering the total time
required to complete the community activity. It may not be realistic to

expect someone who walks at less than 40 percent of normal walking velocity to function independently in the community, becuase it takes too long to complete the task. The ability to negotiate curbs, steps, and ramps is also important in the assessment of functional community ambulation.

An area that is often overlooked by physical therapists when evaluating patients in physiologic response to exercise or activity. It is not necessary to have a sophisticated exercise laboratory to objectively evaluate work performed and physiologic response. Monitoring of heart rate, blood pressure, and dyspnea level is done while the patient performs a specified activity such as walking. ECG telemetry may also be used to detect cardiac abnormalities.[52] The patient's response is assessed. If an elderly lady has a heart rate of 180 beats per minute after one trip down the parallel bars at a walking velocity of 20 percent of normal, it is doubtful that she will perform that activity for prolonged periods. In addition to the above-mentioned clinical tools, other useful signs and symptoms include chest pain, claudication, and complaints of fatigue. The measurements observed during the evaluation can then serve as a baseline for initiating a treatment program and reassessing progress.

The difficult part of the evaluation process is putting all of the pieces together: past medical history; physical, psychologic, and social findings; and clinical knowledge of the effects of aging, disuse, and disability in order to determine realistic goals and treatment plans.

GOALS

Goals give direction and purpose to treatment and, generally speaking, for the older adult, serve to minimize functional losses associated with aging, disease, and disability while maximizing remaining capabilities. However, within this broad definition, lie many more specific short- and long-term aims which vary considerably depending on the individual and the influence of those responsible for his or her success or failure: the patient, the patient's family, the physical therapist, and other health care workers.

THE PATIENT

What does the patient want? Little can be accomplished without the patient's cooperation. Mutual goals which are acceptable to both the older adult and the therapist may require negotiation. Establishing rapport initially generates a trust relationship which encourages the patient to plan constructively with the therapist.

The older adult must first understand the goal, agree that it is important, and be able to relate the treatment to the goal. Hearing or mild
cognitive deficits, frequently seen in the older population, make it more
difficult to accomplish this step. The therapist must encourage the patient's
participation in the planning and check often for understanding.

Goals also must be based on objective findings from the physical
examination and the patient's past functional status.

FAMILY OR SIGNIFICANT OTHERS

Family goals must be integrated into treatment from the onset. Questions such as these must be pursued: Are the children willing to take the
parent into the home and provide physical care, if necessary? Are the
children able to supply daily contacts necessary to allow the mother to
remain in her home? Is the wife strong enough physically and emotionally to assist with the care of her husband? Are the family dynamics
contributing positively or negatively to the best interest of the older
adult? Negative family dynamics need to be approached by many
members of the multidisciplinary team and in a variety of ways. The
goals established by the physical therapist will vary depending on the
answers to these types of questions.

One area in which the physical therapist can be of assistance is in the
area of family teaching. Goals directed toward training the family in
ways to therapeutically offer more or less assistance to the older adult
may resolve some conflicts between the family and the patient or among
family members.

Although these considerations may apply to patients in general, many
subtle differences exist in the older patient population which affect goal
setting when considering the family. By the time older adults have
reached 65 or 70, many of their significant others or family members
have died or are ill themselves. Thus the number of persons available to
assist has decreased. Secondly, the attitude of family and others may be
that the life of the older adult is almost over. Thirdly, children may deny
that a parent is not as functional as he once was. An unwillingness to
accept the functional decline of a parent may be due to the childrens'
inability to face the eventuality of the parent's mortality. Fourthly,
children have many other responsibilities such as their own children and
jobs which prohibit them from assisting an aged parent.

Although physical therapists may not be able to do much about these
factors, they need to be aware of these dynamics. When the patient lacks
significant others, the therapist may need to assume greater responsibility in making decisions, in coordinating care provided by other
agencies, or in guiding the patient in making decisions. Otherwise, the

physical therapist needs to (1) be aware of why the family is behaving in a certain way, (2) practice greater patience in dealing with the family, and (3) set goals which include patient and family education in order to maximize the rehabilitation of the older adult.

THE PHYSICAL THERAPIST

Physical therapists need to be aware of their own attitudes toward aging when establishing goals for the older adult. Unlike Japanese and Indian cultures where the wisdom of elders is greatly respected, our society has focused on its youth and has stressed productivity. Therefore, physical therapists in the United States may have a tendency to prefer to work with young and middle-aged patients who have potential for leading "productive" lives after rehabilitation. Therapists who feel that older adults have little to offer society may see little purpose in rehabilitating them. Therefore, the therapist may set very limited goals or may even deny treatment. On the other hand, the physical therapist who understands little of the effects of aging, disuse, and multiple medical problems may set goals too high and expect too much too fast from the older adult.

The elderly, who are not suffering from severe dementia, can and do learn effectively. Although approaches may need to be modified to adjust for certain declines which occur with aging, goals which require learning should still be attainable. The time required to meet these goals may be longer.[39,43]

Realistic functional goals are very important for retaining the interest and cooperation of the older adult. Endurance training with emphasis on normal gait characteristics and normal velocity is a realistic goal for the older adult with mild emphysema who wants to return to playing 18 holes of golf. On the other hand, treatment to attain 120 degrees of knee flexion for a patient with arthritis who walks limited distances with a cane and does not do her own housework is unrealistic. Goals to increase strength and range of motion should coincide with the functional level that is realistic for that individual.

THE HEALTH CARE TEAM

The multidisciplinary team is a definite asset in dealing with the multifaceted problems of many older adults. These concerns include such things as dietary deficiencies, psychosocial problems, and limited finances. Although these concerns may fall outside the realm of physical therapy, many of these patient problems directly affect the treatment provided by the therapist. A person with an inadequate diet may have limited energy to devote to an exercise program. Likewise, a patient suffering from an adverse reaction to a medication or one who is filled with anxiety because of a financial or psychosocial problem will not be able to give full attention to physical therapy. The physician, nurse, occupational therapist, social worker, psychologist, psychiatrist, dietitian, pharmacist, and audiologist are great assets to the total care of the older adult. Without the assistance of one or all of these health experts, physical therapy goals may be hampered or the duration of rehabilitation lengthened.

TREATMENT

Physical therapists treat older adults who have a variety of disabilities and functional capabilities. At one end of the spectrum are the individuals who receive maximum assistance with functional needs in a hospital or nursing home. At the opposite end of the spectrum are those who live independently and receive individual or group treatments as outpatients. Therefore, physical therapists must be prepared to treat geriatric patients with a variety of physical and functional problems and in a variety of ways. This section on treatment focuses on special considerations of treating the older adult in the following four categories:

1. Preventing disuse
2. Maximizing function in the older adult with chronic disease and disability
3. Preventing falls
4. Maximizing function in the older adult with progressive disability

PREVENTING DISUSE

It is unlikely that physical therapy per se contributes anything to reversing the direct effects of aging. However, the disuse that accompanies the sedentary lifestyle commonly adopted by an older adult can be positively influenced through physical therapy intervention. Bedside exercises, transfers, sitting, and ambulation should be started as soon as they are medically and orthopedically feasible, following an illness.

Loss of joint mobility and decreased strength secondary to musculoskeletal dysfunciton, including the residual of many neuromuscular disorders, are primary causes of loss of function in the elderly.[33] Knee flexion contractures not only cause a disadvantage biomechanically during gait, but also increase the energy requirements for walking. Loss of hip extension range leads to compensatory knee flexion and a forward posture at the trunk. The strength losses described previously that occur in the hip extensor-abductor muscles and ankle plantar-flexor muscles of many elderly may be because they no longer challenge these muscles. Many no longer walk fast, climb stairs, or walk up inclines.

Lyons and colleagues demonstrated in an EMG study of the gluteus medius and gluteus maximus muscles that fast walking and stair climbing increased the intensity and duration of electrical activity in these muscles.[34] The person who usually walks slowly and does not use curbs or stairs does not challenge these muscles and may suffer a decline in strength. This can lead to increasing difficulty in rising from chairs, ascending stairs, and doing other functional activities requiring strength in the extensors of the lower extremities.

Preventing loss of joint mobility and strength is a must in working with the elderly. Regular exercise will help increase or maintain strength, improve or maintain joint function, and increase strength of the bones. Exercising the hip and knee extensors by working in limited arcs of motion which are critical to a certain activity can help improve function. For instance, functional treatment for training a patient to rise from a chair might consist of resisting hip and knee extension in the final arc of motion. This can be done by using ankle weights or isokinetic equipment.[32] Having the patient repeatedly move up and down on the balls of the feet while standing, practice stair climbing, or get in and out of a bathtub are other means of providing functional treatment to increase strength and mobility.

Exercise programs for general conditioning and endurance training are excellent ways to prevent functional losses due to disuse in both the healthy elderly and those with disabilities. These programs can be done either individually or in a group setting. Unfortunately, endurance training for the elderly is sometimes neglected by physical therapists.

Studies by several investigators support the effectiveness of exercise programs to improve cardiopulmonary responses in the elderly.[2,15] deVries[15] as well as Amundsen and colleagues[2] demonstrated a significant increase in the oxygen-carrying capacity of older subjects following exercise programs. Of special interest is the fact that deVries found this significant improvement not only in the 59 patients who participated in a more aggressive exercise program, but also in a group of seven subjects who participated in a modified program. The modified program did not permit jogging or a heart rate in excess of 120 beats per minute. His study also demonstrated significant improvement in vital capacity and systolic and diastolic blood pressures in both groups.[15] Although the number of subjects in the modified exercise program was small, the results suggest that, for this age group, important physical benefits can be derived from a program as light in intensity as moderately paced walking.

The subjects in the study by Amundsen and colleagues were separated into two groups. One half did calisthenic exercises while the other half did a walking and stair-climbing program. Both groups demonstrated a significant increase in their oxygen-carrying capacity. Many older adults with whom physical therapists work are unable to jog or walk fast. The results of these studies are of special interest because they suggest that exercises such as calisthenics and walking are sufficient to bring about conditioning in those elderly who are not very active.

However, the physical therapist must exercise caution when implementing an endurance program for the older adult. He or she must be aware of the normal and abnormal cardiovascular responses to exercise.[3,30,52] Patients must be assessed medically by the physician prior to being placed on the program. These programs usually incorporate the use of walking, jogging, or biking to stimulate the cardiovascular systems. Physiologic monitoring by means of heart rate, blood pressure, and observation for symptoms will assist the physical therapist in establishing a program and adapting it to the tolerance of the individual. Telemetered ambulatory ECG monitoring allows the therapist to more precisely monitor the function of the heart during functional activities.

Several resources outline methods for establishing exercise and endurance programs[2,16,30] These programs need to be modified in accordance with the physical and medical status of the patient involved. In general, however, the cardiovascular and pulmonary systems in the elderly do not respond as quickly to an increase in activity as do the systems of the young. Therefore, the older adult will take longer to reach steady state at any given work load. The elderly also have a decreased maximum heart rate. For example, an older person exercising at a heart rate of 120 beats per minute is working harder than a young person exercising at a heart rate of 120 beats per minute.

The physical therapists at Rancho Los Amigos Medical Center conducted an endurance program consisting of conditioning exercises followed by an individualized group walking program. Subjects were over 60 years of age and had at least one chronic disease. The treatment was given 3 times a week as part of a 5-hour-a-day multidisciplinary outpatient program. Ambulation data on 25 patients collected during a 3-month period were reviewed. Average attendance was once per week. The best distance for each individual during the first month was compared against the best distance for that same individual during the third month. Seventeen of 25 (68%) patients increased their total distance walked. The average increase was 430 m. Eleven out of the 25 patients (44%) increased their walking velocity.

Of the 17 patients who improved in distance, only five were able to ambulate for 350 m at 40 to 50 percent normal velocity the first month. At the end of 3 months, this number had increased to 12, representing a greater than 50 percent increase in the number of individuals having adequate endurance and walking velocity to ambulate fairly comfortably in the community. This change may have been due to improvement in the cardiovascular system, improvement in lower extremity strength, or increased self-confidence in one's own physical ability, or other reasons. Regardless of the cause, clinically these individuals demonstrated functional improvement after being in the multidisciplinary outpatient program over a 3-month period.

MAXIMIZING FUNCTION IN THE OLDER ADULT WITH CHRONIC DISEASE AND DISABILITY

In the elderly, aging and disuse can be compounded by pathologic changes such as cerebral vascular accidents, arthritis, diabetes, respiratory disorders, hypertension, and cardiac disease. The primary goal of rehabilitation is to restore function. If this is not possible, potential capabilities are maximized by teaching the patient to function effectively within the limits of the disability. Traditional treatment approaches for specific disabilities are described in many textbooks and in the literature and will not be addressed here. Many of these treatment techniques can be used as effectively with the elderly as with the young. However, this section will focus on special considerations the therapist must be aware of when treating the older adult who has a specific disability.

Since the older adult frequently has medical problems in addition to the effects of aging and disuse, the physical therapist must consider more than just the primary diagnosis. A secondary diagnosis may dictate alterations of the treatment techniques used. For instance, osteoporosis or painful arthritis joints may preclude aggressive stretching of a contracture. Although a patient may have been admitted for a stroke, hypertension or history of a myocardial infarction warrants close monitoring of heart rate and blood pressure, before, during, and after activity. A secondary diagnosis of diabetes will require special attention to the patient's eating schedule and observation for insulin reaction. The therapist must also be alert to the patient's skin condition and footwear. Suitable shoes provide support, adequate space for foot and toe deformities, and protection from the environment.[17]

Medications are a second consideration. The elderly receive more drugs than any age group and are particularly vulnerable to deleterious effects from them. Elderly patients exhibit a decreased capacity to eliminate drugs through the kidney.[12] Digoxin, a drug frequently prescribed to increase the contractility of the heart muscle, is excreted through the kidney. Build-up of the medication can occur due to decreased renal elimination, causing a toxic reaction.[12,26] Other drugs, such as propranolol, are metabolized more slowly by the elderly.[25] Again, this leads to an accumulation of the drug in the body tissue over time.

Side effects from drugs are weakness, fatigue, vertigo, symptomatic postural hypotension, depression, and confusion.[12] Physical therapists should be aware of what medications the patient is taking. Adverse physical and mental changes should be reported quickly to the physician.

In addition, cardiac glycosides such as digitalis can cause cardiac arrhythmias. Sinoatrial block and extreme sinus bradycardia also occur, especially in the elderly.[25] The physical therapist may be the first to note the ECG change while monitoring the patient with telemetry.

Thirdly, loss of mobility and strength must be prevented in the patient with a disability as well as in the deconditioned elderly. Exercises and endurance programs discussed earlier in this chapter are also relevant for the older adult with a disability.

Finally, psychosocial aspects must be considered as well as physical factors. Lewis lists three psychosocial complications that have an impact on rehabilitation of the older person: depression, hypochondriasis, and organic brain syndrome.[31] She advocates encouraging depression patients to discuss their problems and suggests that the therapist engage the patient emotionally, mentally, and physically. For hypochondriasis the older adult should be encouraged to be as independent as possible in spite of the pain. Two suggestions for working with the patient with organic brain syndrome are to assist the patient by simplifying the environment and to use touch to help orient the patient to time and place.

PREVENTING FALLS

Potentially avoidable environmental factors account for 40 to 50 percent of falls in the elderly.[41] Underlying medical problems probably account for the remaining 50 to 60 percent.[50]

The older adult is at greater risk of falling as a result of minor environmental hazards than is a younger person. Factors which contribute to this are poor vision, decreased strength, and slower reaction time due to loss of neural function both centrally and neuromuscularly. Physical therapists can assist in preventing falls in the following ways:

1. Home visits should include an environmental inspection to reduce hazards. Recommendations should be made to the patient or family regarding hazards such as loose throw rugs, slippery floors, stairs without rails or adequate lighting, furniture blocking door-

ways, lack of grab bars and other safety assists in the bathroom, or bedrooms remote from the bathroom necessitating the need for a bedside commode.

2. The therapist should educate the patient with poor vision on ways to compensate for visual deficits.
3. Strengthening weak muscles can provide reserve strength which can be called upon to correct loss of balance.
4. Coordination exercise done with or without music, balance activities, and a program to improve endurance may assist in slowing the decline in reaction time.

Upper extremity aids are sometimes helpful in increasing safety and preventing falls. Canes and walkers can substitute for weak muscles or impaired balance. Frequently older adults are fearful of crutches, and therefore their use may not be beneficial. In some cases upper extremity aids cannot be used because the patient is unable to use them correctly. They may only add to his or her instability and confusion.

Other causes of falls are vertigo, postural hypotension, disorders of eyes and ears, medications, and cardiovascular disorders.[19,50] A sudden change in the patient's balance, functional ability, or cognition may be due to transient ischemic attacks, an adverse reaction to medications, or cardiac arrhythmias. Such changes should be reported to the physician. A sudden onset of confusion is not an indication of dementia and should not be ignored; dementia comes on slowly.

Falls in the elderly can be devastating to them both psychologically and physically. Every attempt should be made to prevent their occurrence.

MAXIMIZING FUNCTION IN THE OLDER ADULT WITH PROGRESSIVE DISABILITY.

Parkinsonism, supranuclear palsy, and Alzheimer's disease are progressive diseases of the nervous system which are found in the older population. Since performance frequently fluctuates and always eventually declines, goals which strive for lasting improvement in patients with these diagnoses cannot be achieved. Physical therapy will not alter the course of these disease processes. However, intervention may prolong functional capabilities and delay the need for physical assistance by the family.

The family may tend to shelter the individual with progressive disease. Family members may fear that the older adult will fall, or they may be uncertain how much independence to allow him or her. The decline due to disuse which results may cause the individual to lose function more rapidly than is warranted by the disease process. Individual or group treatments, including exercises and ambulation, will prevent deconditioning from occurring. Treatment should include educating the family on means of prolonging function.

Upper extremity aids are useful in certain stages of the disease process to increase safety and stability. Raised toilet seats, grab bars in the bathroom, and shower or tub benches will enable the patient to remain independent longer or decrease the amount of assistance necessary. This may enable the patient to remain in the home longer than would have been possible without the intervention.

CONCLUSION

Physical therapy for the older adult offers a challenge to the talent and creativity of those involved. Effective programs are those administered by therapists who are knowledgeable about the aging process, skilled in team interaction, and cognizant of the special considerations needed for the older adult undergoing rehabilitation.

REFERENCES

1. Adams, G.M., and deVries, H.A. (1973). Physiological effects of an exercise training regimen upon women aged 52 to 79. *J. Gerontol., 28,* 50.
2. Amundsen, L.R., et al. (1983). Cardiac considerations and physical training. In O. Jackson (Ed.), *Clinics in physical therapy: Physical therapy of the geriatric patient* (pp. 188–201). New York; Churchill Livingstone.
3. Amundsen, L.R., and Nielsen, D.H. (1981). Normal and abnormal cardiovascular responses to acute physical exercise. In L.R. Amundsen (Ed.), *Clinics in physical therapy: Cardiac rehabilitation* (pp. 1–9). New York: Churchill Livingstone.
4. Astrand, P.O. (1987). Exercise physiology and its role in disease prevention and rehabilitation. *Arch. Phys. Med. Rehabil., 68,* 305.
5. Astrand, P.O. (1977). *Textbook of work physiology.* New York: McGraw-Hill.
6. Badenhop, D.T., et al. (1983). Physiological adjustments to higher-or lower-intensity exercise in elders, *Med. Sci. Sports Exerc., 15,* 496.
7. Bierman, E.L., and Brady, H. (1980). *Our future selves: Report of the Panel on Biomedical Research.* Washington, D.C.: National Advisory Council on Aging. NIH publication No. 80-1445, 1980.
8. Boone, D.C., and Azer, S.P. (1979). Normal range of motion of joints in male subjects. *J. Bone Joint Surg., 61,* 756.
9. Bortz, W. (1982). Disuse and aging. *JAMA, 248,* 1203.
10. Brown, M.B., Batten, C., and Porell, D., (1978). Efficiency of walking after total hip replacement. *Orthop. Clin. North Am., 9,* 364.

11. Brown, M. (1987). Selected physical performance changes with aging. *Top. Geriatr. Rehabil., 2,* 68.
12. Chapron, D.J. (1983). Drugs: an obstacle to rehabilitation of the elderly. In O. Jackson (Ed.), *Clinics in physical therapy: Physical therapy of the geratric patient* (pp. 127–147). New York: Churchill Livingstone.
13. Cohen, J., et al. (1987). Establishing criteria for community ambulation. *Top. Geriatr. Rehabil., 3,* 71.
14. Cress, M.E., and Schultz, E. (1985). Aging muscle: Functional morphologic, biochemical, and regenerative capacity. *Top. Geriatr. Rehabil., 1,* 11.
15. deVries, H.A. (1979). Physiological effects of an exercise training regimen upon men aged 52 to 88. *J. Gerontol., 25,* 335.
16. deVries, H.A. (1979). Tips on prescribing exercise regimens for your older patient. *Geriatrics, 34,* 75.
17. Edelstein, J.E. (1988). Foot care for the aging. *Phys. Ther., 68,* 1882.
18. Frankiel-Learner, M., and Vargas, S. (1986). Functional community ambulation: What are your criteria? *Clin. Manage., 6,* 12.
19. Gordon, M. (1982). Falls in the elderly: More common, more dangerous. *Geriatrics, 37,* 117.
20. Gutmann, E., and Hanzlikova, A. (1972). *Age changes in the neuromuscular system.* Bristol; *Scientechnica* 1972.
21. Harper, C.M., and Yvonne, M.L. (1988). Physiology and complications of bed rest. *J. Am. Geriatr. Soc., 36,* 1047.
22. Jackson, O.L. (1979). Functional assessment of the aged. *Allied Health Behav. Sci., 2,* 47.
23. Johnson, J. (1982). Age related differences in isometric and dynamic strength and endurance. *Phys. Ther., 62,* 985.
24. Kauffman, T.L. (1985). Strength training effect in young and aged women. *Arch. Phys. Med. Rehabil., 66,* 223.
25. Kleiger, R.E. (1983). Cardiovascular disorders. In F.U. Steinberg (Ed.), *Care of the geriatric patient* (pp.   ). St. Louis, Mosby.
26. Kramer, P. (1987). Influence of aging on drug distribution and response. *Top. Geriatr. Rehabil. 2,* 1.
27. Larsson, L., and Karlsson, F.J. (1978). Isometric and dynamic endurance as a function of age and skeletal muscle characteristics. *Acta Phys. Scand., 104,* 129.
28. Larsson, L. (1978). Morphological and functional characteristics of the aging skeletal muscle in man: A cross-sectional study. *Acta Phys. Scand., 457,* 1036.
29. Larsson, L. (1982). Physical training effects on muscle morphology in sedentary males at different ages. *Med. Sci. Sports Exerc., 14,* 203.
30. Lewis, C.B. (1984). Effects of aging on the cardiovascular system. *Clin. Manage., 4,* 24.
31. Lewis, C.B. (1984). Rehabilitation of the older person: a psychosocial focus. *Phys. Ther., 64,* 517.
32. Lewis, C.B. (1984). What's so different about rehabilitating the older person? *Clin. Manage., 4,* 10.
33. Liang, M.H., et al. (1983). Management of functional disability in home-bound patients. *J. Fam. Pract. 17,* 429.
34. Lyons, K. et al. (1983). Timing and relative intensity of hip extensor and abductor muscle action during level and stair ambulation. *Phys. Ther., 63,* 1597.

35. Montgomery, J., et al, (1983). *Physical therapy management of patients with hemiplegia secondary to cerebrovascular accident* (pp. 11–15). Rancho Los Amigos Hospital, Downey, CA.
36. Mortani, T., and DeVries, H.A. (1980). Potential for gross muscle hypertrophy in older men. *J. Gerontol. 35*, 672.
37. National Center for Health Statistics. (1980). *Health United States 1978*. U.S. Dept. of Health, Education, and Welfare publication No (PHS) 79-1232. Washington D.C.: Government Printing Office.
38. *Observational gait analysis handbook*. (1989). Pathokinesiology Service and Physical Therapy Department, Rancho Los Amigos Hospital, Downey, CA.
39. Orgren, R.A. (1983). On teaching older adults. *Geri-topics*, Spring 14.
40. Orlander, J., et al. (1978). Skeletal muscle metabolism and ultrastructure in relation to age in sedentary men. *Acta Phys. Scand., 104*, 249.
41. Overstall, P.W. (1978). Falls in the elderly: epidemiology, etiology, and management. In B. Isaacs (Ed.), *Recent Advances in Geriatric Medicine* (pp. 61–72). New York; Churchill Livingstone.
42. Payton, O.D., and Poland, J.L. (1983). Aging process: Implications for clinical practice, *Phys. Ther., 63*, 41.
43. Peterson, D.A., and Orgren, R.A. (1983). Older adult learning. In O. Jackson (Ed.), *Clinics in physical therapy: Physical therapy of the geriatric patient* (pp. 65–81). New York: Churchill Livingstone.
44. Posner, J.D., et al. (1986). Exercise capacity in the elderly. *Am. J. Cardiol., 57*, 52C.
45. Raab, D.M., and Smith, E.L. (1985). Exercise and aging effects on bone. *Top. Geriatr. Rehabil., 1*, 31.
46. Raven, P.B., and Mitchell, J. (1980). The effects of aging on the cardiovascular response to dynamic and static exercise. In M.L. Weisfeldt (Ed.), *The Aging Heart*, (pp. 269–296). New York: Raven Press.
47. Redden, W.G. (1981). Respiratory system and aging. In E.L. Smith, and R.C. Serfass (Eds.), *Exercise and aging: The scientific basis* (pp. 89–108). Hillside, NJ: Enslow Publishers.
48. Rikli, R., and Busch, S. (1986). Motor performance of women as a function of age and physical level. *J. Gerontol. 41*, 645.
49. Robinett, C., and Vondran, M. (1988). Functional ambulation velocity and distance requirements in rural and urban communities. *Phys. Ther. 68*, 1371.
50. Rubenstein, L.Z., and Robbins, A.S. (1984). Falls in the elderly: A clinical perspective, *Geriatrics 39*, 67.
51. Saltin, B., et al. (1968). Response to exercise after bed rest and after training. *Circulation 38* (Suppl. 7), 1.
52. Schoneberger, B. (1981). *Guidelines for physiological monitoring in physical therapy.* Rancho Los Amigos Medical Center, Downey, CA.
53. Seals, D.R., et al. (1984). Endurance training in older men and women I. Cardiovascular response to exercise. *J. Appl. Physiol., 57*, 1024.
54. Shephard, R.J. (1985). The cardiovascular benefits of exercise in the elderly. *Top. Geriatr. Rehabil., 1*, 1.
55. Shock, N.W., (1957). Physiology of aging. *Sci. Am., 206*, 100–116.
56. Spirduso, W.W. (1980). Physical fitness, aging, and psychomotor speed: A review. *J. Gerontol., 35*, 850.
57. Spirduso, W.W., and Clifford, P. (1978). Replication of age and physical activity effects on reaction and movement time. *J Gerontol., 33*, 26.

58. Waters, R.L., et al. (1978). Energetics: Application to the study and management of Locomotor disabilities, *Orthop. Clin. North Am., 9,* 351.
59. Waters, R.L., et al., (1988). Energy expenditure following hip and ankle arthrodesis. *J. Bone Joint Surg. 70,* 1032.
60. Waters, RL, et al. (1982). Energy cost of walking in lower extremity plaster casts. *J. Bone Joint Surg., 64,* 896.
61. Waters, R.L., and Lunsford, B.R. (1985). Energy expenditure of normal and pathologic gait: Application to orthotic prescription. In *Atlas of orthotics* (pp. 151–159). St. Louis: Mosby, 1985.
62. Yerg, J.E., et al. (1985). Effect of endurance exercise training on ventilatory function in older individuals, *J. Appl. Physiol., 58,* 791.
63. Young, A. (1986). Exercise physiology in geriatric practice, *Acta Med. Scand. Suppl., 711,* 227.

CHAPTER 10

Deconditioning
HILARY SIEBENS

One of man's unique attributes is his vertical posture during stance and gait. When upright posture and physical activity cannot be maintained, multiple physiologic changes occur. A person becomes "deconditioned," and less "physically fit." Although these terms are commonly used, defining them is a challenge. Robert Darling pointed out that "fitness has established meaning only in terms of the task to be accomplished."[8] Physical fitness for the weight lifter is not comparable to physical fitness for the master-level marathoner. Achieving fitness through training or conditioning is a very different process for each of these athletes. Likewise, the process of deconditioning is different. Changes will occur in multiple organ systems—the cardiovascular, musculoskeletal, and nervous systems—and to varying degrees. Deconditioning is probably best defined as the multiple changes in organ system physiology that are induced by inactivity and reversed by activity. The type of changes depend on prior fitness level and the degree of superimposed inactivity.

Medical interest in deconditioning developed in the middle of this century. Until then, activity and inactivity were unstudied and unspecific factors in medical treatment. In hospitalized patients, chart orders progressed from B.R. (bed rest) to C. & B. (chair and bed) to U. & A. (up and about) (Mark Altschule, M.D., personal communication, 1988). A series of articles appeared in the *Journal of the American Medical*

Association in 1944 on the "abuses" and the "evil sequelae" of bed rest.[19] The British surgeon Norman Browse wrote *The Physiology and Pathology of Bed Rest* in 1965, one of the first, and still excellent, books on this subject.[3] During the last 25 years the understanding of immobilization has grown, especially through the development of the space program.

Exercise has not been viewed as an important factor in health until recently. Up to the 1950s the rate-of-living theory was in vogue. According to this theory, the body would be worn out faster and life shortened by expending energy during exercise.[18] However, studies in the last 25 years have shown that regular, strenous exercise does not shorten life span.[34] Therefore exercise is increasingly viewed as beneficial for both the primary and secondary prevention of disease.[1]

There are several challenges to understanding the interaction between inactivity and health in older persons. The first is that aging itself causes some changes resembling the consequences of inactivity. However, studies on exercise programs in the elderly have helped separate the consequences of sedentary lifestyle from the aging process itself.[4,5,35,] It is heartening that in fact older persons *can* improve their flexibility, strength, and aerobic capacity as can young people. It now appears that some "aging" effects are the consequences of inactivity. The second challenge in studying inactivity is trying to separate the effects of deconditioning from disease.[2] Many elderly who are deconditioned may have concurrent illnesses. Recent studies, primarily in young subjects, do clarify some of the effects of inactivity alone, that is, bed rest, on human physiology and functional performance.

A third challenge is understanding the relationship between physiologic decline and functional loss. Is the inability to climb stairs in an 87-year-old primarily from cardiovascular deconditioning, hip extensor and guadriceps weakness, or impaired balance secondary to a sedentary lifestyle? Is this the beginning of a new disease process? Is this normal aging? An important concept is that "threshold" values of physiologic function may exist.[39] Below these thresholds someone may suddenly lose an essential functional skill.

An understanding of the consequences of deconditioning will be obtained as more is learned about how physical activity and inactivity affect the healthy, and diseased, older person. Many themes and data address the deconditioning process. This review covers a select few that pertain especially to rehabilitation of the elderly.

PHYSIOLOGY OF INACTIVITY

Deconditioning can result from many different levels of inactivity. For the sake of simplicity and clarity, two clinically important categories of inactivity are discussed in this chapter. The first is acute inactivity such as bed rest. The second is chronic inactivity: a sedentary lifestyle lacking routine aerobic exercise. Each of these types of inactivity is discussed in reference to the various functions affected.

NEUROLOGIC FUNCTION

Deconditioning of the nervous system has not been evaluated as intensely as other organ systems. This may be related to the complexity of the nervous system and the crudeness of assessment techniques. In younger persons any changes that occur are relatively slight. In the elderly, however, especially with concurrent illness, the consequences of inactivity may be particularly dangerous.[25]

Bed Rest

Bed rest has been compared to the experience of sensory deprivation. In a study of extreme immobilization with subjects unable to move during the day, followed by bed rest at night, occipital lobe frequencies on EEG were substantially decreased in awake subjects.[41] These changes also occur in sensory deprivation studies. Exercise prevented some of these changes.[40] Performance on several intellectual tests deteriorated including verbal fluency, color discrimination, and reversible figures. In another sensory deprivation study, young subjects lay on a bed in an experimental hospital setting.[12] Tapes played periodically simulated the effects of brief, disjointed conversations. The subjects' perception of time intervals became distorted during the brief 3-hour test. In addition, several subjects described hallucinatorylike experiences. Social isolation also made the subjects uncomfortable. Frequent complaints included feeling lonely and longing for some sign of recognition from the investigator. It is rather dramatic that these feelings occurred in perfectly healthy young people during only 3 hours of bed rest.

Other emotions occur during prolonged bed rest in healthy young subjects such as anxiety, irritability, and a depressed mood.[11,32] Reactions were more intense in subjects who were not allowed to exercise compared with those allowed to perform moderate work on a total body ergometer, in bed, 3 times a day.[32]

Bed rest also affects the EEG pattern of sleep. In subjects on bed rest a larger portion of sleep is spent in deep, stages 3 and 4 slow-wave sleep.[31] This is even more pronounced in subjects who are not permitted light supine exercise. Rapid eye movement (REM) sleep periods increase as well. A clinical correlate may have been the increased mental lethargy that was observed during the day. Interestingly, in fit subjects, the onset of stage 3, deep slow wave sleep is sooner, and stage 3 longer, than in unfit subjects.[15] The clinical implications of these findings are not yet clear but may be important in the elderly.

Thermoregulation is also altered by bed rest.[14] Oral and skin temperatures decline in young persons. These may be of greater clinical importance in the elderly who already have decreased thermoregulatory responses.

Several nervous system changes occur which directly affect motor performance. Significant balance decrements occur after 2 to 3 weeks of bed rest.[16,38] Muscle strengthening during bed rest did not prevent this deterioration. Recovery occurred in 3 to 5 days. Permitting visual cues by keeping the eyes open improved the relearning rate and overall performance scores. Central brain processing, as tested by coordination, can decline after bed rest.[38] Pattern tracing skill tests coordination. The frequency and duration of stylus marks that are incorrect during a trial of pattern tracing are measured. Performance on this test deteriorated 10 percent after 3 weeks of bed rest and resolved within 4 days of resumed activity.

Chronic Inactivity

The neuropsychologic consequences of a chronic level of inactivity, as in a sedentary lifestyle, are not easy to determine. The Greeks of course advocated that a sound body was necessary for the presence of a sound mind. Shephard in reviewing the literature suggests that physical activity of moderate intensity makes a person feel better, leading to better intellectual and psychomotor development.[36] Mechanisms may include increased arousal, improved self-esteem and body image, as well as decreased anxiety, stress, and depression.

Balance function is affected by chronic inactivity. Postural sway is known to increase with aging. Inactivity may contribute an additional increase in sway. Balance was better in active compared to inactive elderly women.[29] Results were similar in both moderately active women who played golf and more active women who 3 times a week exercised for at least 30 minutes hard enough to perspire. In another study, a 12-week training program improved standing balance on one foot.[13]

A sedentary lifestyle is also associated with prolonged reaction times.[5,29,37] When comparing active young versus older persons, 8 percent of decrements in reaction and movement times were from age alone whereas a 22 percent decrement was present when nonactive young and old groups were compared. Spirduso has proposed that exercise prevents the cycle in which disuse decreases brain metabolism leading to decreased blood flow and neuronal loss.[37]

Inactivity, then, has several effects on the nervous system. Acutely, during bed rest, some cognitive changes can occur including distortion of time perception and decrements in some intellectual tests. Mood changes occur as well. Consequences on cognitive and emotional function of chronic inactivity may include a better sense of well-being. Balance is impaired after both acute and more chronic inactivity whereas prolonged reaction times are associated thus far only with chronic inactivity.

CARDIOVASCULAR FUNCTION

Alterations in cardiovascular function are the hallmark of deconditioning. The well-conditioned individual responds to submaximal work without significant rise in pulse and blood pressure. In contrast, the deconditioned individual faced with a slight to moderate workload experiences a marked increase in vital signs. Maximal workloads elicit similar increases in blood pressure and pulse rate in both trained and untrained individuals. However, the return of blood pressure and pulse rate to resting values, the recovery rate, is much slower in deconditioned persons.

Bed Rest

The most fundamental change with bed rest is an increase in resting heart rate starting by the end of the first week.[11,33,38] Even though the body remains at rest, the work of the heart is increased as indicated by a higher heart rate. By the end of 3 weeks morning heart rate can increase by 21 percent and evening heart rate by 33 percent, averaging one beat per 2 days of bed rest.[38] Other investigators have documented lesser increases in resting heart rate, about four beats per minute.[33] Six weeks of exercise were required before resting heart rate returned to baseline.[11]

While resting heart rate increases with bed rest, total blood volume decreases 5 to 6 percent after several weeks of bed rest.[11,26,33,38] Plasma volume decrements are usually greater than red cell mass decrements. Such a change could have significant import for older persons. The mechanism behind the loss in red cell mass is unclear. The reductions in blood volume do not correlate with the development of orthostatic hypotension in young subjects but further study is needed to see if the elderly are similarly spared this change.[26]

Orthostatic hypotension occurs as soon as 1 week in young subjects.[11,26,33,38] This, and other cardiovascular signs of deconditioning, also occur after 1 week of chair rest.[21] Orthostasis resolves slowly, over weeks, even when the recovery period includes heavy exercise.[11,33,38]

Besides the deterioration of the cardiovascular system at rest, any level of work becomes more strenuous. At submaximal exercise levels, heart rates increase 10 to 20 percent and stroke volumes decrease.[33] Delayed recovery rates also indicate an increased cardiac and metabolic stress. In healthy subjects, at submaximal workloads, the pulse rate return to baseline in less than 2 minutes and the systolic blood pressure returns in 4 minutes or less. After 6 weeks bed rest, 3 to 6 minutes were required for the pulse rate and 5 to 7 minutes for the systolic blood pressure to return to baseline.[11]

In deconditioned individuals, maximal oxygen uptake decreases 15 to 30 percent at maximal work rates.[9,33] Closely related to the decrement in maximum oxygen uptake are reduced stroke volume and cardiac output in the face of an unchanged maximal heart rate. The recovery of these impaired responses to submaximal and maximal exercise is slow. Moderate training programs lasting 4 to 6 weeks are needed to reverse only 3 weeks of bed rest.[11,33,38]

In one of the few studies of older men, mean age 50 years, maximal oxygen uptake decreased 15 percent during upright testing after 10 days of bed rest.[9] Oxygen uptake at submaximal upright workloads was approximately 10 percent less after bed rest despite a higher heart rate. These peak oxygen uptakes returned to baseline by 30 days, the first time that subjects were retested. Interestingly, recovery rate was similar for subjects who returned to their usual activities as well as for those who participated in an aerobic exercise program.

The cardiovascular system changes markedly during bed rest. The alterations are noted even without activity by an increase in resting heart rate. Merely standing can be accompanied by orthostasis. Any stress on the heart, as in exercise, elicits a higher heart rate and a decreased stroke volume. These factors contribute to the overall decrease in maximal oxygen uptake.

Chronic Inactivity

The cardiovascular consequences of chronic inactivity are similar to the changes noted after acute bed rest. Resting heart rates are higher. At submaximal workloads, heart rates and blood pressure are higher than in physically fit individuals performing the same workload. Maximal oxygen uptake is lower than in individuals who exercise aerobically. The well-documented decline of maximal oxygen uptake with age is half as great in physically active people as compared with sedentary persons.

The recovery rate of vital signs is prolonged. Unfortunately, this easily followed parameter has not been routinely reported in recent studies of physical fitness and exercise programs in the elderly.

RESPIRATORY FUNCTION

Bed rest has a relatively small effect on pulmonary function in healthy subjects.[11,33] Chronic inactivity may cause some reversible decrement in vital capacity, and exercise training may lead to more efficient respiratory mechancis.[35]

MUSCLE FUNCTION

Skeletal muscle constitutes the largest organ system by mass in the body. More than any other organ system is physiologic capabilities are closely tied to levels of activity.

Bed Rest

Bed rest imposes inactivity nonuniformly in muscle groups. Functionally, neck extensors and the antigravity muscles of the legs are exercised the least. Arm, back, and abdominal muscles may be used considerably during positional changes and basic care activities. During several weeks of bed rest in young men, grip, abdominal, and back muscle strength did not change.[11,38] Arm flexors and shoulder muscle strength decreased 6 percent. Tibialis anterior strength decreased 13 percent and gastrocsoleum strength 20 percent. Muller reported a loss of strength of 1.0 to 1.5 percent per day during 2 weeks of bed rest in a young man.[28] The exact muscles were not mentioned. The amount of strength lost by the elderly during bed rest is unknown.

Chronic Inactivity

The twentieth-century lifestyle requires less physical exertion which precludes routine maintenance of muscle strength. In young persons, maintaining muscle strength requires only one submaximal contraction of 10 seconds' duration at 20 percent of the muscle's initial strength.[28] The amount of exercise required to maintain strength in older persons needs to be determined.

The 33 percent decrement in strength with aging is at least partially due to inactivity. Training programs increase strength.[35] From the response to strengthening in the elderly, part of the weakness with inactivity is from a less efficient recruitment of motor units.[27] Aging as well is associated with a loss in the number of muscle fibers, a phenomenon not seen with deconditioning alone.[35] There is a loss of motor neurons while peripheral metabolic pathways are preserved in the muscle.

CONNECTIVE TISSUE AND JOINT FUNCTION

Extremes of immobilization clearly lead to a decreased range of motion secondary to connective tissue changes. There is no evidence yet that bed rest per se in healthy subjects leads to clinically relevant changes in flexibility which in turn would lead to decreased fitness. The chronic inactivity of a sedentary lifestyle may have an effect. Some decrements in flexibility are reversed by exercise programs.[35] Interestingly, flexibility was similar in one study comparing moderately active and extremely active women.[29] Maintaining good flexibility may be possible through a mild, reasonable exercise program.

BOWEL AND BLADDER FUNCTION

Lack of fitness or deconditioning per se do not appear to directly impair defecation or urination. None of the studies of bed rest in young subjects reported on bowel or bladder dysfunction. Bedpans were used in some of these studies. Bed rest may affect older people more. Browse points out that in the physiologic position for defecation, squatting, the perineal musculature must relax while the intraabdominal pressure is raised. The lack of privacy and the awkward position on a bedpan may preclude relaxation of the perineal muscles for defecation. This could start the cycle of suppressed urge followed by progressive accumulation of feces in the rectum.

While acute bed rest may lead directly to constipation, the effect of chronic inactivity is less clear. In constipation, it is difficult to sort out effects solely related to decreased physical activity from dietary and functional problems. Bladder function, as affected by chronic inactivity, has yet to be evaluated.

METABOLIC FUNCTION

Bed Rest

The major metabolic changes with bed rest include increased excretion of calcium starting on day 2 of bed rest and peaking in the fourth week of a 6-week bed rest period.[11] Calcium losses stabilize by the fifth week of recovery. Negative nitrogen balance can start by the fifth day of bed rest. The protein degradation, occurring primarily in muscle, is equivalent to 1.7 kg muscle mass over 6 weeks of bed rest. During the recovery phase, losses stop by the second week, gains are above control, and then subsequently return to control values by 6 weeks. Accelerated loss of calcium has important implications with regard to the high incidence of osteoporosis in older females.

Chronic Inactivity

Aging is associated with loss of lean body mass and a gain in body fat.[5,35] Some of these changes are related to inactivity. Active elderly show lesser degrees of these changes, and exercise programs in sedentary elderly persons can modify them.

TREATMENT APPROACHES TO THE DECONDITIONED PATIENT

Deconditioned persons perform less physical work than they could if they were physically fit. For example, the self-selected walking speed in the elderly is related to fitness level.[17] Since maximum aerobic capacity is decreased, walking speed is adjusted to comfort levels. Improved fitness can lead to faster walking speeds. When disease and physical disability are added, the consequences could be disastrous. The quadriceps strength in a deconditioned 80-year-old women is poor, yet she can toilet herself without adaptive equipment. If she develops an acute exacerbation of osteoarthritis with acute knee pain, it may reflexly inhibit quadriceps strength even more. The patient may then suddenly be unable to toilet herself in her bathroom, threatening her independent living.

Intuitively it would appear plausible that an elderly person who is more physically fit will experience less functional decline. While this hypothesis has yet to be established, encouraging physical fitness in the elderly seems appropriate. The risks are small and generally preventable.[10,22,35] The cardiac risks are minimized by obtaining a careful history and performing a complete physical examination. An exercise program that is not overly stressful is also needed. The more common problem of musculoskeletal injuries is avoided by proper stretching and warm-up calisthenics.

FATIGUE

Understanding and correctly managing patients' sensation of fatigue is essential in any exercise treatment program. Fatigue, a word understood by every layman, lacks precise definition. Darling likens the concept of fatigue to the concept of pain.[7] Both must be considered from physiologic and psychologic points of view. Physiologic types of fatigue include "muscle" fatigue from prolonged use of a local muscle group, "circulatory" fatigue associated with elevated blood lactate levels during prolonged work above 50 percent of maximum aerobic capacity, and "metabolic" fatigue in exercise which depletes glycogen stores. General fatigue, which is related to subtle factors like interest, reward, and motivation, might be viewed as opposite to arousal.

Given these definitions, it is easy to understand why a deconditioned person can experience fatigue. From a treatment perspective it is essential to determine what sensation the patient is describing as fatigue. Elevated vital signs and progressively weak muscle contractions suggest that rest is needed. A vaguer complaint of fatigue in the absence of these changes would not necessarily be a basis for reducing exercise. In fact, poor aerobic fitness may be related to an otherwise healthy patient's complaint of fatigue.[20]

TREATMENT OF ACUTE DECONDITIONING

The acute deconditioning that results from bed rest should be prevented at any cost. Patients should be out of bed, except for nighttime sleep, as much as possible. Sitting in and of itself is an exercise for frail patients. Patients should have appropriate footwear as well as sufficiently warm clothing available to help keep them comfortable when out of bed.

Assessment

Assessment for the presence and degree of deconditioning is not routine in most hospitals. It is relatively straightforward unless major cardiopulmonary disease or physical disability are present. An elevated resting heart rate, above around 84 beats per minute, is the first indication of a deconditioned cardiovascular status unless other explanations are possible, that is, fever, anemia, anxiety, dehydration, arrhythmias, or hyperthyroidism. The presence of orthostasis likewise indicates deconditioning unless medications, low blood volume, or a disease of the autonomic nervous system are present. To these static measurements is added the heart rate response to a physical examination. The examination includes a manual muscle test, and observation of bed mobility, transfers, and gait. Significant deconditioning is present if the physical examination elicits an increase of greater than 10 to 20 beats above a nonelevated resting heart rate. A practical point of comparison is that the heart rate during normal gait was 89 in a group of 246 elderly men and women with a mean age around 72.[17] Finally, a physical therapist's observations are invaluable in helping a physician assess physical fitness. Symptoms, endurance, and vital sign responses during therapy are easily noted by the therapist and help identify the degree of deconditioning.

Treatment

For the patient who must be kept at bed rest, the reverse Trendelenburg position of the bed at night may help decrease the amount of orthostatic hypotension that will develop.[23] The role of this maneuver merits further research.

Treatment of acute deconditioning starts with stretching exercises to improve any deficits in range of motion and to help improve body awareness. This is important for external shoulder rotation, hip extension, knee extension, and ankle dorsiflexion—the motions most likely to become limited from disuse during bed rest. Initial stretching can be supervised by the nursing staff, trained family, or a physical therapist. The patients can perform these exercises independently as soon as possible.

The next step is establishing adequate sitting tolerance by increasing the frequency and duration of sitting. If orthostatic hypotension is a problem, the traditional treatments usually work—elastic hose, elevated head of bed at night (with the whole bed tilted, not just the top half), and progressive mobility training. Strengthening exercises are the next step followed by ambulation with or without an assistive device.

For the severely deconditioned patient, early mobilization should be done by a physical therapist who monitors the patient's symptoms and vital signs. A practical guide for target heart rate is 20 beats above the resting heart rate if the latter is not excessively elevated. If the patient tolerates this over 1 to 2 days, the target could be increased to resting plus 30 (Keith Robinson, M.D., personal communication, 1988). These guidelines have not been rigorously studied but appear to work well clinically. Guidelines for ambulation frequency likewise do not yet exist but ambulation to mild fatigue 3 times a day seems reasonable. If deconditioning is the main limitation to exercise tolerance, patients should improve initially almost daily. If muscles are extremely weak, these may delay progress initially until strength is sufficient to ambulate. If progress stops before the patient reaches his pre–bed test tolerance level, evaluation for medical, neurologic, or orthopedic problems could be indicated. A rule of thumb is that reconditioning can take up to twice as long as the period of deconditioning in the absence of additional major debility from an acute illness. This guideline can serve as a general rule but clearly needs more rigorous evaluation to assess its accuracy.

Prevention of deconditioning can be hard in patients with acute illnesses. A guideline can be that, unless there is reason to expect medical problems, a gradual exercise program can be tried once the patient has stable resting vital signs.

It can be difficult to know when a deconditioned patient is ready for discharge from the acute hospital. If the patient is to live alone, a practical guideline suggests that a patient can leave when ambulation is independent. When a caregiver is available, whether in the home setting or in an alternate care setting, the patient may leave when ambulation with a stand-by assistance by a caregiver is accomplished. In the home setting, the patient should be ambulating 3 times daily to the point of mild fatigue. At the same time the home program must include basic stretching and strengthening exercises.

TREATMENT OF CHRONICALLY DECONDITIONED ELDERLY

Assessment

Assessment of deconditioning in chronically inactive persons is the same as in acutely deconditioned persons. The clinical exercise test may need to be more extensive, including stair climbing and walking for longer distances. In more formal testing, simple submaximal tests like the 12-minute and 1-mile walk tests are available.[22,30,35]

Treatment

Numerous reviews and Chapter 9 in this book discuss training programs for the able-bodied elderly.[6,22,30,35] Several key points merit emphasis. The physician-patient relationship should be a close one if an exercise program is to be successful.[10] Patients need careful screening and follow-up to establish an appropriate exercise program and to prevent complications. For the patient to make exercise routine and part of a lifestyle change, the program definitely needs to be convenient, varied, fun, and not overly strenuous.

There is considerable debate on target heart rates in older persons to achieve cardiovascular training effects. Relatively low levels of exercise, including walking, can be sufficient.[22,30,35] Walking therefore should be encouraged. This idea is not new or original. The first volume of *The Journal of Health* advocated the same concept in 1830.

Patients may still benefit from a simple exercise program, prescribed and followed by a physician during routine office visits, even if aerobic capacity does not change.[24] Patients are instructed to exercise only to the point of slight effort and to never feel overloaded or distressed. They perform stretching and strengthening exercises and walking or a jog-walk combination. These programs may help with other aspects of fitness, like flexibility, balance, arousal, and the self-confidence to remain independent. At the very least, low-level exercise programs are not harmful and may be the only level of exercise a sedentary person will accept. As older sedentary adults become more aware of physical limitations, they may be more willing to start slow, comfortable exercise.

DECONDITIONING IN PHYSICALLY CHALLENGED OLDER ADULTS

Compared to the able-bodied population, older persons who are physically challenged from impairments like stroke, amputation, and spinal cord injury are at even greater risk of becoming, and remaining, deconditioned. Fortunately, research is evaluating methods of testing, and training, elderly persons who cannot walk. In the next 10 years appropriate exercise regimens will undoubtedly be developed.

CONCLUSION

Acute loss of physical fitness is an immediate threat to any elderly person who becomes ill. The deconditioned state is easily diagnosed from a careful bedside examination and treatment can be straightforward. Untreated acute deconditioning is a very likely source of treatable functional loss in adults.

A chronic state of poor physical fitness may well be a major threat to the health and functional independence of the elderly, especially those over 75. In the next 10 years, improved exercise therapy for the acutely and chronically deconditioned elderly may well be the most simple, safe, and beneficial intervention in health care of the older population.

REFERENCES

1. Astrand, P.O. (1987). Exercise physiology and its role in disease prevention and in rehabilitation. *Arch. Phys. Med. Rehabil., 68,* 305.

2. Bortz, W.B. (1982). Disuse and aging. *JAMA, 248,* 1203.
3. Browse, N. (1965). *The physiology and pathology of bed rest.* Springfield, IL: Thomas.
4. Bruce, R.A. (1984). Exercise, functional aerobic capacity, and aging—another viewpoint. *Med. Sci. Sports Exerc., 16,* 8.
5. Buskirk, E.R. (1985). Health maintenance and longevity; exercise. In C.E. Finch and E.L. Schneider (Eds.), *Handbook on the biology of aging* (pp. 894–931). New York: Academic Press.
6. Clark, B.A. (1985). Principles of physical activity programming for the older adult. *Top. Geriatr. Rehabil., 1,* 68.
7. Darling, R.C. (1971). Fatigue. In J.A. Downey and R.C. Darling (Eds.), *Physiological basis of rehabilitation medicine* (pp. 199–208). Philadelphia; Saunders.
8. Darling, R.C. (1947). The significance of physical fitness. *Arch. Phys. Med., 40,* 140.
9. DeBusk, R.D., et al. (1983). Exercise conditioning in middle-aged men after 10 days of bed rest. *Circulation, 68,* 245.
10. DeVries, H.A. (1971). Prescription of exercise for older men from telemetered exercise heart rate data. *Geriatrics, 26,* 102.
11. Dietrick, J.E., Whedon, G.D., and Shorr, E. (1948). Effects of immobilization upon various metabolic and physiologic functions of normal men. *Am. J. Med., 4,* 3.
12. Downs, F. (1974). Bed rest and sensory disturbances. *Am. J. Nurs., 74,* 434.
13. Emes, C.G. (1979). The effects of a regular program of light exercise on seniors. *J. Sports Med., 19,* 185.
14. Greenleaf, J.E., and Reese, R.D. (1980). Exercise thermoregulation after 14 days of bed rest. *J. Appl. Physiol., 48,* 72.
15. Griffin, S.J., and Trinder, J. (1978). Physical fitness, exercise, and human sleep. *Psychophysiology, 15,* 447.
16. Haines, R.F. (1974). Effect of bed rest and exercise on body balance. *J. Appl. Physiol., 36,* 323.
17. Himann, J.E., et al. (1988). Age-related changes in speed of walking. *Med. Sci. Sports Exerc., 20,* 161.
18. Holloszy, J.O. (1983). Exercise, health, and aging: a need for more information. *Med. Sci. Sports Exerc., 15,* 1.
19. *JAMA* (1944). *125,* 1075.
20. Kohl, H.W., Moorefield, D.L., and Blair, S.N. (1987). Is cardiorespiratory fitness associated with general chronic fatigue in apparently healthy men and women? *Med. Sci. Sports Exerc., 19,* (S6).
21. Lamb, L.E., Stevens, P.M., and Johnson, R.L. (1965). Hypokinesia secondary to chair rest from 4 to 10 days. *Aerospace Med., 36,* 755.
22. Larson, E.B., and Bruce, R.A. (1987). Health benefits of exercise in an aging society. *Arch. Intern. Med., 147,* 353.
23. MacLean, A.R., and Allen, E.V. (1988). Orthostatic hypotension and orthostatic tachycardia. *JAMA, 259,* 2720.
24. Millar, A.P. (1987). Realistic exercise goals for the elderly; Is feeling good enough? *Geriatrics, 42,* 25.
25. Miller, M.B. (1975). Iatrogenic and nursigenic effects of prolonged immobilization of the ill aged. *J. Am. Geriatr. Soc., 33,* 360.
26. Miller, P.B., Johnson, R.L., and Lamb, L.E. (1964). Effects of four weeks of absolute bed rest on circulatory functions in man. *Aerospace Med., 35,* 1194.

27. Moritani, T., and deVries, H.A. (1980). Potential for gross muscle hypertrophy in older men. *J. Gerontol., 35*, 672.
28. Muller, E.A. (1970). Influence of training and of inactivity on muscle strength. *Arch. Phys. Med. Rehabil., 51*, 449.
29. Rikli, R., and Busch, S. (1986). Motor performance of women as a function of age and physical activity level. *J. Gerontol., 41*, 645.
30. Rippe, J.M., et al. (1988). Walking for health and fitness. *JAMA, 259*, 2720.
31. Ryback, R.S., Lewis, O.F., and Lessard, C.S. (1971). Psychobiologic effects of prolonged bed rest (weightless) in young, healthy volunteers (study II). *Aerospace Med., 42*, 529.
32. Ryback, R.S., et al. (1971). Psychobiologic effects of prolonged weightlessness (bed rest) in young healthy volunteers. *Aerospace Med., 42*, 408.
33. Saltin, B., et al. (1968). Response to exercise after bed rest and after training. *Circulation 38* (Suppl. 7), 1.
34. Schneider, E.L., and Reed, J.D. (1985). Modulations of aging processes. In C.E. Finch and E.L. Schneider (Eds.), *Handbook on the biology of aging* (pp. 51–53). New York; Academic Press.
35. Shepard, R.J. (1978). *Physical activity and aging.* Chicago, Year Book.
36. Shephard, R.J. (1983). Physical activity and the healthy mind. *Can. Med. Assoc. J., 128*, 525.
37. Spirduso, W.W. (1980). Physical fitness, aging, and psychomotor speed: a review. *J. Geromtol., 35*, 850.
38. Taylor, H.L., Henschel, J.B., and Keys, A. (1949). Effects of bed rest on cardiovascular function and work performance. *J. Appl. Physiol., 2*, 223.
39. Young, A. (1986). Exercise physiology in geriatric practice. *Acta Med. Scand. Suppl. 711*, 227.
40. Zubek, J.P. (1963). Counteracting effects of physical exercise performed during prolonged perceptual deprivation. *Science, 142*, 504.
41. Zubek, J.P., and Wilgosh, L. (1963). Prolonged immobilization of the body: changes in performance and in the electroencephalogram. *Science, 140*, 306.

CHAPTER 11

Falls and Instability in the Older Person

KENNETH BRUMMEL-SMITH

Falls are frequently reported by older persons. Even when falls do not lead to injury the person may develop such a fear of falling that his or her mobility or continued independent living may be endangered. With injury the person may suffer serious primary or secondary complications. The rehabilitative approach, which emphasizes function, is an ideal method for addressing the problems of the person that falls. This chapter discusses the epidemiology of falls, the complications commonly encountered, the reasons for the high rate of falling among the older population, and the various causes of falling. Finally, an approach to the workup and intervention of falls is presented.

EPIDEMIOLOGY OF FALLS

Accidents are the fifth leading cause of death in the older population. Falls make up the largest percentage of accidents in this age group. While young children may fall more frequently than old people, the injury rate, particularly for serious injuries, is higher among the elderly. The "old-old," those aged 75 years and more, have the highest rate of both falls and fall-related injuries. For the purposes of this discussion, all references, unless stated otherwise, refer to the older population.

For those persons living at home it is thought that the rate of falls is approximately 0.5 fall per year.[35] However, the rate may actually be higher due to unreported episodes that are forgotten.[10] There appears to be about a 5 percent injury rate and about 1 in 40 will be hospitalized as a consequence of falling.[7] Of those hospitalized many will not be alive 1 year later.

Nursing home residents have an even higher rate of falling. The average rate of falling is about two falls per year.[37] The rate may be higher due to the high rate of disability found in institutionalized elderly or the fact that such incidents are more accurately reported. From 10 to 25 percent of such falls are associated with significant injury.[17] For those over age 85, one out of every five fatal falls occurs in the nursing home.[3] In one study, 2.4 percent of falls resulted in hip or other fractures.[2] It is clear that falls are a major risk to the patient living in a long-term care institution.

The acute hospital is also a site of frequent falls. Patients there experience about 1.5 falls per person per year. Many of these may be related to medication effects or the result of the illness for which they were admitted. Frequent falls in the acute hospital may lead to a cascade of disasters that ultimately ends with the patient being admitted to a long-term care institution from the acute hospital. Hence, the prevalence of falls is high regardless of the living situation of the older person. The risk of such falls is similarly high.

CONSEQUENCES OF FALLS

Unfortunately, the person that presents with an adverse consequence of a fall may have been falling for some time. The fall for which he or she is being treated may be only the last in a series of falls. Therefore, the potential for adverse consequences is high and should be conceptualized in terms of a holistic approach.

Medical consequences are the most obvious ones. Fractures of the hip, forearm, ribs, or vertebral column affect about 5 to 10 percent of fallers. Hematomas and lacerations are common due to age-related changes in skin, collagen, and elastic fibers or underlying disease. Medical consequences are often the reason for hospital admission which then may expose the person to further iatrogenic complications.

The person may also experience profound psychologic consequences of falls. Most studies that have looked at psychologic associations with falls have attempted to show the relationship of the person's psychologic state and the risk of falls. Few investigators have analyzed the psychologic reactions to having fallen. The fear of falling is commonly reported by the elderly. Such fear may lead to a decreased sense of self-confidence. Depression is frequently seen in functionally disabled persons though the evidence that depression itself causes falls is weak.[4] Attention problems associated with anxiety are also seen following falls.

It is in the area of social functioning that falls may take their greatest toll. Increasing dependency is also one of the most common fears of older persons. Social withdrawal, with its attendant risks of poor nutrition and physical functioning, may develop following falls. The person's ability to live safely in the home may be questioned by the family or discharge planners, paving the way to long-term care institutionalization. The person may be admitted to an acute hospital for the diagnostic evaluation where the risk of falling may be actually higher.

The final common pathway to negative consequences is in the realm of functional losses. As a result of immobility from the complications of a fall the person may develop serious problems such as skin breakdown, pneumonia, and deep venous thrombosis. Even without immobility the person may restrict his or her activity leading to losses in strength, joint mobility, and reflexes. These changes initiate a vicious spiral whereby the person's compensatory reactions to a noninjurious fall increase the risk of a later, more serious fall.

PREDISPOSITION TO FALLS

Because of the many normal changes of age the older person is particularly disposed to falling. Although it is difficult to distinguish clearly between those changes that are specifically due to aging and those that are strongly associated with age, the changes noted below are commonly encountered in aged rehabilitation patients.

Sensory changes occur frequently in older persons. Vision plays a major role in maintaining stability both at stance and while undergoing movement. Aging-associated decreases in visual acuity, visual fields, depth perception, and glare tolerance have been reported.[15] Contrast sensitivity, the ability to distinguish differences in brightness, decreases with age.[9] Vestibular function, especially in response to sudden movement, may also decline with age.[40] Proprioception likewise decreases with age. Large increases in postural sway occur when ankle proprioception was experimentally eliminated.[46] Changes in touch and vibration have also been reported but their relationship to falls is unknown. Similarly, though nerve conduction velocity decreases with age it is unknown whether this is the major factor associated with the observed decrease in older persons' ability to "right" themselves after losing balance.

Musculoskeletal changes are frequently found in the elderly. A general decrease in muscle strength and muscle contraction rate are found.[45]

More important than the isolated changes noted above is the fact that the visual, neurosensory, and musculoskeletal systems must work in perfect concert in order to maintain balance or respond to falling episodes. Postural sway is the result of such an integrative process. Sway has been shown to increase with age.[39] Increased sway is associated with a lower "mobility index" and a greater risk of falling.[19] Increased sway is more commonly seen in women.[16] Thus, proper balance requires a complex interaction among multiple organ systems ina dynamic fashion. The integration required to effect this working relationship is extremely complex. Even small perturbations in sensation, processing, or reaction may have significant effects and lead to a fall.

Gait changes also affect the older person. Like balance, gait requires a complex interaction among multiple organ systems. Walking is basically controlled falling. As males age they tend to develop a flexed posture, the gait develops a wider base, and the step length decreases. These changes can take on the appearance of a parkinsonian posture. Elderly females are found to have a narrower-based gait that appears more waddling, also with short steps. Both genders are seen to have shorter steps, decreased velocity, decreased height of foot pickup, and a decreased arm swing. Furthermore, more irregular steps are seen.[23] Gait velocity plays an important role in maintaining stability. The highest rate of falls is found in those patients with intermediate velocities (50–60% of normal). High gait velocity and very low velocities are both associated with fewer falls. Many older persons, even without a primary gait problem, may have low velocity due to underlying cardiac or pulmonary diseases.[8]

Finally, there are a host of common conditions found in the elderly that may increase the predisposition to falling though not actually cause the fall itself. Neurologic disorders such as neuropathy, stroke, or Parkinson's disease influence gait and accommodation mechanisms. Cardiac conditions such as chronic congestive heart failure and exercise-induced angina may limit mobility and affect righting reflexes. Underlying arthritis or prior fractures may limit joint mobility. Dementia may reduce attention to the environment. Generalized deconditioning, particularly after a long illness or hospitalization, may also increase the chances of a fall.

ACCIDENTAL FALLS

Accidents and environmentally related falls are the most common types of falls. A review of the available literature reveals that almost 37 percent of all falls are due to accidents.[37] However, accidents usually occur in the presence of underlying conditions that increase the chance that an "accident" will occur. The main associations between accidents and underlying conditions are pathologic gait problems (such as Parkinson's disease or arthritis) and visual-motor inattention, such as that seen in persons with depression, dementia, or drug usage.

Environmental hazards are frequently found in the homes of older persons. Hazards may promote falling through a variety of mechanisms. In the older person with decreased visual acuity, poor lighting may promote falling over objects on the floor while structurally unsound steps may provoke a fall in anyone. Loose throw rugs or area rugs may contribute to tripping in the person with decreased toe clearance. Even shag-type carpeting may enhance the risk of a fall in the Parkinson's patient. Falls often occur during normal periods of being in transition of position, for instance, when arising from the toilet or bed. This occurrence is particularly true when there is underlying hip weakness or truncal instability. A person's self-designed compensatory adaptations may actually increase falling. For instance, the person that consistently reaches for objects for stability when walking may fall while leaning to grab the side of the table.

Over 85 percent of all deaths due to stair accidents occur in the elderly. The use of stairs by older persons has recently received attention.[1] Seventy-five percent of stair accidents occur while descending the stairs and most are in the second half of the flight. By using videotaped observations of 32,000 stair users Archea was able to describe the process by which humans use stairs.[1] He found there are two tests that a person uses when preparing to descend stairs: the visual test and the kinesthetic test. The visual test occurs first and allows the person to make judgments about the support railing, size and length of the steps, and any unusual features. Following the visual test the person carefully steps down to corroborate kinesthetically the information gained from the visual test. Kinesthetic testing diminishes with each successive tread. In effect, if in the first few steps the information gleaned from the two tests is concordant, the person goes on "automatic pilot" for the bottom half of the stairs. Hence, stair accidents may occur when there is a poor or misinterpreted visual test, a disorder in the senses that perform the kinesthetic test, or when an unforeseen complication (a loose board) develops.

From the prior discussion it is clear that simply ascribing the cause of a person's fall to an "accident" does a great disservice to the patient. Rather, the interface between each patient and his or her environment should be investigated.

FALLS WITHOUT SYNCOPE

Nonaccidental falls that are not associated with syncope account for probably 20 to 25 percent of falls in the elderly. Drop attacks, the sudden loss of strength in the legs, were frequently reported in the older literature to cause falls.[38] However, in more recent reports they appear to be the cause of falls in only about 10 percent of cases.[37] There is controversy as to the existence of a drop attack as a true clinical entity at all. The person experiencing a drop attack usually describes falling without warning or any apparent cause and no associated changes in consciousness. Once on the floor the person can sometimes "reactivate" weak legs by pressing his or her feet against the wall or floor. The cause of this condition is unknown but it is presumed to be related to a paroxysmal decrease in blood flow to the midbrain or reticular activity system.

Orthostatic hypotension frequently affects the older person, with as many as 30 percent of the population being affected.[5] The risk of developing orthostatic changes (a fall of 20 mm Hg systolic or 10 mm Hg diastolic blood pressure when standing up) rises with hypertensive states and advancing age. With underlying cerebral insufficiency such a drop in blood pressure may be enough to induce a fall with syncope. Even without syncope the patient may lose his or her balance. Particularly prone to this condition are those with neuropathy or diabetes, hypertension, Parkinson's dehydration, and users of certain drugs. Excessive use of alcohol may also play a role in developing hypotension.

There is a growing body of literature documenting the relationship of the use of various drugs to falls. Long-acting sedative-hypnotics and barbiturates appear to be the greatest offenders.[36] Other psychotropic drugs such as antidepressants and antipsychotics may promote falling through their sedative, anticholinergic, or extrapyramidal side effects.[11] Antihypertensives may cause orthostatic changes,[28] while other cardiac drugs, such as calcium channel blockers and nitrates, may reduce blood pressure in normotensive persons. Antiparkinsonian medications may also cause hypotension. Finally, digoxin may increase carotid sinus responses as can methyldopa and beta blockers.[25] Hence, the list of potential drugs contributing to a falling episode is long and the medication regimen must be carefully evaluated. In addition, the method by which the drugs are used should also be analyzed. Certain drugs, particularly those with rapid onset of action, may be more likely to cause symptomatic problems. Dosage schedules and drug combinations may promote falls.

Neurologic problems may also contribute to falling. A number of neurologic diseases significantly increase unsteadiness and reduce reactive responses to loss of balance. Parkinson's disease, through both its effect on postural control and abnormal gait, is frequently associated with falls. A hemiplegic gait, especially if combined with a significant toe drag, can easily lead to a trip. Cervical spondylosis, when accompanied by lower extremity weakness and hyperactive reflexes, may present as a falling problem. Cerebellar lesions that produce motor control disorders can contribute to falls. Any ataxic gait, especially when associated with normal pressure hydrocephalus and decreased attention, may lead to a fall.

Clinically, a large number of older people complain of "dizziness" when describing their falling episodes. True vertigo is relatively rare and implies a disorder of the central or peripheral vestibular system. Light-headedness, which most laypersons call dizziness, can have multiple causes such as orthostatic hypotension or cardiovascular disorders. Careful questioning is required to distinguish the two. When uncertain a workup to search for central causes such as cerebellar or vertebrobasilar infarction is indicated.[30]

The evidence linking psychologic causes to falls is less exact. However, it seems reasonable to conceive that psychologic factors could play a role in enhancing the risk of a fall. For instance, depressed persons often complain of problems with attention and concentration. The chronic use of alcohol as a self-treatment for loneliness may increase the risk of a fall by promoting depression, or through physiologic sequelae such as hypotension, ataxia, decreased attention, or nutritional effects. There is some evidence that there may be premonitory falls related to occult cancer.[18] Finally, the fear of falling commonly follows a falling episode and may increase the risk of a fall itself.

FALLS WITH SYNCOPE

Falls with syncope are relatively uncommon. Although one study has reported syncope to account for 13.3 percent of falls,[6] most studies report the rate to be closer to 1 percent of all causes.[37] Although most patients can report a loss of consciousness following a syncopal episode, many older persons cannot recall the details about a fall, leading the clinician to suspect syncope. Hence, many patients undergo extensive hospital evaluations.

Because of the well-known association between cardiovascular problems and syncope, such an evaluation is often centered on cardiac monitoring. Cardiovascular causes may account for as many as 50 percent of the causes of syncope in the elderly. However, establishing a causal link between an arrhythmia detected on monitoring and a fall is more difficult. Arrhythmias occur frequently in older persons. Paroxysmal atrial tachycardia affects 9 to 13 percent of the elderly,[13] sick sinus syndrome and atrioventicular block are not uncommon, and ventricular ectopia may affect up to 50 percent of this population.[26] Such rhythm disturbances are usually short-lived and revert spontaneously. Because of their high prevalence it would seem that arrhythmias probably cause falls only when associated with decreased cerebrovascular blood supply or if they persist for some time. The correlation between the arrhythmia and symptoms (such as dizziness or syncope) is low, probably on the order of 2 to 15 percent.[34] Furthermore, there are no controlled studies that have demonstrated that treatment of arrhythmias found on monitoring will decrease the occurrence of further falls. Simply treating an arrhythmia found on monitoring is associated with a high rate of adverse effects.[34] Hence, further studies are needed to clarify those patients that are falling due to their rhythm disturbances.

Other cardiac causes may contribute to falls. Atypical presentations of myocardial infarctions are common in the elderly. Approximately 8 percent of elderly patients with a myocardial infarction present with syncope.[32] Aortic stenosis is the most common valvular abnormality found in older persons and also presents frequently with syncope. Finally, hypertrophic cardiomyopathy is commonly associated with syncope, often exacerbated by the administration of a diuretic.[34]

Vasovagal syncope is probably more commonly seen in the elderly as well. A number of conditions which are more frequently found among the older population predispose those persons to such attacks. Benign prostatic hypertrophy may promote a vasovagal attack while the older man is standing at the toilet straining to urinate. Chronic laxative abuse may lead to bowel dysfunction and fecal impaction. A syncopal episode may then develop while the person attempts to defecate. Syncopal episodes following forceful coughing spells can also occur.

The most common type of transient ischemic attack, that in the middle cerebral artery distribution, is not usually associated with syncope. Sudden interruptions of blood supply in the vertebrobasilar artery distribution are, however, associated with fainting spells. This syndrome is also characterized by nausea and vomiting, visual disturbances, and vertigo. It is uncertain how frequently syncope occurs in vertebrobasilar transient ischemic episodes. In the person with underlying atherosclerotic changes or severe osteoarthritic changes of the cervical spine, such episodes may be precipitated by looking up to reach for something on a high shelf.

Lastly, the diagnosis of a possible seizure disorder should be entertained in the person presenting with syncope and falls. Most seizures in the elderly present in the same manner as in younger persons. However, only 50 percent of elderly epileptics have abnormal electroencephalograms.[20] Furthermore, 40 percent of normal elderly have abnormal EEGs.[20] The use of antiseizure medication, particularly barbiturates, is associated with significant side effects in older persons and may themselves increase the risk of a fall.

DIAGNOSTIC EVALUATION OF THE PERSON WHO FALLS

HISTORY

In spite of its limitations the most important component of the diagnostic evaluation is the history. Each older person should be asked whether he or she has experienced any falls recently, as part of the review of systems. If the patient is being evaluated specifically for falls, he or she should be asked about any previous falls. An open-ended question, such as, "Tell me about the other falls you've had . . .," can encourage the person who is embarrassed to speak more freely. Each falling episode should be carefully assessed as different causes may coexist and precipitate falling by different mechanisms.

Patients tend to leave out important details when describing their falls so the clinician must be more directive in questioning. A useful method is to ask the patient to recount chronologically exactly what was happening before, during, and after the fall. The patient can then be prompted to become more detailed in his or her account with a statement like, "And then what happened?" It is also helpful to review when medications were taken in reference to the fall. If the history indicates a relationship to movement or change of position the patient should be directed to attempt to demonstrate those actions. The patient should be asked specifically about premonitory symptoms (such as lightheadedness or vertigo), loss of consciousness, or incontinence. Past medical problems that are associated with falls should also be investigated.

MEDICATIONS

The patient's medications must be reviewed as well as the dosing schedules. The patient should be shown the medication and asked, "What time of day do you take this one?," rather than simply taking the information from the instructions on the bottle. The ideal location for such an assessment is in the patient's home. Patients may forget to bring their medications to the clinic or office and they usually won't bring in medicines that have been given to them by friends or family. Over-the-counter medicines should also be listed.

PHYSICAL EXAMINATION

A complete physical examination should be performed. Certain elements of the examination deserve mention. When taking the patient's vital signs supine and standing blood pressure and pulse should be measured. If orthostatic changes are suspected the measurements should be repeated after 1 and 5 minutes. The patient's vision should be assessed. If syncope is considered in the differential diagnosis, the use of carotid sinus massage while the patient is being monitored may be attempted. This maneuver should be used only in those patients with no clinical evidence of cerebrovascular disease. The patient lies supine while the carotid artery is gently massaged for 5 seconds. A positive test is seen in those patients with a greater than 50 percent slowing of their baseline sinus rate or a 50 mm Hg drop in blood pressure. Less significant drops in blood pressure are considered positive if associated with symptoms.[26] The extremities should be evaluated for musculoskeletal problems with special emphasis on functional joint range of motion. The feet should be examined for lesions and deformities. The patient's shoes may provide clues to gait problems. A back examination for range of motion and flexibility is also important.

A complete neurologic examination is essential. The presence of underlying cognitive deficits that may affect the patient's ability to attend to the environment often go undetected.[33] A search for signs of focal weakness, muscle atrophy, or fasciculations should be made. Manual muscle testing may be unreliable and more functional assessment of muscle strength can be accomplished by having the patient walk first on the toes and then on the heels in order to detect subtle, unilateral weakness. Peripheral sensation to touch, vibration, and proprioception should be tested. Cerebellar tests of both upper and lower extremities should also be done. The extremities should also be tested for increased tone, rigidity, or cogwheeling. Tone in the lower extremities is best tested with the patient is standing.

GAIT EVALUATION

One of the most important components of the physical examination is an evaluatoin of the patient's gait. Pathokinesiology laboratories have been developed to accurately assess gait disturbances. Recently two scales for clinical assessment of gait have been validated against this more complex method of analysis.[29,42] The "get up and go test" is one method suitable for use in primary care settings. The patient is instructed to stand up from the chair without using his or her hands, walk 15 m down the hall, turn around, come back, and then stand still. While standing still with the eyes closed a gentle push on the sternum can be given to test righting reflexes. Finally, the patient is directed to sit down without using the hands.

Each component of the test should be analyzed carefully. Inability to arise from the chair without the assistance of the hands is indicative of hip extensor weakness. Steps should be regular with the length of the stride about one length of the patient's foot. One can evaluate toe clearance by squatting down and looking for light visible beneath the swing foot. Step symmetry can be observed and irregular steps, either shorter than normal or laterally displaced, can be noted. A tendency to veer, loose balance, or hold on to surrounding objects may be apparent. While turning, loss of balance or the presence of a stiff, en bloc disjointed turn should alert the clinician to the possibility of underlying neurologic disorders such as Parkinson's disease.

SWAY AND BALANCE

While standing with feet together and eyes closed the patient should be evaluated for excessive sway. Some minimal sway is normal with aging[39] but gross sway visible on this examination is associated with increased risk of falls.[33] First, the patient is viewed from the side for evidence of anteroposterior sway, then from the rear for lateral sway. The former would usually indicate problems in the musculoskeletal or peripheral nervous system while the latter is associated with central neurologic problems. Finally, while braced to stop a potential fall, the examiner gently pushes on the patient's sternum to test the righting reflex. Normally patients will either rebalance immediately or throw a foot back quickly to catch themselves.

Because persons come in contact with a number of obstacles such as crosswalks, stairs, curbs, and ramps during a normal day, additional testing may be warranted.[24] In a more detailed assessment velocity determination over a 300-m walk will identify those patients who can be considered community ambulators.[8] Physiologic measurements such as blood pressure and pulse responses are also helpful. If the patient uses a walking aid, such as a cane or walker, the gait should be evaluated both with and without the aid. Proper sizing of the aid should also be checked as well as safety features such as the rubber tips, tightness of joints, and functioning of any wheels. The use of a wheelchair should also be evaluated if the history indicates falls from the chair. The patient's knowledge of safety measures (e.g., setting the brakes properly), and the fit and stability of the chair, are important features to observe. The newer lightweight chairs may tip over backward more easily when used by older persons.[44]

FUNCTIONAL ASSESSMENTS

Other functional examinations may also be administered. Self-report of functional activities may be unreliable so a series of physical tests that simulate normal daily activities has been developed. It must be remembered that even though the patient may be able to perform the test, that does not mean he or she can perform the activity in the home. Other assessment instruments such as the Katz ADL (activities of daily living) scale[21] and the Duke-OARS IADL (instrumental ADLs) scale[12] may be used. If there has been a history of falls in the bathroom or while arising from the bed, functional tests duplicating the maneuvers are helpful.

LABORATORY AND DIAGNOSTIC STUDIES

Decisions regarding laboratory or investigational studies depend on information gathered in the history and physical examination. Some general guidelines can be followed. A complete blood count, chemical screen, urinalysis, and thyroid function tests should be ordered. If premonitory falls are suspected, stools for occult blood and the sedimentation rate may be helpful. If the physical examination or history reveals a potential cardiopulmonary etiology, a chest x-ray and ECG should be obtained. When a history of incontinence with the falls is found, an EEG should be considered. A Holter monitor should be considered in the patient with syncope, palpitations, or pulse irregularities. Because of the high incidence of clinically insignificant rhythm abnormalities in the elderly, treatment should be reserved for those with high-grade ventricular ectopia, sustained supraventricular tachycardia, or severe bradycardia.[37] Electronystagmography should be considered in cases of vertigo. Hence, the diagnostic workup should include an in-depth history and physical and targeted laboratory and diagnostic studies.

ENVIRONMENTAL ASSESSMENT

An assessment of the patient's home or living situation should be a routine component in the workup of the patient with falls. Hazards in the patient's environment may account for 40 to 50 percent of accidental falls.[27,31] Occupational or physical therapists, nurses or nurse practitioners, or physicians can evaluate the home environment. In the nursing home or hospital the environment assessment should be part of the "incident report." A systematic approach to examining the environment will usually reveal potential hazards.

The examination begins with the entryway. Inadequate lighting, loose steps or rails, cracked sidewalks, and clutter should be noted. Inside the house the rooms should be checked for loose rugs or torn carpets, unstable furniture, electric cords in walkways, and clutter. Stairways should be examined for lighting, visibility of the nosing (the edge of the step), and the quality of the railing and floor covering. Loose linoleum or water spills may be found in the kitchen. The bathroom may need adaptive equipment installed such as raised toilet seats or arm frames for the toilets, grab bars for the toilet and bath, and bath or shower benches. If a bench is installed a handhold shower hose facilitates bathing. The beds and chairs should be assessed for height and ease of exiting. Properly positioned the patient should have greater than a 90-degree angle at the knees when sitting down.

During the home visit the patient's commonly worn shoes can also be inspected. Storage facilities for medications can be assessed while the medicines are reviewed. Food storage can likewise be evaluated and frequently used items can be moved to lower shelves. Telephone usage in an emergency or the potential need for a "lifeline" system may also be discussed. The patient or the caregiver can be provided with one of many available lists[37,41,43] for assessing and modifying the home at that time along with specific recommendations based on the home visit findings.

INTERVENTIONS

MEDICAL

Medical interventions are directed toward those causes of falls found during the diagnostic evaluation. Unfortunately, in a significant percentage of patients no specific cause will be discovered. Even in those patients where a specific inciting problem is discovered the clinician may face difficult value decisions regarding treatment. For instance, the finding of a potentially dangerous arrhythmia may lead the clinician to initiate antiarrhythmic therapy with digoxin. But digoxin may itself increase the risk of falls by enhancing carotid sinus sensitivity or by its toxic effects. For that reason, the rehabilitative approach that emphasizes enhancement of function should place the medical interventions in the context of the patient's total health care needs.

PSYCHOLOGIC

A significant number of patients will develop strong fears of falling, particularly if a previous fall resulted in injury. An opportunity to discuss these fears will often limit their effect on further functioning. Some patients may need more intensive therapy and a few may require the use of desensitization programs or hypnosis to begin a rehabilitative exercise program.

SOCIAL AND ENVIRONMENTAL

In addition to the home environment assessment, many patients benefit from enhanced social contacts. Recreation programs, arrangement for transportation services, and volunteer telephone call programs are but a few of the methods used to maintain active contacts with other people.

FUNCTIONAL

If limitations of range of motion, decreased muscle strength, coordination deficits, and limitations in ADLs or IADLs, or gait deviations are detected during the physical examination, consideration should be given to physical or occupational therapy referral. Specific strengthening programs as well as balance and gait training may be beneficial even when the cause of the falls is not found. The patient may also be able to overcome the fear of falling when helped to practice activities and movements under the watchful eye of the therapist.

Physical therapists can conduct detailed evaluations that more clearly identify biomechanical problems that interfere with a safe gait. Occasionally they may employ computer-assisted pathokinesiology examinations that help to identify which type of assistive device may be most beneficial. They also can design outpatient or home exercise programs to enhance strength and promote balance. Occupational therapists can identify unsafe behaviors or maneuvers that the patient may be using in the home. A home visit may be performed by either therapist to better assess safety and equipment needs.

Clinicians may wish to make many modifications based on such an assessment but a great deal of tact is required in discussing such recommendations. The patient may not have the financial resources to buy recommended products or the skills to install them. Local volunteer organizations such as the Retired Senior Volunteer Program or others may be able to assist. The patient may feel that the recommendations are an intrusion on their independence or personal values. Demonstrating sensitivity to these concerns and explaining the reasons for the recommendations will often result in a mutually satisfying solution.

SUMMARY

Falls and instability are major problems for the elderly. Reports of falls and instability on examination should lead to an aggressive investigation as to their cause or causes. Such an investigation should take a functional approach emphasizing the underlying medical problems that may be contributing to the patient falling, the psychologic reactions to these disturbances, and the hazards in the patient's social situation.

Rehabilitation interventions may help to decrease further falls even when specific causes are elusive.

REFERENCES

1. Archea, J.C. (1985). Environmental factors associated with stair accidents in the elderly, Clin. Geriatr. Med., 5, 555.
2. Baker, S., and Harvy, A.H. (1985). Fall injuries in the elderly. *Clin. Geriatr. Med., 1*, 501.
3. Baker, S., et al. (1984). *The injury fact book.* Lexington, MA: Lexington Books.
4. Blazer, D. (1982). The epidemiology of late life depression. *J. Am. Geriatr. Soc., 30*, 587.
5. Caird, F.L., Andews, G.R., and Kennedy, R.D. (1973). Effect of posture on blood pressure in the elderly. *Br. Heart J., 35*, 527.
6. Camm, F.L., et al. (1980). The rhythm of the heart in active elderly subjects, *Am. Heart J., 99*, 598.
7. Campbell, A.J., et al. (1981). Falls in old age: a study of frequency and other related factors. *Age Aging, 10*, 264.
8. Cohen, J.J., et al. (1987). Establishing criteria for community ambulation. *Top. Geriatr. Rehabil., 3*, 71.
9. Cohn, T.E., and Lasley, D.J. (1985) Visual depth illusion and falls in the elderly, *Clin. Geriatr. Med., 1*, 601.
10. Cummings, S.R., Nevitt, M.C., and Kidd, S. (1988). Forgetting falls: The limited accuracy of recall of falls in the elderly. *J. Am. Geriatr. Soc., 36*, 613.
11. Davie, J.W., Blumenthal, M.D., and Robinson-Hawkins, S. (1981). A model of risk of falling for psychogeriatric patients. *Arch. Gen. Psychiatry, 38*, 463.
12. Duke University Center for the Study of Aging and Human Development (1978). *Multidimensional functional assessment: The OARS methodology,* 2nd ed. Durham, NC: Duke University.
13. Fleg, J.L., and Kennedy, H.L. (1982). Cardiac arrythmias in a healthy elderly population: Detection by 24 hour Holter ambulatory electrocardiography, *Chest 81*, 302.
14. Garcia, C.A., Tweedy, J.R., and Blass, J.P. (1984). Underdiagnosis of cognitive impairment in a rehabilitation setting. *J. Am. Geriatr. Soc., 32*, 339.
15. Goldman, R. (1986). Decline in organ function with aging. In I. Rossman (Ed.), *Clinical geriatrics* (pp. 23–59). Philadelphia: Lippincott.
16. Hasselkus, E.R., and Shambles, G.M.: Aging and postural sway in women. *J. Gerontol., 30*, 661.
17. Hogue, C. (1982). Injury in late life: I. Epidemiology, II. Prevention. *J. Am. Geriatr. Soc., 30*, 183.
18. Howell, T.H. (1971). Premonitory falls. *Practitioner 206*, 666.
19. Isaacs, B. (1985). Clinical and laboratory studies of falls in old people. *Clin. Geriatr. Med., 1*, 513.
20. Katz, R.I., and Harner, R.N. (1984). Electrocephalography in aging. In M.L. Albert (Ed.), *Clinical neurology of aging.* New York: Oxford University Press.
21. Katz, S., et al. (1963). Studies of illness in the aged. The index of ADL: A standardized measure of biological and psychosocial function. *JAMA, 185*, 94.
22. Klass, D.W., and Daly, D.D. (Eds.). (1979). *Current practice of electroencephalography.* New York: Raven Press.

23. Koller, W.C., Glatt, S.L., Fox, J.H. (1985). Senile gait. *Clin. Geriatr. Med., 1,* 661.
24. Lerner-Frankiel, M., Vargas, S., and Brown, M. (1986). Functional community ambulation: What are your criteria? *Clin. Manage. 6,* 12.
25. Lipsitz, L.A. (1985). Abnormalities in blood pressure homeostasis that contribute to falls in the elderly. *Clin. Geriatr. Med., 1,* 637.
26. Lipsitz, L.A. (1983). Syncope in the elderly. *Ann. Intern. Med. 99,* 92.
27. Lucht, U. (1971). A prospective study of accidental falls and injuries at home among elderly people. *Acta Socio-Med Scand., 2,* 105.
28. Macdonald, E.T., Macdonald, J.B., and Phoenix, M. (1977). Improving drug compliance after hospital discharge. *Br. Med. J., 2,* 618.
29. Mathias, S., Nayak, U.S.L., and Isaacs, B. (1986). Balance in elderly patients: The "get up and go" test, *Arch. Phys. Med. Rehabil., 67,* 387.
30. McClure, J.A. (1986). Vertigo and imbalance in the elderly. *J. Otolaryngol., 15,* 248.
31. Mofitt, J.M. (1983). Falls in old people at home: Intrinsic versus environmental factors in causation. *Public Health 97,* 115.
32. Muntz, G.S., and Kotler, M.N. (1981). Are you overlooking IHSS in your elderly patients? *Geriatrics 36,* 95.
33. Overstall, P.W., et al. (1977). Falls in the elderly related to postural imbalance. *Br. Med. J. 1,* 261.
34. Pathy, M.S. (1967). Clinical presentation of myocardial infarction in the elderly. *Br. Heart J. 29,* 190.
35. Perry, B.C. (1982). Falls among the elderly living in high rise apartments. *J. Fam. Pract. 14,* 1069.
36. Ray, W.A., Griffen, M.R., and Shaffner, W. (1987). Psychotropic drug use and the risk of hip fracture. *N. Engl. J. Med., 316,* 363.
37. Rubenstein, L.Z., et al. (1988). Falls and instability in the elderly, *J. Am. Geriatr. Soc., 36,* 266.
38. Sheldon, J.H. (1960). On the natural history of falls in old age. *Br. Med. J., 2,* 1685.
39. Sheldon, J.H. (1963). The effect of age on the control of sway. *Gerontol. Clin., 5,* 129.
40. Stelmach, G.E., and Worringha, C.J. (1985). Sensorimotor deficits related to postural stability: Implications for falling in the elderly. *Clin. Geriatr. Med., 1,* 679.
41. Tideiksaar, R. (1986). Preventing falls: Home hazard checklist to help older patients protect themselves. *Geriatrics 41,* 26.
42. Tinetti, E.M. (1986). Performance-oriented assessment of mobility problems in elderly patients. *J. Am. Geriatr. Soc., 34,* 119.
43. United States Consumer Product Safety Commission. (1985). *Home safety checklist for older consumers.* Washington, D.C.: United States Consumer Product Safety Commission.
44. Unpublished study by L. Axtell (1987). Clinical Gerontology Service, Rancho Los Amigos Medical Center, Downey, CA.
45. Woollacott, M.H., Sumway-Cook, A., and Nashner, L. (1986). Aging and postural control: Changes in sensory organization and muscular coordination. *Int. J. Aging Hum. Dev., 23,* 97.
46. Woollacott, M.H., Sumway-Cook, A., and Nashner, L. (1982). Postural relexes and aging. In J.A. Mortimer, F.J. Pirozzolo, and G.J. Maletta (Eds.), *The aging motor system.* New York: Praeger.

CHAPTER 12

The Impact of Technology on Geriatric Rehabilitation

DENNIS R. LA BUDA

In recent years there has been a shift from a narrow perspective on rehabilitation on geriatrics to a more comprehensive gerontologic approach. As a result, attention is beginning to be focused on the fundamental differences between (and therefore basic strategies to be employed for) the "well elderly," who are just beginning to experience limits to their abilities, and those older persons who are disabled and are entering into the rehabilitation system. It is important to focus on strategies that will maintain the highest level of function for as long as possible, and to compensate in both the macro- and microenvironments where possible, to forestall developing disabilities from becoming excessive for older persons.

There are, of course, many approaches to responding to the need to maintain function. At the Stein Gerontological Institute (SGI), the concentration has been on the impact of technology, specifically hard technology, that is, *products*, as opposed to soft technology, that is, *systems* or *services*.[6] The thrust of this chapter is an attempt to examine the potential impact of hard technology on rehabilitation services.

AN AGING SOCIETY

John Naisbitt coined the term *megatrend*. According to Naisbitt, a megatrend is "a major transformation in society."[20] These trends are of such a

209

magnitude that they affect all other trends. These trends may be social, political, economic, scientific, or demographic. As we move forward into the twenty-first century, there are two such megatrends that are converging and the impact of that convergence is already being felt. First, our population is growing older, both in median age as well as in sheer numbers. "The older population itself is getting older. In 1986 the 65–74 age group (17.3 million) was eight times larger than in 1900, but the 75–84 group (9.1 million) was 12 times larger and the 85+ group (2.8 million) was 22 times larger."[3] Of these growing numbers, the 85+ cohort is the fastest growing of all. This population traditionally is in greatest need of services.

Most older persons have at least one chronic condition and many have multiple conditions. In 1984, about 6.0 million (23%) older people living in the community had health-related difficulties with one or more personal care activities (19% of men, 25% of women) and 7.1 million (27%) had difficulty with one or more home management activities (18% of men, 33% of women). Less than half who had difficulty with personal care but most of those who required aid in home management were receiving at least some personal help. The percentages needing and receiving help increased sharply with age.[2]

With other factors such as the decline in the birth rate and high divorce rates, there may develop a trend toward fewer family members to care for the growing elderly population. The demand on formal support services (traditional human service systems) to supplement this deficiency in the number of informal caregivers, that is, family members, can never be adequate to serve such a large population of frail elderly.

As a consequence, rehabilitation will be necessary to maintain the highest level of functioning and ease the demand on the more traditional form of intervention and service. The Veterans Administration has realized this phenomenon and has named it "the demographic imperative."[9] The VA is now admitting into its long-term care system veterans of World War II. During the 1990s it will begin responding to the needs of the veterans of the Korean conflict, and in the first decade of the next century the Vietnam veterans. When the system begins to take in the Vietnam veterans, the majority of both the World War II and Korean veterans will still be alive and aging. This means that in a short 20 years, the VA will have to respond to three levels of aging veterans. Strained to respond to the demands placed on it in 1989, alternatives to traditional health care services must be found and the VA is looking to technology as part of the answer.

THE EXPANSION OF TECHNOLOGY

The second megatrend of the twentieth century is the virtual explosion of scientific discovery and the resulting technologic innovations. In an article published in the *National Journal* in 1983, Bruce Merrifield discussed science and technology in this century.[18] He contends that scientific discovery followed a relatively stable, slow growth process in the period from 10,000 B.C. to A.D. 1,900. However, this changed dramatically in the twentieth century. More scientific discoveries occurred in the first 80 years of this century than in the preceding 11,000 years. In fact, 90 percent of what we know about our world was discovered in a 30-year period ranging from the early 1950s to the early 1980s. That knowledge base will likely double again in the next 10 to 15 years.[18] Given that scenario, a crescendo of the technology explosion should occur in the early years of the next century and intersect, if not collide with, a second phenomenon, the advent of the aging of the "baby boomers." Clearly, aging and technology are two megatrends that will continue to interact and impact one upon the other and the ramifications will affect us socially, economically, politically, and in many other areas.

TECHNOLOGY AND DISABILITY

In order to properly plan for old age we need to examine where we are now. Historically, the disability community and the aging community have not identified with one another, nor have they worked closely together. Rehabilitation has traditionally been hard technology–intensive, for example, concerned with prosthetics and assistive devices. Gerontology, or aging, has been soft technology–intensive, for example, concentrated on formal and informal support services or skilled nursing facilities where physical and occupational therapy are ancillary to nursing care. These fundamental differences in focus have created equally significant differences in approach to providing supportive environments for those who need them. Rehabilitation is disability-specific and follows very much a medical model. The individual is diagnosed and the treatment prescribed emanates from the individual's problems. On the other hand, "long-term care providers, including nursing homes and informal caregivers such as family and friends, have not generally used available technologies to facilitate caregiving and improve quality of care."[5]

This dichotomy is further exacerbated by the difference between specialities in how they describe technologic devices. Vanderheiden, an occupational therapist, talks about "appliances," which he refers to as technology-independent items such as eyeglasses, hearing aids, and pacemakers; and "tools," which he suggests are user-dependent and include items such as prostheses, communication aids, and mobility aids. His rationale, appropriately, is that the user does not have to acquire skills to operate eyeglasses or a pacemaker, but does need to learn how to use a prostheses or a communication aid.[23] Paul Haber, a physician with the VA, contrasts "medical technologies," which are life-sustaining, that is, drugs, pacemakers, glasses, (in other words, Vanderheiden's appliances), with "ecological technologies,"[10] which are life-enhancing, such as electric can openers, prosthetics, and remote controls (Vanderheiden's "tools"). I prefer "assistive devices," for those items necessary for effective functioning, to "enabling products," Vanderheiden's "tools," or Haber's "ecological technologies." The last-named are items that require some skill to use, are not necessary, but which enhance effective functioning. Whatever they are called, the point is that *technologic innovation and development will affect the practice* of geriatrics and rehabilitation.

GERIATRIC REHABILITATION AND MARKET FORCES

The impact of technology on the practice of geriatric rehabilitation seems like an obvious point, so why is it important? When tied to aging it becomes significant because of the commercial implications. This is becoming evident in the proliferation of publications and programs directed toward this group. One report states, "Older persons account for a disproportionately large share of total discretionary spending power, according to a joint study of The Conference Board's Consumer Research Center and the U.S. Bureau of the Census."[17] A recent successful trade newsletter is entitled *The Mature Market Report*. Aptek International, a subsidiary of the National Center for Appropriate Technology, was created to develop business opportunities to respond to the needs of the frail elderly and the disabled.

Those who create and disseminate technologies and products will be seeking markets. The implications for the older market are clear. The potential exists for manufacturers to create technologies which have clear rehabilitation implications and to market them directly to an older population, without consulting rehabilitation professionals, and without incorporating appropriately supervised testing or evaluation. Further, if companies are successful in their marketing, the nature of rehabilitation, and therefore the practice of the rehabilitation professional, could be dramatically affected by what happens in the marketplace. If rehabilitation professionals are not involved in the research and development phases of new product development there could be serious consequences, both for the practitioner and the end user.

TECHNOLOGY AND THE FUTURE

RECORD KEEPING

How far out and how far away are these future technologies? An illustrative example is the laser card. The laser card utilizes the same technology as the compact disc player. It is the size of a standard credit card. Marketed by Drexler Technology Corp. of Mountain View, California, the card was used in initial trials by Blue Cross/Blue Shield of Maryland. The laser card can hold up to 60 pages of information and can be configured up to two megabytes. It can record entire medical records, x-rays, digitized computed tomography (CT) scans, pharmaceuticals, etc. Recording of prescription medications can preclude drug interaction or drug overdoses because this information would be available to the pharmacist. These cards will become "living medical histories" allowing subsequent generations access to the medical life histories of their ancestors. Of course, these cards will carry all financial and health insurance information making billing and processing automatic. They will also eradicate the necessity of ever filling out another medical form in one's lifetime.

While the laser card is impressive, it is already being outmoded by the "smart card." Created by Intelmatique, a French corporation, and getting attention from American BellCore, this credit card has a built-in microcomputer capable of being "programmed for multiservice capabilities and the magnetic strip enables the card to be compatible with existing equipment."[22] Because the card contains its own microprocessor, when attached to communications equipment it will allow remote monitoring and adjustment of biomedical equipment. A physician or therapist with the right equipment and a telephone line will be able to respond to the needs of a patient anywhere, eliminating the need to be present physically to effect changes. Both the laser card and Intelmatique's smart card, called Smart and Striped, are currently commercially available.

COMPUTERS

A technology that is becoming increasing prevalent in our lives is the computer. Much work has been done in rehabilitation circles utilizing computers, especially in communications. However, there has been much speculation about the applicability and acceptance of computer technology by older persons.[16] With the advent of publications such as *Computers for Kids Under 60*, and projects such as SeniorNet, a national computer community of seniors (IFF newsletter), there is now no question that computer technology is accepted by older persons and can play a role in all aspects of their lives. Maintaining independence need not be an exception. The work of the Aspen Institute, with funding from the Markle Foundation, is showing the merger between computers and telephone communications. The reader may have seen the American Telephone and Telegraph Co. advertisement, "Suddenly there are 250 million more computers in America," with a picture of a telephone.[1] The importance of this integration lies in the development of medical hotlines, customized "reminder" services for such things as medication needed, even computerized systems which allow patients to call a computer to analyze the effect of and, if necessary, adjust drug dosages.

Space age technology is being applied through the National Aeronautics and Space Administration's technology transfer program in innovations such as electronic monitoring systems, which track wandering patients who are victims of Alzheimer's and related diseases. Other systems will alert a nurse when a patient is getting out of bed, or, for the incontinent patient, will alert the nursing staff that toileting needs to take place. The Long-Term Care Foundation is looking to develop a prototype "smart" nursing home, probably with many of the features of the National Association of Home Builder's Smart House, which holds tremendous promise for monitoring both physical conditions and behavior to assist the occupant in remaining independent, safe, and secure in the home.[7]

ROBOTICS

The final testing stage is a robot designed for use in long-term care facilities. In addition to alleviating many tedious tasks, robots can be used in the home to assist with basic activities of daily living (ADLs), thus enabling a person to remain more independent. In a therapeutic and rehabilitation environment a robot can provide assistance with passive physical therapy exercises and even feeding. However, many problems still remain to be solved in robotics. There needs to be a refinement of sensing systems for the robot so that it does not hurt the human using it. The robot needs its own "tools" and work environment within which to function. In an experiment conducted at SGI employing a robotic arm to cut and juice an orange, it was discovered that if the oranges were not of a particular size the end manipulators could not accomplish the task. Obviously, future robots will need to not only be more sensitive, but more adaptable. Given the resolution of these difficulties, these machines will become powerful tools for rehabilitation. However, it has long been acknowledged that "high technology" may not always be the best solution. Robots are controlled by computers, and computers are controlled by humans. The difficulty starts when the technology begins to run humans. Repeatedly, we have learned that the more complicated technologies become, the easier they must be to use.

THE UTILIZATION OF TECHNOLOGY

As on the larger social level, there are differences in approach and sometimes friction between generations related to allocation of resources.[21] This may continue to be a growing phenomenon in the years to come and may grow out of inherently different approaches to rehabilitation between the young and the old. For the young, rehabilitation is vocationally oriented, the objective being to compensate for the disability and, to the greatest degree possible, restore normal functioning. The end objective is independence and with that comes the ability to earn a living, so this approach is driven by vocational needs. In some cases, such as in the VA, tremendous sums of money may be spent on an individual to restore his place in society as a productive participant.

In geriatrics the approach is more generalized and disability-oriented. The main outcomes in geriatric rehabilitation are improvements in daily living abilities for their own sake, without reference to a vocational objective. It is basically maintenance with the least discomfort. This is evidenced by the fact that most skilled nursing facilities provide and are reimbursed for physical therapy, whereas occupational therapy is more often an option and is not reimbursed unless specifically prescribed by a physician. With the changing demographics, a new approach must be implemented, one that is a synthesis of the two traditional and related approaches. This must involve attention to design and function, especially of devices to be used in the home.[14] An illustrative example is the use of grab or transfer bars. These may work perfectly well for a young healthy male paraplegic with strong upper body strength and yet be totally useless to a frail older women with the same transfer needs.

Give limited resources, design of products as well as rehabilitation strategies should take the entire spectrum of need into account. Granted, this is not an easy approach, and every response to a given problem often creates new problems. An area which research at SGI has identified as a targeted intervention for older persons is the need to eliminate excessive reaching and bending. One of the tools to resolve this problem is a reacher stick. Improperly designed reacher sticks are fine for strong healthy arms, wrists, hands, and fingers, but when that is not the case, the reacher puts great strain on fingers and wrist. However, modifications to this design, for example, a pistol grip with an extension brace under the forearm, alleviates this problem. The second design is a better design not only for the older person but for everyone who can benefit from the use of a reacher.

As indicated in the beginning of this chapter, a comprehensive gerontologic approach to rehabilitation is needed. While disease, diet, lifestyle and so on may not individually affect function significantly, over time the combination of these factors will affect an individual's ability to manipulate his or her environment. Attention to this fact will allow for earlier and more appropriate technologic interventions, or even preventive intervention. In addition, and again this is a major difference in approach between the young disabled and the elderly, while it seems likely that the disabled would like to have their tools be as attractive as possible, if they allow for restoration of function, esthetics must become a secondary concern. However, for the older persons who can function, albeit with difficulty, if the tool is not esthetically pleasing it is not likely to be acquired or used. This, of course, relates to the issue of design.

SGI conducted a survey questionnaire of 244 persons over the age of 60 (61 men, 183 women) who were screened to be "healthy and independent," meaning that they were living nonassisted in the community. Of those surveyed, 49 percent indicated that they had problems with grocery shopping and 37 percent indicated that they had problems with meal preparation.[8] Although a small sample, these data suggest that there exist significant hidden functional problems among the elderly, problems that could be addressed by traditional approaches used in the rehabilitation community. These problems need to be attended to at an earlier stage, employing strategies which will forestall or eliminate further deterioration to the point where the individual is so debilitated that she or he then comes into the rehabilitation system.

RESEARCH IN TECHNOLOGY

In an effort to better understand not only the limitations of the individual but the limitations of the environment, since 1980 SGI has been conducting human factors research applied to aging. This work has been and continues to be funded by the National Institute on Aging. Research staff have been videotaping older persons on a shopping expedition, preparing meals, cleaning the home, attending to dressing functions, and simulating bathing and grooming tasks. These tapes are returned to the laboratory and interacted to a computer. ADL tasks are broken down into specific coded motions and actions. In addition to a videotaped analysis of ADL tasks the researchers have been measuring environments, creating an ergonomic database, as well as measuring subjects, creating an anthropometric and biomechanic database. With knowledge about the decline of body systems over time, as well as its functional abilities, areas are being identified where the environment can be "fixed" as opposed to concentrating on "fixing" only the person. Evaluation and assessment of the design of household features can suggest ways in which they enhance or detract from normal functioning.

SGI research has focused on two areas of concern within the home; the kitchen and the bathroom. These areas seem to be the interface between dependence and independence. If persons are capable of preparing and consuming meals, and performing toileting and grooming functions, then they usually are able to remain independent. However, when intervention is required to such a degree that the person cannot function without it, independence is lost and that person is at risk of institutionalization. In addition to identifying the kitchen and bathroom as high probability areas for functional breakdown between the individual and the environment, SGI's research has also identified problems associated with excessive bending or reaching. The introduction of "tools" to do the reaching and bending or modification of the environment through the rearrangement of objects will eradicate the need for excessive reaching or bending. Both actions place the older person at risk of falling. In the case of older women, especially those suffering from osteoporosis, the potential for a broken hip or other broken bones, which too often leads to a spiraling downward cycle of health deterioration and reduced function, is ever-present.

In addition to investigating the macroenvironment, that is, the home or apartment, SGI researchers are also investigating issues related to the microenvironment, specifically those related to seating. One such study produced a comparison of the Warren Chair designed by Roger Lieb of Add Interiors, Inc., with conventional seating, specifically traditional recliners, to assess the demands that ingress and egress create resulting from the design of the chair (Fig. 12-1). It was shown that the Warren Chair, due to its design features, for example, the cantilevered seat and back, the forward placement of the arm supports aligning the shoulders above the hands and in vertical alignment with the legs, takes maximum advantage of the sitter's strength (Fig. 12-2). The chair does not have any electrical or electronic components. Its effectiveness is purely a consequence of design considerations. The initial chair has been modified esthetically, now coming in colors as opposed to one shade of brown (sort of the Model T approach) and netting has been added to the seat for increased comfort when sitting for an extended period of time. As a result of this research, SGI is beginning to identify appropriate tools or environmental modifications to respond to commonly experienced functional limitations.

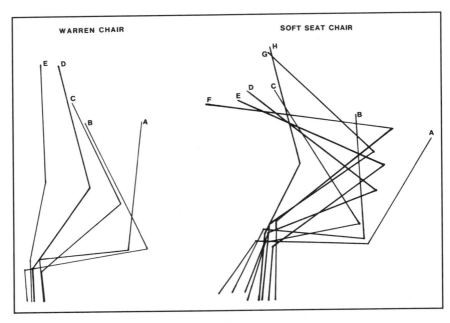

Fig. 12-1. Profiles of types of biomechanical movements involved in chair egress. Egress begins at line A.

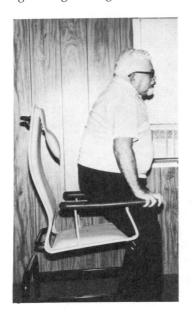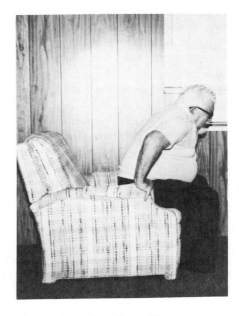

Fig. 12-2. The Warren Chair (A) versus the traditional recliner (B).

TECHNOLOGY AND INFORMATION DISSEMINATION

There is an overwhelming problem of information dissemination related to technologies that can enhance life. Most of these products are marketed through DME (durable medical equipment) supply stores. An older person who may be having some difficulties but who does not consider himself disabled is not likely to walk into a store where the front window is filled with chrome walkers, hospital beds, wheelchairs, and bedpans. On the National Technology and Aging project, older persons were asked, "If you had a lamp that you could turn on and off by simply touching it as opposed to twisting those little knobs, would you buy it?" Overwhelmingly the response was positive and furthermore they stated that they would be willing to pay more than the current market price for such an item. When told that such a thing was commercially available, consistently they were surprised. A questionnaire given to formal caregivers, home health aides, nurses, physicians, and even some occupational therapists revealed that within the professional ranks, there was not a general knowledge of the breadth and magnitude of products which are currently available in the marketplace.

There is a tremendous responsibility for public education in this area.[4] While some mail order companies have found success in the marketplace, others have struggled. There needs to be a campaign to educate the general public about what is available without it being tied to a commercial venture. The federal government of Canada has produced and is disseminating throughout the provinces a series of pamphlets simply entitled, *Independent Living*. Each pamphlet focuses on one task area and identifies strategies and products which can enhance function. Some of the titles are *Food Preparation Aids; Bath, Shower and Transfer Seats; Lifting Aids*, etc. Issued by Health and Welfare Canada, more information on these pamphlets is available from Independent Living, Public Affairs Directorate, Health and Welfare Canada, Ottawa, Ontario, K1A 1B5.

In a more immediate, pragmatic approach to introducing technical interventions into the homes of the elderly, SGI's Technology Center for Independent Living is launching a demonstration called Team Independence. The core of the team will be the pairing of a specially trained social worker with an occupational therapist, the latter sensitized to larger environmental issues. Traditionally, case management, or the brokering of services in the home to assist the frail elderly, is human intervention–oriented. Case managers are usually social workers and their training guides them to utilize human intervention responses to problems. Occupational therapists are trained to enhance function and they do that not only through therapy, but through significant utilization of technology. By teaming these two, when the social worker goes into the home to conduct a psychosocial, economic assessment of the client, the occupational therapist will be conducting a functional assessment of the client as well as evaluating the environment and the associated demands it places on the individual. Therefore, not only will human intervention strategies be employed, as is currently the case, but technologic interventions, be they products or environmental changes, will also be identified.

Another important aspect of this team approach has to do with long-term educational support. In a human intervention situation, there is usually a family member or a home health aide or a chore worker who returns on a regular schedule to intervene and assist. Because the older person begins to rely on this person the intervention is generally integrated into her or his life. All too a technologic intervention is introduced once and then forgotten. An older person is given an electric can opener, for example, shown how to use it, and it is assumed that the problem is resolved. Later, the person may try to use it again, but if it does not work, it is likely to go in a drawer or on a shelf, never to be used again. The problem of opening cans remains unresolved. Follow-up with the technology is needed. The family member or client needs to be asked, "Did you use it? . . . Did it work O.K.? . . . Did you have any problems?" If all is fine, the human support can be withdrawn. If not, more training and support is needed or another technology that is more appropriate can be substituted.

CONCLUSIONS

At this time, there is no empiric evidence that technologic intervention will either reduce health care costs or allow a person to maintain independence for extended periods of time while reducing the need for human intervention. However, there is enough preliminary research to suggest that this could be a plausible scenario. Given the changing demographics, and the social and economic demands for health care for the elderly today, not in the future, this is an area which warrants further serious investigation.

Health care providers we need to learn about technology. This includes not only what exists in the marketplace today, but those innovations and applications that are under development and which will soon become a part of their practice in the future. Due to the overwhelming amount of information which must be dealt with, it will be imperative to formulate and work within the interdisciplinary team approach. Acceptance of new technologies by the elderly is generally not a problem.[13]

Rather, the difficulty lies in lack of knowledge of the existence of helpful technologies, which is an issue we can do something about immediately. The other issue is availability and ability to pay. These are broader social and economic issues that will need to be addressed in the next few years, and at a national level. Finally, research, assessment, and evaluation protocols and systems must be developed that will help the end user as well as the caregivers, both informal and formal, to identify and effectively actuate the use of "appropriate" technologies.

Good design makes good sense for everyone. Design is moving away from institutional chrome or white grab bars and toilet safety rails to color-coordinated products which utilize a variety of materials in their manufacture. Appliance and hardware design has moved from simply esthetic to functional and esthetic, and as the relentless introduction of sophisticated, primarily electronically based, high technologies has spread into the home environment, so also will the nature of living as an older person be significantly different in the future. These forces will also determine which products will be used in rehabilitation, and therefore also define what rehabilitation itself will look like.

For professionals who are working in the rehabilitation area, it is incumbent that they not only understand the demographic phenomena and what they will mean for their professional futures, but also what technology will contribute as well. These megatrends will have an impact with or without the input of rehabilitation specialists. If professionals want to contribute to development, they must not only interact with their peers and colleagues but become involved with those in gerontology, and equally, with those who create and disseminate technology in the health care environment.

REFERENCES

1. American Telephone and Telegraph Co. (1986). Advertisement. *TV Guide.*
2. *A Profile of Older Americans* (p. 13). (1987). Washington, D.C.: American Association of Retired Persons/Administration on Aging.
3. *A Profile of Older Americans* (p. 2). (1987). Washington, D.C.: American Association of Retired persons/Administration on Aging.
4. Clark, M.C., and Gaide, M.S. (1986). Choosing the right device, a capability-demand approach. *Generations*, Fall, 18.
5. Congressional Office of Technology Assessment. (1985). *Technology and aging in America* (p. 188). Washington, D.C.: Government Printing Office.
6. Congressional Office of Technology Assessment. (1985). *Technology and aging in America* (p. 3). Washington, D.C.: Government Printing Office.
7. Czaja, S.J. (1988). Safety and security of the elderly: Implications for smart house design. *Int. J. Technol. Aging, 1*, 49.

8. Czaja, S.J., et al. Problems encountered by healthy older adults performing daily living activities. In press.
9. Eberhardt, D. Together: Meeting the challenge. Presented at Florida's Aging Network Training Conference, Ft. Lauderdale, August 1987.
10. Haber, P.A.L. (1986). Technology: A needed aspect of preserving function. *Geriatr. Consultant*, May/June, 27.
11. Harris, H. (1986). Smart house and aging: Creating responsive living environments through technology. Washington, D.C.; National Council on the Aging.
12. Hiatt, L.G. (1988). Smart houses for older people: General considerations. *Int. J. Technol. Aging, 1*, 11.
13. La Buda, D.R. High technology and its benefits for an aging population. Presented at Hearing, Select Committee on Aging, U. S. House of Representatives, Washington, D.C., May 1984.
14. La Buda, D.R., and Clark, M. (1987). Design that works for the aging. *Innovation*, Summer, 15.
15. La Buda, D.R. (1985). *The gadget book. Ingenious devices for easier living.* Glenview, IL. AARP Books.
16. La Buda, D.R. (1987). Potential of computer technology on the rise. *Perspect. Aging, 16*, 14.
17. Linden, F. (1985). *Midlife and beyond: the $800 billion over fifty market.* New York: Consumer Research Center.
18. Merrifield, D.B. (1983). Forces of change affecting high technology industries. *National Journal*, January, 253.
19. Moore, P. Technology and aging. National conference presentation, Washington, D.C., November 1987.
20. Naisbitt, J. (1982). *Megatrends, ten new directions transforming our lives.* (p. 11). New York: Warner Books.
21. Naisbitt, J. (1982). *Megatrends, ten new directions transforming our lives* (p. 7). New York: Warner Books.
22. *Smart and Striped* (1987). Paris; Intelmatique.
23. Vanderheiden, G.C. (1987). Service delivery mechanisms in rehabilitation technology. *Am. J. Occup. Thera., 41*, 705.

CHAPTER 13

Vision Impairment in Geriatrics

ROBERT N. WEINREB
WILLIAM R. FREEMAN
WILLIAM SELEZINKA

Vision impairment in the aging population is an increasingly important problem. Visual impairment in geriatrics is due largely to one or more of four conditions: (1) cataract; (2) diabetic retinopathy; (3) age-related macular degeneration; and (4) glaucoma.

Cataracts are present when the clear lens within the eye opacifies. If sufficient to cause loss of visual function, it can be treated by lens extraction. With contemporary microsurgical techniques and the availability of intraocular lens implants, cataract surgery has become a safe means for rehabilitating the patient who is visually impaired because of cataract.

Diabetic retinopathy affects both young and elderly persons. It is often asymptomatic and patients may not seek the attention of an ophthalmologist until there is neovascularization with vitreous hemorrhage. With appropriate examination and follow-up, diabetic retinopathy can be diagnosed at its earliest stages and appropriate laser therapy administered.

In this chapter, we consider the two most common irreversible visual impairments in the elderly: age-related macular degeneration and glaucoma. The visual loss with which they are associated and guidelines for rehabilitation of these low vision patients are discussed.

LOW VISION

Low vision is a term describing a serious visual loss which cannot be corrected by medical or surgical intervention, or with spectacles. Visual aids may alleviate the visual disability by use of refractive, nonrefractive, or magnifying devices, but remaining functional vision is still not normal or adequate.

Low vision is not a single condition with predictable manifestations.[2] Therefore, it is necessary to define the type of resulting visual loss, not the underlying condition, in order to properly assist the patient. Low vision affects the patient, not the eye. Vision loss may be classified as central or peripheral. Central loss of vision, the most prevalent type, affects reading and may result from a variety of conditions, including age-related macular degeneration (ARMD). Peripheral vision loss, as found in glaucoma, affects orientation and mobility because the visual field is reduced. Vision loss in these two common geriatric diseases are discussed subsequently. Low vision may be further complicated by such problems as slow dark adaptation (e.g., in ARMD), loss of night vision (e.g., in retinitis pigmentosa), and glare.

The terms "low vision," "visually impaired," or "partially sighted" should be applied to anyone who still has some usable vision, no matter how little. These persons are not blind, though this term is often used. The confusion in terminology may be the result of the legal definition of blindness developed over 50 years ago by the federal government to qualify the visually impaired for special benefits. It was based on 20/200 visual acuity and a central visual field of less than 20 degrees, or a central loss in the better eye reducing vision to 20/200 or less. In reality, at least 85 percent of those classified as legally blind actually have some usable vision and therefore have more potential for low vision training than the totally blind.

SIGNIFICANCE

Over 11 million people in the United States have severely reduced, uncorrectable vision, as noted by a 1977 government health survey.[11] Of these, over 1 million have a visual deficit that interferes with such normal activities of daily living (ADLs) as reading the newspaper. More than 1 million people are totally blind. Seventy percent of the totally blind and severely visually impaired are 65 years of age or older. As the U.S. population ages, it is estimated that over 22 million people will have severely impaired vision by the year 2000. Presently, 26 percent of these persons are 18 to 64 years old and 6 percent are under age 18 years. Of the ten impairments studied by the National Center for Health Statistics for the period 1971 to 1977, visual impairments had the largest increase in rate per 1,000 population. In 1983, there were 2 million people 65 years and older who were unable to see well enough to read the newspaper, and this does not account for those unable to see at a distance. Thus, physicians are encountering more patients for whom there is no effective medical or surgical cure. Two of the most common causes of permanent vision loss in the elderly are ARMD and glaucoma.

AGE-RELATED MACULAR DEGENERATION

The macular area is located approximately 3 mm temporal to the optic disc and is easily visualized with the handheld direct ophthalmoscope. With aging, it may degenerate. ARMD is a common cause of untreatable legal blindness in patients over 65 years old.[5] This condition is characterized by degenerative changes in the retina and underlying supportive structures (retinal pigment epithelium). Because ARMD selectively affects the central macular area, it results in loss of the central 5 to 15 degrees of vision. The earliest changes characteristic of this disease, drusen and pigmentary changes, are often visible with the ophthalmoscope prior to the development of symptoms.

RISK FACTORS AND PATHOGENESIS

The Framingham study[5] showed that drusen and pigmentary degenerative changes in the macular area account for mild visual loss to the 20/30 level in 10 percent of the population over the age of 52. This increases to 30 percent of the population between the ages of 75 and 81. Each year thousands of people have severe bilateral visual loss with legal blindness resulting from ARMD. The disease is more common in whites than in blacks. Known risk factors for the development of ARMD include disease in the contralateral eye; the presence of drusen in the macular area, particularly soft or confluent drusen; blue iris; long-term hypertension; and cigarette smoking.[10]

The degenerative changes which are slowly progressive in these patients also occur elsewhere in the retina but are most pronounced in the macular area. On a microscopic level, the drusen and pigmentary changes seen with the ophthalmoscope are characterized by the accumulation of lipofuscin pigment in the retinal pigment epithelium and Bruch's membrane, and associated degeneration of these supportive structures of the light-sensitive cells of the retina. The pigment epithelium is essential to the proper metabolic function and nutrition of the photoreceptor cells (rods and cones) of the retina. Collagen and elastin become disrupted and calcium accumulates in these structures. Drusen are yellow-to-white rounded lesions which are visible in the macular area of patients with ARMD early in the course of the disease. Large confluent drusen have the highest risk of progression to severe visual loss. These drusen contain periodic acid-Schiff (PAS)–positive hyaline bodies which are sandwiched within the supportive structures of the retina. They may be derived partially from metabolic waste products of the photoreceptor retinal cells in the macular area. The macular area, which is responsible for central vision, is characterized by extremely high metabolic activity. This is the area of the retina which receives the most light and contains the most densely packed array of photosensitive and metabolic supporting cells. It is likely that this high metabolic rate and photo-stress are the reasons why degenerative changes occur so commonly in this area.[12]

The symptoms produced by ARMD are variable. There are two broad types: (1) dry or atrophic macular degeneration and (2) wet or exudative (neovascular) macular degeneration. Dry, atrophic macular degeneration is characterized by the slow painless progression of visual loss. Atrophic macular degeneration accounts for the majority of eyes with ARMD and causes significant visual loss. The atrophic form of macular degeneration is responsible only for approximately 20 percent of severe visual loss attributable to ARMD. Many patients with macular degeneration note decreased color vision and may also note that straight edges appear crooked. This latter condition is termed metamorphopsia and indicates that the macular area is being distorted by a pathologic process. Because these conditions are painless and may only affect one eye initially, persons affected often do not seek medical attention. Instead they ascribe their symptoms to the need for new eyeglasses and often defer medical evaluation.

As atrophic macular degeneration progresses, drusen become more numerous and may take on confluent characteristics. There is loss of pigment in the pigment epithelial cells underlying the retina, resulting in large geographic areas of pigmentary loss. In some persons, the disease is characterized by small patches of pigmentary loss associated with neighboring areas of fine pigmentary clumping. All such changes are easily observed with the direct ophthalmoscope. With fluorescein angiography, the pattern is highlighted as all areas of pigment dropout become hyperfluorescent to the fluorescein dye which passes through the underlying choroidal tissue (Fig. 13-1). Loss of central vision secondary to atrophic macular degeneration is most often moderate. Unfortunately, there is no proven way to prevent loss of vision associated with atrophic macular degeneration.

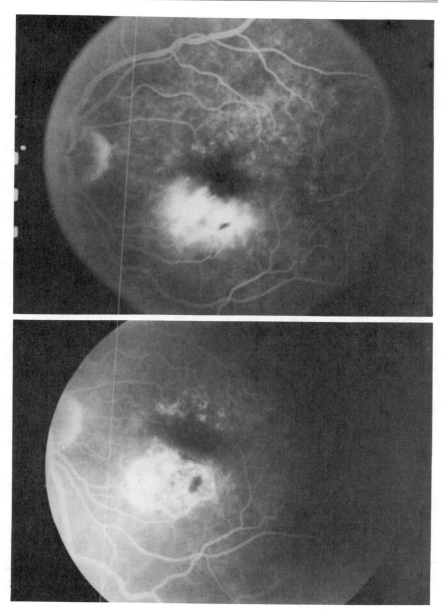

Fig. 13-1. Top: Fluorescein angiogram showing a group of leaking subretinal vessels which have invaded the subretinal space causing visual loss and distortion. Bottom: Same patient 1 month after treatment with krypton red laser. A scar is seen in the area of subretinal neovascularization which has regressed. The subretinal fluid and exudation have resolved and visual acuity has stabilized at 20/20.

Severe scarring associated with hemorrhage in the macular area is associated with the second form of ARMD—neovascular macular degeneration. Neovascular macular degeneration accounts for 80 percent of the severe visual loss attributable to ARMD. Fortunately, this disease is often treatable with laser photocoagulation during its early stages. It is estimated that each year over 130,000 patients in the United States benefit from such treatment. Patients with neovascular macular degeneration also may have associated atrophic macular degeneration. Superimposed on the chronic slow visual loss associated with atrophic macular degeneration is a more rapid phase caused by new and abnormal subretinal vascular invasion with subsequent exudation, leakage, and hemorrhage into the subretinal space. The stimulus for this subretinal membrane remains unknown. However, if the membrane is not directly underneath the ovea and if it is detected early, laser photocoagulation may be effective in halting and even reversing the visual loss that occurs.

In most cases, neovascular macular degeneration characterized by subretinal neovascularization eventually becomes bilateral. Many patients do not present to an ophthalmologist until several weeks after visual loss and are unaware that irreversible visual loss associated with subretinal neovascularization can occur over a matter of several days after the onset of metamorphopsia. For this reason, the first eye to present with subretinal neovascularization is usually not examined until hemorrhage and irreversible scarring have already occurred. Such patients are given an Amsler grid, with instructions to monitor the central vision for distortion or loss of vision in the contralateral eye.

The incidence of subretinal neovascularization (associated with macular scarring and loss of central vision) in persons with one eye already affected is high, approaching 10 percent each year.[8] For this reason, it is important that a patient who has lost central vision secondary to neovascular macular degeneration in one eye is educated about his condition so that the remaining eye can be treated promptly.

VISUAL FUNCTION

Most patients who have lost central vision in one eye function quite well if the other eye retains good central vision. Such patients continue to use both eyes together for tasks that require peripheral vision such as walking, driving, and more gross motor function. They usually retain peripheral stereovision as well. These patients cannot perform functions requiring fine central acuity, such as reading or seeing road signs, with the affected eye. However, the macula in the other eye provides this function and for this reason must be closely monitored. With appropriate education, most patients will report promptly for evaluation if symptoms of subretinal neovascularization develop in the remaining eye.

Unfortunately, many patients develop bilateral central visual loss secondary to atrophic and neovascular macular degeneration. It is important for many reasons to counsel such patients. These patients often fear that they will continue to lose vision until the point of total blindness. This is not the case and patients are relieved when told that visual loss secondary to ARMD is limited to central vision and that they will be able to continue to ambulate, cook, clean, and dress themselves and perform many of the routine ADLs. These patients should have a thorough examination of the peripheral retina and vitreous using indirect ophthalmoscopy and scleral depression to detect any occult peripheral retinal disease. Although this may be overlooked given the severity of the central pathologic changes, retention of peripheral vision is critical for these patients.

Many patients are motivated and can learn to read and perform other activities that require some central vision with the use of magnification aids. These patients learn to use an adjacent area of the retina as their preferred locus of vision and although the area will be not as sensitive to fine detail as the central macular area, patients can learn to read and perform related tasks with magnification.[9] Telescopes may be useful for some persons to aid in the identification of small distant objects, but many patients find them difficult to use. Training patients in the use of such devices requires the patient to be highly motivated and necessitates well-trained personnel. This is done in most eye centers through a low vision clinic. Similar services are available through a variety of organizations for the visually handicapped such as the Braille Institute. It is important to provide such organizations with as much medical information about the patient's remaining vision as possible in order to assist them in the training of these patients.

PREVENTION

Recent research has given new insights into the underlying metabolic and possible toxic processes which may cause macular degeneration of both the atrophic and the neovascular types. Common to the early stages of both types of macular degeneration are morphotic alterations in the photoreceptors and their supporting structures, Bruch's membrane and the retinal pigment epithelium. These cells and structures are subject to intense stress because of their extremely high metabolic rate and exposure to potentially hazardous levels of blue and ultraviolet light. In animal models, exposure to light has been shown to produce structural alterations in the macular area. Blue light and UV wavelengths have been shown to be the most hazardous.[13] For these reasons, it is advisable to protect the macula from these adverse stimuli by wearing sunglasses which filter out the invisible UV portion of the spectrum (wavelengths below 400 nm) and probably the near UV and blue visible wavelengths as well (all wavelengths below 510 nm).[12] It is particularly important to note that use of sunglasses which do not filter invisible UV and near UV wavelengths may not be protective and are potentially harmful. The pupil dilates when visible light is filtered and in so doing, many times the normal amount of invisible UV light enters the eye without any patient discomfort. The effect of appropriate UV and blue filtering sunglasses has not been evaluated in a prospective trial but their use seems reasonable based on our knowledge of the pathophysiology of the disease, particularly in high-risk individuals.

Because of the unknown potential for light-induced molecular damage to the delicate cellular structures in the macular area, there has been considerable interest in antioxidants and vitamin supplements as adjuncts to prevent macular degeneration. In a recent study, some benefit of oral zinc supplementation in prevention of progression of atrophic macular degeneration was shown.[6] There is considerable interest in evaluating this and other nutritional therapies which may modulate the effect of oxidative and photochemical stresses to the macula. Other therapies under consideration include vitamin C, beta carotene, and alpha tocopherol.

GLAUCOMA

BACKGROUND

The glaucomas are a group of conditions characterized by an intraocular pressure high enough to damage the optic nerve with subsequent optic nerve atrophy and visual field loss. Primary open-angle glaucoma is the most common type of glaucoma in the United States and is among the leading causes of blindness in the elderly. It is generally characterized by: (1) an intraocular pressure consistently above 21 mm Hg; (2) an open, normal appearing anterior chamber angle with no apparent ocular or systemic abnormality that might account for the elevated intraocular pressure; and (3) a typical glaucomatous visual field and/or optic nerve head damage.

RICK FACTORS AND PATHOGENESIS

There is widespread agreement that the prevalence of primary open-angle glaucoma increases with age. It is unusual to diagnose it before the age of 40, and most cases are diagnosed after age 65. The risk factors for primary open-angle glaucoma include race (it is more prevalent and develops at an earlier age in blacks), diabetes mellitus, family history, and myopia (nearsightedness). Elevation of intraocular pressure in primary open-angle glaucoma is due to obstruction of aqueous humor outflow. In other words, the resistance to fluid leaving the eye is increased. The precise mechanism of this is not understood.

TREATMENT

When primary open-angle glaucoma is diagnosed, treatment to reduce the intraocular pressure is initiated with eyedrops. A number of drugs have been formulated as eyedrops to treat glaucoma. These include beta-adrenergic blocking agents (e.g., timolol and betaxolol), parasympathomimetic agents (e.g., pilocarpine and carbachol), and adrenergic agonists (e.g., epinephrine).

Progression of glaucoma is monitored by measuring intraocular pressure, evaluating the optic disc, and examining the condition of the visual field. If eyedrop treatment is inadequate, an oral carbonic anhydrase inhibitor (e.g., acetazolamide) may be used.

Both eyedrops and oral carbonic anhydrase inhibitors are associated with considerable side effects, particularly in the aged. Eyedrops can pass through the nasolacrimal duct and into the nose. They are absorbed rapidly into the bloodstream through the nasal mucosa and hence can be associated with significant systemic toxicity. In the case of beta-adrenergic blocking agents, this can lead to bradycardia, hypotension, central nervous system depression, and even respiratory failure in susceptible individuals. Oral carbonic anhydrase inhibitors also have significant side effects, including nausea, fatigue, malaise, weight loss, paresthesias, and others. Failure to satisfactorily ameliorate the deterioration of the visual field with medication, or intolerance to its administration, may be followed by laser treatment. With this therapy, known as laser trabeculoplasty, the outflow obstruction is often relieved. Finally, conventional surgery is indicated if the condition still is not stabilized. In this procedure, a microscopic fistula is placed in the sclera to lower intraocular pressure.

VISUAL FUNCTION

Loss of vision in primary open-angle glaucoma occurs only late in the disease. Preservation of central vision allows most patients to continue their daily activities with little loss of function. However, preservation of central vision also leads to a diagnostic dilemma since most patients are asymptomatic and may not be aware that they have glaucoma. Although an occasional patient may become aware of a scotoma (blind spot) in the field of vision, the disease can only be diagnosed with a thorough examination. In most patients with primary open-angle glaucoma, subjective loss of vision is found to be due to associated cataract (lens opacity) or ARMD.

LOW VISION EVALUATION

Low vision is evaluated in terms of visual acuity, visual fields, and other aspects of perception such as contrast sensitivity, color recognition, and sensitivity to bright light or glare. Equally important in low vision evaluation is the determination of the visual needs of the patient to perform his or her basic daily tasks, at home, on the job, or socially. This is accomplished by asking specific screening questions.[3]

1. How would you describe your reaction to vision loss?
2. How does your vision loss affect the various aspects of your life, such as job, leisure time, and social loss?
3. What visual activities do you miss the most?
4. How are you managing to keep your accounts?
5. How are you managing to prepare meals and cook?
6. Are you staying home more?
7. Are you seeing your friends?
8. Do you feel there are changes in any areas of your life that are hard to manage?

It is useful to assess whether a patient has the ability to determine where objects are located as well as identify them. Perhaps vision is good enough to read, but inadequate to get about the house or neighborhood, or vice versa. One should think in terms of function, albeit residual, not disease. Even if a disease is untreatable, one can still do something to improve both visual function and the quality of life.

COORDINATING SERVICE FOR THE VISUALLY DISABLED

Once a new social stage is set for the patient by the diagnosis of visual impairment, a physician can assist in improving the quality of life. The use of rehabilitation services should be encouraged.[4] If a patient recognizes that his visual condition is irreversible and untreatable, as in ARMD, he is more likely to accept his visual status and start on a path toward successful rehabilitation.[1] The patient has to understand that, although he has limited vision, he can learn to use what remains; this provides hope. With vision rehabilitation services, which are not only for the totally blind, and by adapting and using visual aids, a productive life can be continued.

It is imperative to recognize that there is no standardized approach to coping; every person is unique, not only in the nature of his or her disease, but also in the dynamic and complex adaptation process. Furthermore, there must be a realization that the disability is a social disease (affects the way people interact), a shared state (family members' lives change), and that psychosocial rehabilitation (teaching the patient to interact with the world) is the responsibility of everyone.[7] Referrals may be job-related, school-related (special education), or for family counseling.

To achieve this end, it is easier to teach participatory realization and training when there is better sight and also when patients are able to better deal with their fears. A low vision assessment may be useful with an ocular problem even if optical aids are not necessary; nonoptical aids may be helpful. For example, sunglasses or visors will reduce light sensitivityin macular disease. Labeling techniques to enhance contrast and solve color recognition problems may also be useful. A bold pen, reflective or light or dark tape to mark the stairs, a dark-and-light cutting board in the kitchen, or a white coffee cup may help. Talking calculators, scales, clocks, watches, blood pressure monitors, and voice-activated telephones are also available. To achieve low vision rehabilitation, it is necessary to understand what this entails.

One begins by supplying information to the rehabilitation agency by letter indicating the diagnosis, prognosis, and so forth, and providing additional information along the way. The agency is requested to report back so as to have an exchange of ideas and information. Return visits to an ophthalmologist after the referral is necessary for continuity of care. Most often, low vision services do not have the expertise to assume follow-up medical care of the patient. After an evaluation of the home and the community, there may be the acquisition of teachers, if necessary, and other direct services including mobility evaluation. The patient may then be referred to a more concentrated program where individualized instruction for his or her needs is provided if that is found necessary. A decision for intensive training for several weeks at a low vision center is made by the rehabilitation team. The rehabilitation counselor is the coordinator of various services. It is a one-on-one relationship. Teacher, social worker, orientation and mobility instructor, psychiatrist or psychologist, occupational therapist, physiotherapist, audiologist (if necessary), and peer counselors participate in the training.

New technology has been introduced during the past 10 years. For example, electronic devices are used in mobility training to alert one if something is in the way. The patient learns safer traveling skills either to be productive or independent. Family and close friends must also be counseled not to take away the independence that is fostered in the patient during this intensified training while being instructed in their proper role.

Various publications exist to assist in rehabilitation. These alert one to the availability of special radio stations (radio reading services), broadcast local newspapers, agencies serving visually impaired that provide volunteer readers, and useful aids (including those employing high technology). Telephone directories or telephone information operators can help one find the services available in one's own area. Many of these may be found under various levels of government listings and many have toll-free numbers. The library, United Way, and National Society to Prevent Blindness are other good sources. Also, there are disease-specific organizations (e.g., glaucoma, retinitis pigmentosa, etc.) that provide specific information.

REFERENCES

1. Cholden, L. (1985). *A psychiatrist looks at blindness*. New York: American Foundation for the Blind.
2. Colenbrander, A., et al. Low vision outline. Joint Commission on Allied Health Personnel in Ophthalmology Course November 1987.
3. Faye, E. (1984). *Clinical low vision*, 2nd ed. Boston: Little, Brown.
4. Hoover, R. (1967). The ophthalmologists' role in new rehabilitation patterns. *Trans. Am. Ophthalmol. Soc. 65*, 471.
5. Leibowitz, H.M., et al. (1980). The Framingham eye study monograph. *Surv. Ophthalmol., 24* (Suppl.), 335.
6. Newsome, D.A., et al. (1988). Oral zinc in macular degeneration. *Arch. Ophthalmol., 106*, 192.
7. Shindell, S. Psychosocial issues of low vision and blindness. Presented at symposium for ophthalmologists, Stanford University Medical Center, Palo Alto, CA, 1988.
8. Strahlman, E.R., Fine, S.L., and Hillis, A. (1983). The second eye of patients with senile macular degeneration. *Arch. Ophthalmol., 101*, 1191.
9. Timberlake, G.T., et al. (1987). Reading with a macular scotoma. *Invest. Ophthalmol. Vis. Sci., 28*, 1268.
10. Tso, M.O.M. (1985). Pathogenetic factors of aging macular degeneration. *Ophthalmology, 92*, 628.
11. United States Public Health Service. (1983). *Vision research, A national plan*. U.S. Public Health Service (NIH) publication No. 83-2471.
12. Young, R.W. (1988). Solar radiation and age related macular degeneration. *Surv. Ophthalmol., 32*, 252.
13. Young, R.W. (1987). Pathophysiology of age-related macular degenerative. *Surv. Ophthalmol., 31*, 291.

CHAPTER   14

Hearing Impairment in Geriatrics

LAUREL E. GLASS

A young woman said, "Youth is a hazardous business." An old woman responded, "Old age is not for sissies!" The "golden years"? While this slogan has helped to modify society's predominantly negative images of the old, it also denies some of the realities of aging. The old body is different from the young body, and change in sensory perception is not the least of the differences.

Few deny that vision changes with age and most know that "people who wear glasses *do* receive passes" (to misquote Dorothy Parker). In fact, if a middle-aged or older adults does not wear glasses, it is assumed she or he is wearing contacts. That hearing changes with age is common knowledge too. Surprisingly, what is not known by most is how very many older people are significantly hearing-impaired or have uncorrectable low vision, nor how handicapping hearing loss or low vision can be, nor how difficult it is to remedy either effectively. This chapter addresses issues of hearing impairment and its remediation and rehabilitation. Vision impairment is discussed in Chapter 13.

Hearing impairment is the third most prevalent chronic condition of elderly people. About half of all hearing-impaired people in the United States are over 65 years old, and the prevalence increases from at least 25 percent of those aged 65 to 74 to almost 40 percent of those over 75. In some surveys of nursing homes, 85 to 90 percent of the inhabitants were seriously hearing-impaired. At present, 7 million elderly people have significant hearing loss. If the rapid growth in numbers of people over 75 persists, more than 11 million elderly people will be significantly hearing-impaired by the year 2000. Moreover, not only the prevalence but the severity of hearing impairment increases with age.[2,14,24,29]

THE ISSUE: HEARING LOSS INTERFERES WITH COMMUNICATION!

Statistics may tell a truth; so may anecdotes, and the latter usually convey the truth more compellingly. The following are all true; each is used with permission; each is only one example of many similar stories.

A medical school professor of pharmacology received numerous teaching awards. However, as her hearing worsened, so did her ability to hear questions within the background noise of a classroom. Students no longer praised; they complained. She was shifted to teaching small graduate seminars; there she did fine until her hearing worsened so much that she could no longer follow the discussion. She was moved to departmental administration and finally urged to take early retirement.

An apprentice welder "passed" as hearing, but panicked and became depressed when he realized that after his graduation to journeyman he would have to receive orders by phone from the construction foreman. He was too hearing-impaired to decode phone messages accurately.

A very competent laboratory technician, whose boss and coworker knew she was severely hearing-impaired, nearly lost her job. Her hospital used a careless system in which staff would come to the laboratory desk and request information or give instructions orally, usually very fast and often while looking away from the person they were addressing. Then, when the wrong information was given or the response was slow, they would complain. The hospital did not fire the hard-of-hearing technician; it changed procedures. Written orders were required in most instances. Communications training was given to the hospital staff. It was made clear that, if oral orders were necessary, they must be given while looking directly at the recipient, spoken more slowly and with clearer enunciation. Not surprisingly, the accuracy of all the laboratory staff increased remarkably, the hearing as well as the deaf.

A severely hard-of-hearing man living in San Francisco's Tenderloin was mugged and nearly raped when he failed to hear a shout of warning and then did not hear his attacker demand money. He was rescued by friends who knew he was deaf.

A profoundly deaf woman began to attend meetings of Self Help for Hard of Hearing People, Inc. (SHHH), an effective information sharing and advocacy group for hard-of-hearing persons. Her sons and their families, though genuinely loving people, complained that she had become too assertive from attending SHHH and asked her to stop going. She requested, for example, that the TV be turned off when people were trying to talk to her in the same room.

A gracious hard-of-hearing woman was unable to understand the question of a young person at her back door; she opened the door, was held at knife point, roughed up, and the house was ransacked.

How safe is hearing impairment? Not very. Neither on the job nor on the street nor in the home.

How uncomfortable is hearing impairment? Helen Keller commented that her blindness separated her from things but her deafness separated her from people.

How handicapping is hearing impairment? It has been described by some as "a glass wall, invisible but forming a barrier."

PERSONAL ADAPTATIONS TO HEARING IMPAIRMENT

Rehabilitation and remediation for the handicaps of hearing impairment rarely occur without the help of someone else. The "other" may be a family member, friend, boss, casual acquaintance, stranger, service delivery professional (e.g., physician, audiologist, otolaryngologist, rehabilitation counselor, teacher, technician)—even an enemy.

RECOGNITION OF HEARING LOSS

Perhaps the hardest task for most hearing-impaired persons is acknowledgment that something is wrong.[7,8,13,15,22] Clusters of reasons for denial have been suggested: the unconscious association of hearing impairment with old age and the unconscious association of old age with failing capacities; self-esteem issues, often including a sense that one is not functioning as well as before and a (usually futile) hope that others don't feel the same way; a genuine feeling (usually not correct) that other people are not speaking clearly anymore. It is also seen by some as a way of temporarily, but successfully, coping, which allows the hard-of-hearing person to keep going without despair when circumstances require it.

UNRECOGNIZED ADAPTATIONS

Unrecognized adaptations often include unconscious lip reading, with the reality that one hears only part of what's said in the next room or in a darkened room; unconscious avoidance of noisy places for important conversations, for example, avoidance of a busy restaurant or the street; speaking less often in groups and saving one's suggestions for a quiet comment later (sometimes rationalized as "wanting to give less experienced folks a chance to speak"); going less often to public meetings even on topics previously of interest; refusing committee leadership with "I'm too busy at work" or "I don't have quite as much energy as I used to." Some symptoms include intense fatigue after a family gathering filled with many conversations going on at the same time; "inappropriately" high anxiety before important business meetings; increased resistance to attending cocktail parties or other crowded gatherings; irritability at home with repeated commands to "Speak up! Quit mumbling!"; more frequent errors in everyday life ("I asked you to get a card for Alice and you bring home the silly cart we decided we couldn't afford"); increasing family complaints (e.g., "John can hear when he wants to"). A frequent comment to audiologists when someone comes for a first hearing test is, "I'm here because my family wanted me to come . . ."

DIAGNOSIS OF HEARING LOSS

The human ear is made up of three parts: the external, middle, and inner ear. Cerumen in the external canal may interfere with hearing; removal of the wax produces a miracle cure. Hearing loss due to middle ear dysfunction may, among other causes, be the result of "glue ear" from fluid coagulation during otitis media, from inhibition of stapes mobility by otosclerosis, and from tumors such as cholesteatoma.[5] Hearing impairment due to such middle ear lesions often can be repaired by surgery.

Hearing impairment due to loss or damage to the cochlear hair cells, the primary sensory receptors of the ear and/or to the nerve cells of the cochlear ganglion, brain stem tracts, and/or cortex is called *sensorineural hearing loss*. Its causes are complex and it cannot be cured. Yet. Cochlear hair cell loss has been demonstrated histologically and seems to be associated with the progressive loss of hearing for high tones experienced by most older people.[11,25] Noise and at least 130 drug and nondrug chemicals have been shown to damage hair cells.[26] Included among the medications is furosemide, a diuretic frequently prescribed for persons over 65 years of age. A decrease in the number of nerve cell bodies in the cochlear ganglion has also been shown, but the cause is not known.[11] Other causes of hearing impairment include Ménière's disease with its symptom complex of vertigo, tinnitus, and hearing loss, and acoustic neuroma with attendant damage to the auditory nerve as it enters the brain stem.

In many states, audiologic testing requires recommendation by a physician. Although this increases the cost to the hearing-impaired person, it also allows a real chance to rule out reparable causes of hearing loss. Audiologic examination assesses how much hearing is lost (measured in decibels at each of several pitches, measured in hertz); these measurements use so-called pure tone stimuli which do not have the over- and undertones characteristic of real-life sound. The audiologist also determines the Speech Reception Threshold (SRT) and the Speech Discrimination Score (SDS). These tests use standardized word lists to measure how loud a word must be for the subject to understand it (SRT) and the extent to which the person understands single-syllable words when they are presented at a loudness just below that which causes discomfort (SDS). Audiologists also test impedance or resistance to the passage of sound waves; this gives one measure of pathologic conditions in the middle ear. In addition, bone conduction is usually measured.

These and other audiologic tests give information about the degree of hearing loss, types of loss, anticipated usefulness of a hearing aid, and rehabilitative needs. A client may be told that he or she has a mild, moderate, severe, or profound loss. With a mild loss, the hard-of-hearing person will have trouble hearing faint or distant sounds. At the other extreme, persons with a severe or profound loss can hear only very loud noises that are nearby; for all practical purposes, they are deaf. Often discussions with the audiologist deal with whether a hearing aid would help, whether it is worth the cost, and what kinds of aids are available.

Differentiation among the several possible causes of hearing loss is usually made by the person's physician plus an otolaryngologist and, usually, an audiologist. Cure of external and middle ear problems usually is the responsibility of the physician and the surgeon. Sensorineural hearing loss, however, is still incurable and persons experiencing it need good advice from the health care professionals on whom they depend.

AURAL REHABILITATION

Practical help from a physician or other health care provider to a person learing to live with hearing loss is a suggestion that he or she participate in an aural rehabilitation program in the area. Aural rehabilitation[1,9] attempts to give the hard-of-hearing person skills that will reduce the communication barrier resulting from the hearing impairment and which will help the hearing-impaired person to adjust to the psychosocial, occupational, and educational impacts of the auditory deficit. Persons are taught how to use and care for a hearing aid. The degree of handicap (undesirable disruption of life) caused by the hearing loss is usually assessed. The Hearing Handicap Inventory for the Elderly

(HHIE), developed by Ventry and Weinstein,[32–34] was standardized on an older population and has been very useful for assessment of hearing handicap in older people. The hard-of-hearing person is helped to develop new strategies for communication, including ways in which he or she can control the listening environment so that it facilitates rather than hinders the understanding of speech. Training in speech reading or sign language or cued speech may be provided (see below.)

LEARNING TO COPE WITH IMPAIRMENT

Feelings of anger, grief, loss, anxiety, decreased self-esteem, isolation, separation, uncertainty, confusion, intense fatigue, stress-related symptoms, and so forth are reported with greater or less intensity by almost every adult who has lost or is losing hearing.[7,8,13,15,18,22] An excellent resource for such persons is the small booklet titled *What Should I Do Now? Problems and adaptations of the Deafened Adult* by Helen Sloss Luey and Myra S. Per-Lee.[18] This booklet is helpful in a myriad of practical ways for people learning to live with hearing loss. In fact, it is so practical and the prevalence of hearing impairment is so high that physicians and other professionals working with older adults might do well to have a number of browsing copies in their waiting rooms.

It is important to recognize that even knowledgeable hard-of-hearing persons may not recognize that their hearing is worse when they are ill, taking certain medications, or are tired, worried, or preoccupied. They may blame themselves for not hearing. Not only do spouse, children, and close friends assert that "Mary can hear when she wants to," but Mary sometimes wonders herself if she could hear if she only tried harder. An important task for service providers working with persons who have recently become deaf or hard of hearing is to make sure the hearing-impaired person understands that the hearing loss is real, not just "in his or her mind" and not just a way to escape from things the person doesn't want to face. Sensorineural hearing loss involves a real damage to the hair cells and/or nerve cells of the auditory system. This is real damage and cannot be wished away.

Especially useful for the hard-of-hearing person is learning how to give others cues about what would make communication easier. For example, instead of saying, "What? What did you say?," the hearing-impaired person can comment, "I'm hard of hearing; could you try that sentence with different words, please?" or "I really want to hear what you have to say so let's turn around and get the light on your face; I'm a lip reader and need all the help I can get." Many hard-of-hearing persons carry a small notebook and a fast pen: "I'm hard of hearing; would you mind writing that?" Or one can say to a family member watching TV,

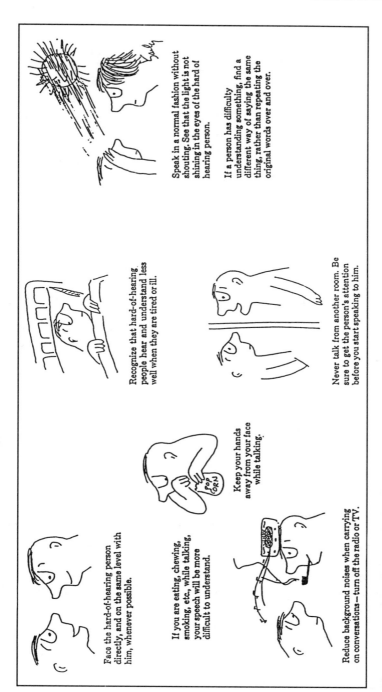

Fig. 14-1. Tips for talking to the hard of hearing. (Reproduced with permission of the Hearing Society for the Bay Area, Inc., San Francisco.)

"Hey! I need to talk with you. Can I turn this thing off while we talk or would you rather I came back later? You know how extra noise confuses me." Simple devices posted in one's office or home, such as the flyer reproduced in Figure 14-1, provide direct, visible reminders to everyone that some behaviors make it easier to hear and some interfere with understanding.

The flyer shown in Figure 14-1 is available in more than 16 languages and copies can be obtained for the price of a postage stamp. One thing is obvious. It requires self-assurance and an inner security to say and do those kinds of things—even though they help immensely in communication with another person. Obviously, some form of assertiveness training is worth the energy for a hard-of-hearing person.

Participation in a group with other hearing-impaired persons can also help one learn to cope. Not least, it is a real relief to be with others who know how it feels and who have experienced the inconvenience and frustration of trying to manage when you don't hear what is being said around you. Also, through self-help groups, opportunities for stress reduction classes (S. Trychin, unpublished) and assertiveness training focused directly on the problem of hearing-impaired person become available. SHHH is one of the fastest growing self-help and advocacy organizations in the United States. SHHH is well led by persons who are themselves profoundly hearing-impaired. Its journal is filled with accurate, current information about people, communication skills (speech reading, sign language, cued speech), assistive listening devices, hearing aids, new instrumentation being developed, legislation, and so on. If an SHHH group is not active in the hearing-impaired person's area, the professional can at least provide the address of the SHHH national office.

SPEECH READING

If formal aural rehabilitation training is not available, training in speech reading, often called lip reading, is advisable.[12,19,20] Classes are available at many community colleges, night schools, extension divisions, churches, agencies working with older persons or focused on hearing and speech, and other organizations. The term "speech reading" is favored over "lip reading" because facial expression and body position as well as mouth movements give cues about what another person is saying. Although only about 40 percent of speech sounds are visible on the mouth, speech reading can provide an excellent supplement for people trying to understand partially heard words. Speech reading classes help the hard-of-hearing person focus attention on all cues that give meaning to what is said. They give information about letters and words which look alike on the mouth but have different meanings. Many hard-of-hearing persons have been supplementing their hearing by lip reading for a long time, but haven't realized it; speech reading classes make that skill more intentional and help the hard-of-hearing person become aware of the need to substitute alternative words when what is "seen on the mouth" doesn't fit the context of the conversation. Not least, participation in a speech reading class brings the hearing-impaired person into contact with others who are experiencing similar difficulties ("It's not easy for them either. Maybe I'm not so dumb!").

SIGN LANGUAGE

Some time ago a Peanuts cartoon showed Woodstock, the bird, talking intensely to Snoopy; in the balloon over his head vertical lines of various lengths and different accents are arranged in patterned clusters. Snoopy, head cocked, listens attentively for three of the four panels; in the fourth, his face is distressed as he says seriously, "It's a difficult language . . ."

Any kind of manual language—whether Signed English, American Sign Language, Cued Speech, or any variation of them—is difficult for people raised to nonmanual, spoken communication. However, knowing at least the manual alphabet can be a real help for hard-of-hearing persons. They often function well in one-to-one situations or in quiet environments. They may also function well in meetings or in casual conversation, even in groups and even with noise pollution, *if* they are cued when the topic of conversation changes. For example, if someone finger-spells or jots down on a small note pad what subject the group is talking about—as it changes—a hard-of-hearing person can often participate comfortably and not feel isolated by his or her impairment. The person providing the cues doesn't need to write, "The thing we are talking about now is . . ."; the hearing-impaired person knows the group is talking about something! Just a finger-spelled or written word or phrase, for example, Jane's promotion, the Olympics, is enough.

If the hearing loss is severe, sign language capability sometimes helps change a hearing handicap into only an inconvenient disability. Signed English is English transferred to the hands and, unlike American Sign Language, it follows English word order, grammar, and syntax. Since Signed English is used with (and by) persons fluent in English, word endings, some tenses, some English grammatical forms, etc., are omitted on the hands and only inferred from context. One can speak (voice) and sign at the same time so that hearing-impaired signers, lip readers, and hearing non-signers can be part of the conversation; no one is excluded. My recommendation is that persons with moderate or more severe hearing losses should start to learn sign language, the simpler the better at the beginning, perhaps with the ABC's of American Sign Language[10] and with simple forms of Signed English[23] or other simplification.[4]

CUED SPEECH

Cued speech is a communication system developed to supplement speech reading and make comprehension of spoken language more exact.[28] Eight hand shapes are used to differentiate consonant sounds and four hand positions are used to differentiate vowel sounds. To learn the symbols requires about 20 hours; to use the symbols well requires many, many hours of practice. Although the method is strongly supported by some, others have found it difficult to use effectively. While relatively few persons use cued speech fluently at the present time, active efforts are being made to extend its use.

TECHNOLOGIES WHICH ASSIST COMMUNICATION

A variety of instruments have been developed which make communication between hearing-impaired and hearing persons easier and more accurate. The two best known are probably the hearing aid and the TDD (Telecommunication Device for the Deaf).

HEARING AIDS

Hearing aids cannot return hearing to "the way it was." This unfortunate truth means that the expectation of many hearing-impaired people (and their families) is disappointed, and this is one reason why many expensive hearing aids end up in bureau drawers, unused. Another reason why hard-of-hearing people don't use the hearing aid they bought is that hearing aids amplify background noise as well as meaningful sound; this can interfere with hearing and can be confusing, irritating, and fatiguing.[2,12,16,29] Nonetheless, almost half (47%) of people who bought hearing aids said they were very satisfied and another 37% said they were somewhat satisfied with their hearing aids.[29] Certainly, training in the use and care of a hearing aid is imperative if a new buyer is to use it optimally. Some hearing aids have a telecoil or telephone or T switch which uses the magnetic field generated by some telphones to amplify the sound. As hearing aids became smaller, the T switch was omitted from many aids. Recently, strong advocacy for T switch hearing aids has begun within many self-help groups and it is possible that the hearing aid industry will begin again to include the T switch in standard hearing aids.

A number of contemporary hearing aids provide some selective amplification of sound, that is, the hearing aid increases loudness at pitches where the hearing loss is greatest, and decreases loudness in pitch ranges where hearing is best. At the same time they are amplifying sound, some hearing aids now have the capability to screen out selected parts of the background noise which interfere with understanding.

Technology is advancing so quickly that several laboratories are now working on a digital aid which could be fitted more precisely to an individual's particular hearing loss, enhance perceptually important sounds, and automatically reduce extraneous noise.[16]

TELECOMMUNICATION DEVICES FOR THE DEAF (TDD)

A TDD allows hearing-impaired persons to use the telephone, even though they cannot comprehend speech transmitted over a telephone.[2,29] Early TDDs were adapted from railroad teletypes and were large and clumsy. Most TDDs now are no larger than a portable typewriter and can be used with most telephones simply by putting the phone handset onto a special holder on the TDD. The instrument sends electronic signals through the phone system to another phone connected to another TDD. The words appear as running text on a light emitting diode (LED) screen and conversational exchange can take place as directly as by voice, though it is slower. In some states, California for example, legislation mandates that a small fee be added to the bill of every telephone subscriber; the funds accumulated are used to make a free TDD available to every severely hearing-impaired person in the state. Initially, few adventitiously hearing-impaired persons knew about TDDs or realized that they were eligible for a free one. That has changed recently due to the efforts of SHHH and other self-help groups.

In addition, California law has established a relay system. The hearing-impaired person calls the relay operator on the TDD; the relay operator, who is hearing, leaves the TDD line open and calls the hearing recipient on voice phone to transmit the hearing-impaired person's message; the voiced response is relayed by the operator via TDD to the hearing-impaired originator of the call. This is slow compared to direct contact by TDD, but it works.

ASSISTIVE LISTENING DEVICES (ALDs)

Assistive listening systems increase access to understandable sound in large rooms or in groups. FM, infrared (IR), and induction loop systems are used most frequently at the present time.[3,30,31] All of them have been used in, for example, auditoriums, churches, symphony halls, and theaters. All have an advantage over traditional loudspeaker systems because they deliver the sound directly from a microphone to a battery-operated receiver worn by the listener; background noise is effectively eliminated and what is essentially one-on-one communication is established between the speaker or performer and the hearing-impaired person. All of these ALD systems have been adapted for use by individuals as personal instruments to supplement hearing.

Loop Systems

These consist of a microphone used by the speaker, a transmitter, and a loop of wire circling the area where there are hearing-impaired listeners; the area may be large or small. Sound from the microphone induces formation of an electromagnetic field within the loop; this can be picked up by a hearing aid with a T switch or by other receivers responsive to electromagnetic signals. The signal is sometimes uneven and reception is often position-dependent. Audio loops once were used extensively, but their usage decreased as other amplification technologies appeared; presently, however, there seems to be a resurgence in the use of loop systems. The loop can be installed anywhere, even in a car, and small loops can be moved easily from site to site.

FM Systems

FM Systems are wireless systems which use FM radio waves to transmit sound from a battery-operated wireless microphone via a transmitter to a small wireless, battery-operated FM radio receiver equipped with earphones. The signal can reach several hundred feet and is not blocked by physical barriers such as walls; therefore its wearer can move from room to room without losing sound. (AM devices are available and AM radio waves for sound transmission; transmission is blocked by walls and is interfered with by the variety of signals which cause static on AM radios.)

Infrared Systems

Infrared systems are wireless systems which require a microphone whose sound goes to a transmitter where it is changed electrically into an infrared light beam. The signal is picked up by a receiver with earphones worn by the listener. The infrared beam cannot pass through walls or other solid objects (e.g., the person sitting in front of a theatergoer). The quality of sound is particularly fine for music and drama and for this reason it is often used in concert halls or for live theater. FM is cheaper; many prefer infrared.

Systems for Personal Use

Amplifying telephone handsets for hearing-impaired users can be exchanged for the regular handset on most modular phones.[6] They give about a 30 percent amplification of sound and every hearing-impaired person probably should have one on his or her telephone. Increasingly, telephones with such amplifier handsets are available in public places like airports, hotels, bus and train stations, public buildings, and so forth. When these are not present, portable amplifiers are available which are small enough to fit into a purse or briefcase and can be slipped over the receiver of a regular telephone handset to provide additional amplification.

Hard-of-hearing persons often need the TV or radio turned louder than is comfortable for hearing members of the family. FM, IR, loop, or hard wire microphones can be placed onto or attached to the TV or radio. The volume of the radio or TV can be adjusted to a comfortable volume for the hearing members; the hearing-impaired listener can then control the sound level by adjusting the volume on the receiver that she or he is wearing.

Another helpful device is a radio with earphones that has been factory-programmed to tune to TV channel frequencies. The radio can be set to the desired TV channel and sound from that channel will reach the hearing-impaired viewer through the radio earphones. Radio volume can be adjusted to the loudness needed by the hearing-impaired person without interfering with the enjoyment of others in the room.

Closed caption decoders significantly increase the pleasure of TV watching by hearing-impaired persons. The number of captioned TV programs has increased greatly during the last 5 years and captioned programs are an enormous source of pleasure and information. Decoders cost about $200.

As noted above, small, portable FM, IR, and audio loop systems have been developed for individual use. In addition to these, hard wire units are available and can be used on a one-to-one basis. In the hard wire system, the speaker talks into a microphone which is attached by wire to a battery-operated receiver which, in turn, is connected by T switch or direct plug-in to the hearing aid of the listener. There are many permutations of this basic concept.

THE FUTURE

Work is proceeding actively toward the development of digital hearing aids whose amplification can be individualized and whose capability will be substantially more flexible than any aid produced by present technology. For modern-day hearing aids, simple, standardized hearing aid controls are being developed which can be manipulated easily by older, less sure, sometimes arthritic, hands. A cheap, readily replaceable ear mold for contemporary hearing aids also is being designed which will benefit many; ill-fitting molds can result in uncomfortable feedback and sound distortion for the hearing aid wearer and can cause hearing aids to emit embarrassing squeals.

More exotic projects are under way. For example, the cochlear implant, though it is still an experimental and expensive procedure, has restored significant amounts of hearing to many of its recipients. It, or the devices derived from it, may one day become truly an "artificial ear."[17,21] In pilot studies, speech detected by a tiny microphone in a pair of eyeglasses has been decoded electronically and transmitted as cued speech symbols visible on one lens of the glasses. Speech transmission via vibrotactile units worn on the arms or trunk of the hearing-impaired person is under active investigation. Interactive video discs are being thought of in relation to the communication and learning needs of hard-of-hearing and deaf persons. The video discs, which are read by laser, can be stopped and queried by the viewer and are programmed to access an enormous menu of networked information from which it can respond appropriately. Speech-to-text-and text-to-speech technologies are also progressing rapidly. Though the primary purpose of their development is not to assist hearing-impaired persons, it is not impossible that they will be adapted for use by the hearing-impaired by early in the next century.

CONCLUSION

Interference with communication is the primary "lesion" created by hearing loss. Loneliness, stress-related tension, fatigue, withdrawal from previously enjoyed activities, deprivation of needed information, anger, lowered self-esteem, depression, loss of easy intimacy—all these happen too often to persons who are adventitiously hard of hearing or deaf, whether they are old or young. Improvement of the communication skills of these persons must be a primary goal of health care professionals who work with them. The prevalence of hearing impairment is high in older adults. Physicians and other health care professionals *do* want each of their patients to have as satisfying a life as possible. No-cost, low-cost, moderate-cost, and high-cost remediations, whether based on advanced technology or on refined human skills, *are* possible. Practical information about the persons, techniques, skills, devices, and procedures available in the area where they live *can* be given to hearing-impaired older persons and *can* help them cope with their hearing impairments.

One hopes that, increasingly, this will happen.

REFERENCES

1. Alpiner, J.G. (1982). Rehabilitation of the geriatric client. In J.G. Alpiner (Ed.), *Handbook of adult rehabilitative audiology* (pp. 160–208). Baltimore: Williams & Wilkins.
2. American Speech and Hearing Association. (1984) The epidemiology of hearing loss: Incidence and prevalence. In P.S. Williams, M.L. Ortenza, and L. Jacobs-Condit (Eds.), *Management of hearing impairment in older adults* (pp 10–25). Rockville, MD: American Speech-Language-Hearing Association.
3. Bergman, M. (1983). Assistive listening devices, Part 1. New responsibility. *ASHA, 25,* 19.
4. Bornstein, H., and Jordan, I.K. (1984). *Functional signs: A new approach from simple to complex.* Baltimore: University Park Press.
5. Davis, H. (1978). Acoustics and psychoacoustics. In H. Davis and S.R. Silverman (Eds.), *Hearing and deafness* (pp. 8–45). 4th ed. New York: Holt, Rinehart & Winston.
6. DiePietro, L., Williams, P., and Kaplan, H. (1984). *Alerting and communication devices for hearing-impaired people; what's available now.* Washington, D.C.: Gallaudet University, National Information Center.
7. Glass, L.E. (1985). Psychosocial aspects of hearing loss in adulthood. In H. Orlans (Ed.), *Adjustment to adult hearing loss* (pp. 167–178). San Diego: College-Hill Press.
8. Herbst, K.G. (1983). Psychosocial consequences of disorders of hearing in the elderly. In R. Hinchcliffe (Ed.), *Hearing and balance in the elderly* (pp. 174–200). Edinburgh: Churchill Livingstone.
9. Hull, R.H. (Ed.). (1982). *Rehabilitative audiology.* New York: Grune & Stratton.
10. Humphries, T., Padden, C., and O'Rourke, T.J. (1981). *A basic course in American sign language.* Silver Spring, MD: T.J. Publishers.
11. Johnsson, L.G., and Hawkins, J.E. Jr. (1979). Age-related degeneration of the inner ear. In S.S. Han and D.H. Coons (Eds.), *Special senses in aging* (pp. 119–135). Ann Arbor, MI: University of Michigan, Institute of Gerontology.
12. Kaplan, H. (1985). Benefits and limitations of amplification and speech reading for the elderly. In H. Orlans (Ed.), *Adjustment to adult hearing loss* (pp. 85–98). San Diego: College-Hill Press.
13. Kyle, J.G., Jones, L.G., and Wood, P.L. (1985). Adjustment to acquired hearing loss: A working model. In H. Orlans (Ed.), *Adjustment to adult hearing loss* (pp. 118–138). San Diego: College-Hill Press.
14. La Plante, M.P. (1988). Data on disability from the National Health Interview Survey 1983–85. An InfoUse Report. Washington, D.C.: U.S. National Institute on Disability and Rehabilitation Research.

15. Levine, E. (1960). Progressive and sudden hearing loss. In E. Levine (Ed.), *Psychology of deafness* (pp. 56–74). New York: Columbia University Press.
16. Levitt, H., et al. (1986). A digital master hearing aid. *J. Rehabil. Res. Dev. 23,* 79.
17. Loeb, G.E. (1985). Functional replacement of the ear. *Sci. Am. 252,* 1104.
18. Luey, H.S. and Per-Lee, M.S. (1983). *What should I do now? Problems and adaptations of the deafened adult.* Washington, D.C.: Gallaudet College, The National Academy.
19. Nitchie, E.H. (1950). *New lessons in lip reading.* New York: Lippincott.
20. O'Neill, J.J., and Oyer, H.J. (1961). *Visual communication for the hard of hearing.* Englewood Cliffs, NJ: Prentice-Hall.
21. Owens, E. (1985). Cochlear implants. In J. Jerger (Ed.), *Hearing disorders in adults* (pp. 221–261). San Diego: College-Hill Press.
22. Ramsdell, D.A. (1978). Psychology of the hard-of-hearing and the deafened adult. In H. Davis and S.R. Silverman (Eds.), *Hearing and deafness* (pp. 499–510). New York: Holt, Rinehart & Winston.
23. Riekehof, L.L. (1983). *The joy of signing,* rev. ed. Springfield, MO: Gospel Publishing House.
24. Ries, P.W. (1985). The demography of hearing loss. In H. Orlans (Ed.), *Adjustment to adult hearing loss* (pp. 3–21). San Diego: College-Hill Press.
25. Schuknecht, H.F. (1964). Further observations on the pathology of presbycusis. *Arch. Otolaryngol. 80,* 369.
26. Sutherland, V.C. (1987). Drug history. In H. Elliott, L.E. Glass, and J.W. Evans (Eds.), *Mental health assessment of deaf clients: A practical manual.* Boston: College-Hill Press/Little, Brown.
27. *Tips for talking with the hard of hearing.* San Francisco: Hearing Society for the Bay Area, Inc., 20 Tenth Street, 2nd floor, San Francisco, CA 94103.
28. Turner, A. (1988). Cued speech: An aid to speechreading. *Shhh Journal.* Special Issue on Alternative Communication, January/February, 8.
29. U.S. Congress, Office of Technology Assessment. (1986). *Hearing impairment and elderly people—A background paper,* OTA-BP-BA-30. Washington, D.C.: Government Printing Office.
30. Vaughn, G.R., and Lightfoot, R.K. (1983). Assistive listening devices, Part 11. Large area sound systems. *ASHA, 25,* 25–30.
31. Vaughn, G.R., Lightfoot, R.K., and Gibbs, S.D. (1983). Assistive listening devices, Part 111. Space. *ASHA, 25,* 33–46.
32. Ventry, I.M., and Weinstein, B.E. (1982). Hearing handicap inventory for the elderly: a new tool. *Ear Hear., 3,* 128–134.
33. Ventry, I.M., and Weinstein, B.E. (1983). Identification of elderly people with hearing problems. *ASHA, 25,* 37–42.
34. Weinstein, B.E., and Ventry, I.M. (1982). Hearing impairment and social isolation in the elderly. *J. Speech Hear. Res., 25,* 593–599.

A MINI-LIST OF RESOURCES*

Self Help for Hard of Hearing People, Inc. (SHHH)
7800 Wisconsin Avenue
Bethesda, MD 20814
Telephone: (301) 657-2248 (Voice)   (301) 657-2249 (TDD†)

National Information Center on Deafness
Gallaudet University
800 Florida Avenue, NE
Washington, D.C. 20002
Telephone: (202) 651-5109 (Voice)   (202) 651-5976 (TDD†)

American Speech-Language-Hearing Association (ASHA)
10801 Rockville Pike
Rockville, MD 10852
Telephone: (301) 897-5700

National Center on Technology and Aging
University Center on Aging
University of Massachusetts Medical Center
55 Lake Avenue North
Worcester, MA 01655
Telephone: (508) 856-3662

---

*From Glass, L.E. (1988). Hearing. In M. Abramson and P.M. Lovas (Eds.), *Aging and sensory change: An annotated bibliography* (pp. 17–23). Washington, D.C.: The Gerontological Society of America.
†Telecommunication device for the deaf.

CHAPTER 15

Evaluation and Treatment of Depression

MICHAEL PLOPPER

The effective rehabilitation of the older patient with chronic, disabling illness often depends upon adequate evaluation and treatment of depression. The presence of depression in the older rehabilitation patient can influence motivation, concentration, intellectual function, memory, and the capacity for learning. Depression also affects energy, sleep, appetite, as well as the course of the physical illness for which the patient is in treatment. Depression may either go unrecognized or be considered a natural consequence of chronic illness, leaving the patient less able to maximize rehabilitation potential, or, in some instances, unable to achieve any benefit within the rehabilitation setting.[3] Much of this unnecessary morbidity could be avoided with a sensible treatment plan geared to the specific needs of the patient.

Although depression is by no means inevitable among older rehabilitation patients, its prevalence is considerably higher than among the general elderly population. In a community study of well-functioning adults over the age of sixty, 20 to 25 percent were determined to be at least mildly depressed.[4] A longitudinal study of stroke patients showed 47 percent of acute stroke patients to have a diagnosable depression.[10] The prevalence of depression had increased to 60 percent by 6 months after stroke.[11] While few other studies of the rate of depression among the disabled elderly have been conducted, these findings are representative of the ubiquitous nature of depression in the geriatric rehabilitation setting.

A number of complicating features make accurate diagnosis and treatment of depression in the older rehabilitation patient a particularly difficult task. Depression may be quite obvious or the patient may complain only of physical symptoms. A depressive episode can recur in an individual with a former history of depression, or it may occur for the first time in an individual adapting to the loss of physical function. The patient's depressed mood may be a direct pathophysiologic consequence of the illness, as in hypothyroidism, or conversely, the depressed mood can itself worsen the course of the patient's illness. Sleep and appetite disturbance may represent vegetative symptoms of depression, or they may be physical symptoms of illness. Memory loss might be secondary to an organic brain syndrome or represent reversible cognitive decline in the depressed patient. Careful evaluation of the older rehabilitation patient must address these issues as well as determine the type of depression the patient manifests, the major precipitants, the patient's capacity for change, and the specific treatment modalities most likely to resolve the patient's depression.

TYPES OF DEPRESSION

The categories of depression described in the *Diagnostic and Statistical Manual of Mental Disorders* (DSM III-R)[1] all have relevance to older rehabilitation patients. These categories include (1) Adjustment Disorder with Depression, (2) Dysthymic Disorder, (3) Major Depression, (4) Dementia with Depression, and (5) Organic Mood Syndrome. Because each of these disorders commonly occurs among older rehabilitation patients and because treatment considerations depend on accurate diagnosis, criteria for diagnosis will be described here.

ADJUSTMENT DISORDER WITH DEPRESSION

As indicated by its name, this disorder consists of a depressive reaction to an identifiable psychosocial stressor, for example, the onset of a disabling physical illness that occurs within 3 months of the onset of the stressor. The reaction consists predominately of a depressed mood which is in excess of a normal or expectable reaction to the stressor and/or impairs occupational or social functioning. The depressed mood must not have persisted longer than 6 months to meet this diagnosis. This disorder is the mildest of the categories of depression and usually remits within weeks to months, presumably sooner if treated. The older rehabilitation patient with no prior psychiatric history or history of depression, with an intact social support system, and who becomes actively involved in the rehabilitation process represents the kind of person whose depression will remit as improved levels of adaptation to physical loss occur.

DYSTHYMIC DISORDER

This disorder, formerly known as depressive neurosis, consists of a chronically depressed mood evident for at least 2 years. During this time the patient has not maintained a normal mood for longer than 2 months at a time. While depressed, the patient will have at least two of the following symptoms: (1) altered appetite, (2) altered sleep, (3) fatigue, (4) low self-esteem, (5) poor concentration or difficulty making decisions, or (6) feelings of hopelessness. The Dysthymic Disorder may be a consequence of a preexisting, chronic physical disorder, such as rheumatoid arthritis, and is then specified as Dysthymic Disorder, Secondary Type. The older rehabilitation patient whose dysthymia predates the onset of chronic physical illness (Dysthymic Disorder, Primary Type) represents the most difficult treatment challenge of the diagnostic categories. This patient's depression may have persisted through much of adult life and he or she responds to any stressor in a depressive fashion.

MAJOR DEPRESSION

This disorder is marked by a more acute onset, a greater severity of symptoms, is more dangerous, and is even likely to culminate in a suicide attempt, particularly in person with a chronic physical illness. At least five symptoms must have been evident for at least 2 weeks, one of which is either a depressed mood or loss of interest or pleasure in nearly all activities. The other symptoms may be altered appetite, usually decreased, with significant weight change; altered sleep, usually decreased; psychomotor retardation or agitation; fatigue; feelings of worthlessness or guilt; poor concentration or indecisiveness; and recurrent thoughts of death or suicide. There may, as well, be associated psychotic features of delusions and hallucinations. A major depression may occur as a single episode or it may be recurrent, with full or partial remission between episodes. In some persons, manic episodes occur, consisting of a euphoric mood, grandiosity, pressured speech, racing thoughts, and poor sleep. When a person has just manic episodes or both manic episodes and major depressive episodes, he or she suffers from Bipolar Disorder.

Although this category represents a more severe form of mood disturbance, it is more amenable to treatment by somatic forms of therapy to be described in a later section.

DEMENTIA WITH DEPRESSION

Older patients with dementia may suffer from depression, particularly early in the course of the dementing process, as they remain aware of loss of cognitive function. In some persons, a depressed mood may be the predominant symptom as they successfully hide or deny memory loss. Dementia with Depression may occur in the patient with Alzheimer's disease, with Multi-Infarct Dementia (due to stroke), with dementia secondary to alcoholism, or any of the many other causes of dementia. Dementia with Depression is to be differentiated from depressive pseudodementia, in which the depressed patient, without true dementia, manifests cognitive dysfunction which resolves as the depression remits.

ORGANIC MOOD SYNDROME

When there is evidence for a specific organic factor which is judged to be etiologically related to the depressed mood, the patient is said to suffer from Organic Mood Syndrome, Depressed Type. Typical organic factors include endocrinopathies, particularly hypo- or hyperthyroidism, excessive psychotropic medications, and cerebrovascular accidents, particularly left hemispheric lesions.[12]

The depressive disorders are to be distinguished from normal fluctuations in mood which are not as severe or as longlasting, nor do they produce interference in social functioning. The first three categories, that is, Adjustment Disorder with Depression, Dysthymic Disorder, and Major Depression differ for the most part in duration and severity. Though Major Depression is considered more severe than Dysthymic Disorder, it is more likely to spontaneously remit and is often more amenable to treatment. Robinson et al. followed their stroke patients for 2 years and found that, without treatment, all those patients initially diagnosed as having Major Depression had shown a remission while, as a group, those patients initially diagnosed as having Dysthymic Disorder were not improved.[9] Both of these disorders respond well to treatment; however, the approaches differ.

EVALUATION OF DEPRESSION

There are several elements necessary for accurate diagnosis of depression and development of the treatment plan for the older rehabilitation patient. A *complete* clinical interview must be conducted and it often is wise to see the patient more than once prior to formulating a diagnosis and treatment plan. A second visit, preferably at a different time of day than the first, provides information as to the persistence and pervasiveness of the patient's mood, whether there is diurnal variation, and whether cognitive function varies. An outside history from an interested family member or friend should be obtained whenever possible, with the permission of the patient, to provide perspective and additional information. Input from members of the treatment team in the rehabilitation setting is essential to answering the questions necessary for an accurate diagnosis and for determining responsiveness of the patient to treatment.

MEDICAL HISTORY AND CURRENT PHYSICAL STATE

It is usually helpful to begin the interview with a focus on the medical, rather than emotional, components of the older patient's illness. The patient may feel more comfortable talking about medical symptoms and history and appreciate that the interviewer understands what he or she has experienced. By reviewing past illnesses and hospitalizations, as well as the illness for which the patient is in treatment, the interviewer can begin to understand how the patient has responded to physical illness. The person who suddenly develops a disabling illness in late life, and who has had little former experience with physical illness, may show a more depressive response than one who has had former serious illnesses and hospitalizations. The latter patient has been in the position of being reliant upon physicians, nurses, therapists, and family members, and therefore has coped, hopefully successfully, with enforced dependency. The interviewer, therefore, while attempting to accurately diagnose the patient's depression, should also be formulating an understanding of the patient's usual coping mechanisms in order to conduct more meaningful psychotherapy when treatment commences.

Masked Depression

In many older rehabilitation patients, depression may present without strong emotional display but rather with physical complaints, often multiple, which "mask" the depression.[5] The older patient may minimize or frankly deny emotional distress while expressing great discomfort with headache, back pain, abdominal pain, or any number of other complaints. The interviewer is faced with the task of validating these symptoms for the patient while trying to determine whether they represent *depressive equivalents* or, instead, manifestations of the patient's physical illness. If the symptoms are of an intensity or duration which are out of keeping with the physical illness, they more likely represent depressive equivalents. The same is true if the illness improves or stabilizes and the somatic complaints persist. For the patient in whom the approximate date of onset of a depressed mood may be determined, the depressed mood may predate the onset of somatic symptoms. Most often, and even with the patient denying a depressed mood, there is evidence through outside history or the patient's clinical presentation that the patient is depressed. The patient may *look* depressed. Sad facies, slowed physical movements out of keeping with the patient's disability, poor eye contact, lack of attention to hygiene or dress, all point to depression. A final determination as to whether somatic complaints represent depressive equivalents may have to wait until treatment has commenced and the depression remits, the patient then reporting improved physical as well as emotional well-being.

Vegetative Signs

The presence of vegetative and physical signs of depression have important ramifications for treatment and merit careful evaluation. These signs may again be difficult to differentiate from the physical sequelae of the patient's illness or from side effects of a variety of medications. Altered sleep is a consequence of nearly any serious physical illness and at the same time is a hallmark symptom of Major Depression. Late-night insomnia and awakening in the middle of the night are common in both physical illness and depression, while early morning awakening, that is, arising 1 to 2 hours earlier than normal on a regular basis, is more specific for a major depression. Altered appetite should be accompanied by measurable weight loss or gain in order to be considered significant. Fatigue, constipation, and loss of libido are common but relatively nonspecific vegetative symptoms. Psychomotor retardation is an important sign in Major Depression but must be differentiated from the bradykinesia of parkinsonism, fatigue, or the consequences of stroke or congestive heart failure. Psychomotor agitation in the depressed patient is most often accompanied by complaints of anxiety and behavior such as pacing or hand wringing rather than the less organized motor restlessness seen in head injury or following cerebral hemorrhage.

MEDICALLY INDUCED DEPRESSION

As mentioned earlier, when a specific organic factor is judged to be the cause of the patient's depressed mood, the proper diagnosis is Organic Mood Disorder. This determination is rarely easy to make and most often a patient presents primarily with a depressed mood, usually with vegetative symptoms, and one or more physical illnesses. In addition to the disorders mentioned earlier, pancreatic carcinoma and certain viral infections may present with depression and little apparent physical dysfunction. Excessive or inappropriate use of any psychotropic medication may produce depression and a careful analysis of all medications the patient may be taking, including over-the-counter medications, is necessary.

PERSONAL HISTORY AND PRESENT MENTAL STATE

The patient's personal history should include inquiry into possible prior depressive episodes, treated or untreated, or other psychiatric disturbance. If the patient has had former treatment, an exploration of what has worked or not worked, particularly regarding antidepressant medication, helps narrow the choice of treatment modalities. The patient should be asked about a family history for depression or alcoholism, as each may predispose the patient to depression. A description of the patient's personal habits including diet, smoking, exercise, and particularly alcohol consumption, is essential to the development of a treatment plan. Alcohol is a major contributor to depression in late life, and, if the patient is alcoholic, all other forms of treatment will be of no value until the patient achieves sobriety.

Mood

Whether or not the patient has difficulty expressing his or her distress in emotional terms, an exploration of the patient's feeling tone is necessary. If reluctant early on, he or she may be more inclined to discuss emotional factors after a full description of physical symptoms has been completed. More important than the patient applying the right terms to his or her feeling tone is the notion that the patient and treating person understand each other and what it is the patient wants to change. For the purposes of diagnosis, a sense of low self-esteem, anhedonia, and particularly, a sense of hopelessness, leave little doubt as to the presence of depression. The patient should be asked whether his or her mood or functioning varies over the course of the day on a predictable basis, that is, reflective of a diurnal variation in mood. Most often the patient will find that the mornings are the most vulnerable time. This diurnal variation is a good predictor of a Major Depression that will respond to antidepressant medication. A depressed older patient should always be asked about suicidal ideation because the older person with physical illness is more likely than any other category of patients to actually commit suicide.[2]

Cognition

The older depressed patient may complain of memory loss, and in some patients, this may be the chief complaint. Unless the presence of depression is carefully looked for, the patient may be mistakenly diagnosed as having an organic brain syndrome. The process of differentiating this so-called depressive pseudodementia from the patient with true dementia includes a careful history and mental status examination.[13] The patient with pseudodementia may complain more of memory disturbance, whereas the demented patient will often try to hide dysfunction. The depressed patient may not try very hard on cognitive testing whereas the demented patient will struggle to perform. The depressed patient may give a more variable performance on repeat testing while the demented patient demonstrates more consistent cognitive loss. By history, the depressed patient's cognitive decline may be more acute and the depressed mood often predates the onset of cognitive loss. There may be a prior history of depressive episodes and/or family history of depression with the depressed patient. Often the depressed patient's apparent decline in memory can be attributed to poor concentration and inattention, leading to misplaced items or the forgetting of the content of a television show or newspaper article. As mentioned earlier, dementia and depression may coexist and this further complicates the differential diagnosis.

Personality and Coping Mechanisms

The interviewer, after evaluating the foregoing information, should have some idea of how the patient copes with his or her physical disability and its attendant loss of function. The presentation of depression will manifest itself differently in individuals with different personalities and coping mechanisms, and therefore an understanding of these unconscious defensive strategies help in accurate diagnosis and treatment planning. The patient may utilize *denial* as a coping mechanism and therefore have difficulty dealing with the reality of the loss of function. Some measure of denial, particularly early in the rehabilitation process, may, however, help the patient to put forth maximum effort in physical rehabilitation. Usually, unless denial is the predominant method of coping for the patient, there is a gradual meddling of hope and reality that allows the patient to come to terms with physical disability. For those in whom denial is an unhealthy defensive strategy, there may be excessive use of depressive equivalents to explain their dysfunction, impeding rehabilitation efforts. Headache or bowel pain, for example, may prevent them from participating fully in therapies.

Some patients may unconsciously utilize *projection* as a coping or defense mechanism, and rather than deal with their own loss of mastery or control secondary to physical disability, will blame others for usurping that control. These patients may have great difficulty forming a therapeutic alliance with caregivers and may sense rejection at every turn. Power struggles may ensue as patients insist on controlling interactions. While it is helpful to give all patients in rehabilitation some measure of control and choice in their rehabilitation efforts, these patients may need particular strategies to remove areas of conflict and allow more realistic coping with loss.

Other patients, when placed in a position of enforced dependency, may utilize *regression* as a coping mechanism and become excessively dependent, forcing caregivers to do for them and slowing the process of rehabilitation.

A certain measure of regression is healthy when one is physically ill and placed in the care of others, allowing temporary and partial dependency without conflict. The excessively dependent patient, however, poses a particularly difficult treatment challenge.

Dealing with these mechanisms and the promotion of healthier strategies are discussed in the next section.

TREATMENT OF DEPRESSION

The effective treatment of the depressed older rehabilitation patient requires a multifocal approach, including psychotherapy, family and social intervention, and somatic therapies when indicated. Medication usually does not work as well alone as it does when combined with psychosocial intervention.

PSYCHOTHERAPY

Older persons, in general, represent good candidates for psychotherapy,[8] and depressed older rehabilitation patients are no exception. All but severely demented patients may benefit from psychotherapy of one form or another. Obviously, intensive psychodynamic psychotherapy is unrealistic in the rehabilitation setting, but time-limited focused psychotherapy tailored to the specific needs of the patient can be quite useful. In a sense, any caregiver who talks to the patient engages in psychotherapy, and therefore all members of the treatment team should be aware of the identified problems of the patient, the goals, and the treatment plan as to the patient's depression.

A number of important themes emerge during the process of psychotherapy with older rehabilitation patients. With the onset of disabling illness in late life, patients must deal with adjusted family roles and body image changes, which, for some, are overwhelming. Patients are forced to accept a measure of dependency on spouses or children and must be assisted to tolerate this change in role while attempting to restore function. Patients must be helped to accept physical change without shame and to maintain a level of intimacy with spouses. The meaning of the functional loss should be explored openly with patients so that they may adequately grieve the loss while still restoring function. Some persons have difficulty tolerating the notion that something they used to do well will now not be done as well. A stroke with hemiparesis has a different meaning to a tuna fisherman who may be far more troubled by loss of physical vigor than to an accountant, who may be more concerned about visual agnosia or apraxia.

Patients should be helped to understand coping mechanisms, which may have been maladaptive, and shift to healthier strategies if they are able. More adaptive coping mechanisms include *anticipation*, or realistic planning for inner discomfort, rather than denying future difficulties. For patients unable as yet to do this, *suppression*, or a conscious decision to postpone attention to a conflict or problem, would be a healthier approach than the unconscious process of denial. *Humor* can help patients bear the unbearable. Sometimes "gallows humor" initiated by patients is a useful substitute for despair, uncomfortable as it may be to some caregivers. *Sublimation* allows patients to channel aggressive impulses through valued substitutes. The retired business executive, used to the competition and pleasure of golf every day, who is suddenly disabled by a stroke, will need to find a meaningful substitute for release of energy and aggression. *Altruism* gives patients the opportunity to focus less on their own losses and express or act upon concern for others. Generally, patients do best when they utilize coping mechanisms they are used to, rather than what treating persons imagine would be good for them. An active process of identifying what has worked for patients in their vocational and family lives as well as when faced with illness, and then enhancing these strategies, provides a framework for conducting psychotherapy with depressed older rehabilitation patients.

FAMILY INTERVENTION

Families must be helped to cope with the patient's dysfunction and altered role within the family. Sometimes, families do too much and inhibit autonomy in patients. Others, particularly families in denial, will overwhelm patients with "never-say-die" enthusiasm. In the process of therapy with families or others in the support system, it is important to allow patients the choice of whom to include or exclude from the process. Old family conflicts tend to re-emerge at times of crisis, and families often need guidance so as to minimize interference and to be allies in patients' rehabilitation. The process of helping families cope with older patients in rehabilitation is dealt with in Chapter 19.

SOMATIC THERAPIES

Antidepressant medications are useful in many older depressed patients. However, they should be used with caution. Antidepressants have a narrow lethal-to-therapeutic dosage ratio, often produce troubling side effects, and in some patients don't work. The only patients in whom they are rarely of value are those with Adjustment Disorder. Most other patients, including those with Organic Mood Disorder,[6] may show response and therefore deserve a trial unless their use is contraindicated. Generally, patients with Major Depression or patients with more significant vegetative signs are most likely to respond to antidepressants. Patients with Dysthymic Disorder may be less likely to respond; however, they also often deserve a trial.

The choice of which antidepressant to utilize depends more on the side effect profile than on any other consideration, unless the patient has shown past responsiveness to a particular medication. Among the tricyclic antidepressants, the secondary amines, such as nortriptyline and desipramine, have less anticholinergic side effects such as dry mouth, urinary retention, and constipation than do the tertiary amines, such as amitriptyline and doxepin, and are therefore preferred in this population. Orthostatic hypotention and sedation are also less likely to occur with the secondary amines. Trazadone has little anticholinergic effect, but is sedating. The monoamine oxidase inhibitors, such as phenelzine, have little use in this population due to their possible hypertensive effect and the need for a strict low tyramine diet. Fluoxetine produces minimal sedation or anticholinergic effect; however, there is as yet little clinical experience with this drug in this population.

Older patients should be started at one-third to one-half the usual adult dose of any of these medications and titrated upward slowly. Plasma levels may be used with nortriptyline, desipramine, and trazadone for determining a therapeutic level or potential toxicity. Any of these medications may take 3 or 4 weeks before significant clinical response occurs, sometimes leading to treatment failure secondary to premature termination of medication.

Lithium carbonate is of most value with Bipolar Disorder, but may be useful as a potentiator of the action of antidepressants. Strict attention to plasma levels is necessary, however, because of the possibility of lithium toxicity. Thyroid extract may also potentiate the action of antidepressants.[7] Electroconvulsive therapy (ECT) is gaining a resurgence in popularity for patients with severe, unresponsive depressions for the simple reason that it is often effective. Temporary memory disturbance does occur with ECT; however, this is lessened by unilateral treatment.

Benzodiazepines, hypnotics, and opioid analgesics should be used with caution and for brief periods of time in this population due to their potential for physical dependence and for their depressant effect.

In general, depressed older rehabilitation patients are quite responsive to treatment. Depression can be removed as a barrier to effective rehabilitation by a sensible treatment plan geared to patients' specific needs and capacity for change.

REFERENCES

1. American Psychiatric Association. (1987). *Diagnostic and statistical manual of mental disorders*, 3rd ed., rev. Washington, D.C.: American Psychiatric Association.
2. Dorpat, T.Z., Anderson, W.F., and Ripley, H.S. (1968). The relationship of physical illness to suicide. In H.L. Resnik (Ed.), *Suicide behaviors: Diagnosis and management* (pp. 209–219). Boston, Little, Brown.
3. Fiebel, J.H., and Springer, C.J. (1982). Depression and failure to resume social activities after stroke. *Arch. Phys. Med. Rehabil., 63,* 276.
4. Gianturco, D.T., and Busse, E.W. (1978). Psychiatric problems encountered during a long-term study of normal aging volunteers. In A.D. Isaacs and F. Post (Eds.), *Studies in Geriatric Psychiatry* (pp. 1–16). London; Wiley.
5. Lesse, S. (1983). The masked depression syndrome—results of a seventeen year clinical study. *Am. J. Psychother. 37,* 456.
6. Lipsey, J.R., et al. (1984). Nortriptyline treatment of post-stroke depression: A double blind study. *Lancet 1,* 297.
7. Louie, A.K., and Meltzer, H.Y. (1984). Lithium potentiation of antidepressant treatment. *J. Clin. Psychopharmacol., 4,* 316.
8. Nemiroff, R.A., and Colarusso, C.A. (1985). *The race against time: Psychotherapy and psychoanalysis in the second half of life.* New York: Plenum Press.
9. Robinson, R.G., Bolduc, P., and Price, T.R. (1987). A two year longitudinal study of post-stroke depression: Diagnosis and outcome at one and two year follow-up. *Stroke, 18,* 837.
10. Robinson, R.G., et al. (1983). A two year longitudinal study of post-stroke mood disorders: Findings during the initial evaluation. *Stroke, 14,* 736.
11. Robinson, R.G., Starr, L.B., and Price, T.R. (1984). A two year longitudinal study of post-stroke mood disorders: Prevalence and duration at six months follow-up. *Br. J. Psychiatry, 144,* 256–262.
12. Starkstein, S.E., Robinson, R.G., and Price, T.R. (1988). Comparison of patients with and without poststroke major depression matched for size and location of lesion. *Arch. Gen. Psychiatry, 45,* 247.
13. Wells, C.E. (1979). Pseudodementia. *Am. J. Psychiatry, 136,* 895.

CHAPTER 16

Treating Mental Health Conditions in the Rehabilitative Setting

DOMINICK ADDARIO

Demographic, economic, clinical, and humanitarian considerations impact on the care of the elderly. No single area of medicine illustrates this impact more than mental health issues. Proper assessment, diagnosis, and treatment of behavioral illnesses determine rehabilitation potential and outcome. This chapter presents an overview of pertinent problems and approaches to elderly patients with mental health problems. The topic of depression is more fully covered in Chapter 15.

DEMOGRAPHIC ISSUES

Nearly 25 percent of a cross section of community-dwelling elderly have symptomatic mental illness, including 10 percent with significant depression and 5 percent with dementia.[10] Studies have shown that 20 percent of older persons living at home receive psychotropic medication. Of that 20 percent, only 1 percent were under the care of a psychiatrist for counseling.[11]

At the other end of the spectrum, estimates of the American Health Care Association show that approximately 5 million Americans 65 and older need nursing home care. At present growth that figure will be 18 million persons by the year 2040. Today, 20 percent of persons 85 years old and above reside in nursing homes or hospitals for the chronically ill.[8] Common problems leading to nursing home admissions are falls, inability to care for oneself, confusion, bone fractures, stroke, incontinence, and behavioral difficulties. It is clearly apparent that primary or secondary psychiatric factors such as dementia, depression, paranoia, and/or psychosocial breakdown in caregiver systems play a major role in institutional placement.

A study using a standardized interview by Rovner et al.[13] at Johns Hopkins found that 94 percent of a random sample of residents at a large, intermediate care nursing home had mental disorders according to DMS-III-R criteria.[2] Primary Degenerative Dementia (56%) and Multi-Infarct Dementia (18%) were the most common diagnoses. Demented and nondemented patients with delusions and hallucinations were more likely to have associated behavioral disorder. Mood disorder with and without dementia involved 28 percent of the population. Only 6 percent had no psychiatric diagnoses.

In between these two populations, a cross-sectioned sample of older persons and those residing in nursing homes, is a third group with significant mental health problems and needs. This group consists of older individuals with chronic physical illness and disability. Mental problems are high in this group and often go unrecognized.

Humanistic, pragmatic, and economic implications of proper diagnostic and treatment approaches to mental health problems serve to enhance rehabilitation potential while reducing behavioral disturbance, psychiatric morbidity, and the likelihood of institutionalization.[19]

ISSUES AFFECTING RECOGNITION, DIAGNOSIS, AND TREATMENT

Older persons do not receive adequate treatment for behavioral health problems. Why does the problem of adequacy of treatment exist? The following are causative factors in the delay of treatment of diagnosis on the part of the patient, family, and health care provider.

1. Factors in the elderly patient causing delay in care:
   a. Cognitive factors preclude the elderly patient's awareness that there is need.
   b. Elderly patients associate growing old with discomfort and unhappiness and cannot differentiate existential stereotypes of aging

with emotional illness, such as depression.

c. Elderly persons fear that psychiatric diagnosis will lead to pejorative labels by health personnel and further their sense of disenfranchisement from society.

2. Factors in families causing delay in diagnosis and teatment of mental health problems[17]:

a. Families often share the same misbeliefs of aging and often mistakenly interpret psychiatric illness as old age.

b. Families often need to maintain an idealized view of the parent, fostering denial of psychiatric illness in favor of somatic diagnoses, mistaking "weakness" for illness.

c. Families fear that a diagnosis of a psychiatric problem will threaten them with having to assume a parental role in the care of an intimidating elderly parent who may not relinquish authority, even at time of need.

d. Families fear that acknowledging an emotional illness such as depression might implicate them as a causative or contributing factor, and thus choose to ignore the signs.

3. Factors in professionals causing delay in diagnosis and treatment of mental health problems:

a. Professionals may view psychiatric symptoms as part of aging and neglect to treat.[5]

b. Professionals have historically little training with elderly patients, and in diagnosing mental health problems.

c. Professionals may incorrectly perceive mental problems in older persons as being treatment-resistant and/or having a poor prognosis and fear being defeated in their attempts to help, so they don't try.

d. Professionals avoid counseling the elderly patient if issues such as aging, loss of spouse, and loneliness trigger the professional's own sense of vulnerability.

e. Professionals avoid helpless feelings in elderly patients (often as part of psychiatric illness) due to projected anger at the patient arising from the threat to the professional's own omnipotence.

f. Professionals feel pressured by the demands of others to try "quick" remedies, such as drugs first, often before correct diagnosis of behavioral symptoms has been made.

ASSESSMENT GUIDES TO DIAGNOSIS

Mental health problems are frequently misdiagnosed in older persons and thus go untreated or poorly treated. Proper assessment requires following some simple rules.

1. *Rule of threes.* Obtain a good history of the patient's functional level 3 days, 3 months, and 3 years prior to the current assessment. Onset factors also aid in diagnosis. For instance, insidious decline suggests Primary Degenerative Dementia (Alzheimer type); subacute changes suggest possible depression or cerebrvascular problems; acute changes suggest medical illness leading to behavioral change, such as diuretic-induced hyponatremia, or an acute viral illness.[18]

2. *Past medical history.* Many medical conditions have profound behavioral effects. Illnesses causing pain, such as degenerative arthritis, can cause insomnia. Parkinsonism and other illnesses have a high incidence of secondary depression. Medications (e.g. levodopa) can induce a chemically based paranoia.

3. *"Bag test."* Especially in outpatients, knowing all prescribed and over-the-counter medications is critical to proper evaluation. Request outpatients to put all such medication in a bag and bring it in for the evaluation. This approach tells what medications they are taking; it also reveals their attitudes and knowledge about their medications. Many patients have been on medication for 2 or 3 years. If asked whether it helps, many say no, suggesting a blind compliance. Medicines tell how many physicians they see, and if six different vials with six different physicians' names are present, poorly coordinated care, mistrust, or "doctor shopping" is evident. It also suggests that the patient is managing his or her own case. It is then necessary to decide which medications are lifesaving, and which are simply symptomatic. Usually about 50 percent of the medications are simply for symptomatic treatment.

4. *Quiet.* Always examine a patient's mental state and conduct the interview process in a quiet room, allowing for a therapeutic alliance to develop through interest, empathy, and trust. A noisy, distracting, and nonprivate environment greatly limits obtaining pertinent information and making accurate observations of mental function.[1,6]

5. *Family interview.* All too often patients are evaluated either in facilities or on an outpatient basis, and a history from the family is not obtained. Once permission of the patient is obtained, interview of the family is essential. First, assess caretaking skills of those who are helping. If there has been burnout, alienation, hostility, or a history of conflict between patient and caretaker, things rarely get better. If relationships were good before the illness was diagnosed, and tended to create cohesiveness, there may be few significant problems; but if families were problematic and conflict-laden before the illness, it will rarely improve after. Elderly patients who

refuse to accept the forced dependency in the sick role can sabotage the caretaker through power struggle.
6. *Treatment history.* It is important to assess all previous mental health problems as well as treatments. Many patients will be unable or unwilling to discuss previous problems at the initial interview with a new physician. Some patients may not relate their previous mental health problems in today's terms. Knowing the level of previous care is important. Has the patient seen someone who is interested in geriatrics? You can get an appraisal of a previous physician's care by discussing the case with him or her. If you receive a superficial level of interaction about the patient, you can suspect that the patient may not have had a thorough previous evaluation. If a patient is adoring and testifies how wonderful it is that you are seeing him or her, going on to criticize previous treating physicians they have seen, sooner or later the scene will probably repeat itself. Avoid the defeat and hostility that follows and understand the problems in delivering appropriate care to such a patient.

MENTAL STATUS EVALUATION AND TREATMENT ISSUES

Care in assessing the older person's mental health problems is essential. Older persons often display illnesses differently from younger persons, often have multiple contributing factors, and often respond to treatment differently. The following paragraphs give suggestions for both assessment and treatment of conditions frequently seen in rehabilitation settings.

COGNITIVE DYSFUNCTION

Cognitive dysfunction refers to impairment of mental alertness, confusion, impairment of recent memory, and impairment of orientation. Use of the mini-mental status questionnaire (MMS)[6] standardizes the evaluation, and is easy to use. Because the MMS test has simple questions and can offend more defensive patients, or be very difficult for patients of limited functioning, explain the series of questions to be asked, saying that some are simple and some more difficult. It is useful to quantify your assessment with such a tool so that weeks or months later it helps assess exactly your mental function in a standard way. It is essential to evaluate every patient because the incidence of hidden cognitive problems is very high.

The treatment of patients with dementia is covered in Chapter 25. Basically, it centers about a patient with Alzheimer's disease of over 3 years duration who presented for treatment with acute confusion. Medical evaluation demonstrated a recent anemia associated with bleeding from diverticulosis. The reestablishment of a normal hematocrit led to stabilization of this patient's cognitive status. A patient with a previous history of Multi-Infarct Dementia developed acute confusion and paranoia. Observation by nursing staff of a seizure led to a diagnosis of postictal paranoia and confusion. Control of the seizure disorder, which had been induced by scars on the brain from previous strokes, led to control of the patient's mental status difficulties.

Alzheimer's patients often show significant regression in hospital or rehabilitative settings. This is frequently the result of separation from a familiar environment. Familiarization of the patient with his environment in the presence of supportive family and staff, as well as familiar objects such as bed pillows and personal pajamas and clothing, can be extremely helpful. Objects such as pictures, clocks, and so forth, as well as biographic data easily accessible at the bedstand or posted above the bed, assists the staff in carrying on a conversation and orienting the patient, as well as in developing a closer working relationship with the patient.

At present, primary cognition-enhancing medications are limited. The treatment of secondary manifestations, such as psychosis and depression complicating the illness in Alzheimer patients, continues to be the primary thrust of psychopharmacologic intervention. Studies show that as high as 30 to 50 percent of Alzheimer patients are suffering from associated mood and delusional symptoms. Appropriate control of these symptoms leads to a much enhanced level of functioning, with the patient often able to return home.

DELIRIUM

Delirium is an acute mental disorganization often associated with dementia, but at times often occurring in patients without preexisting cognitive impairments. Episodes of delirium are often brief, lasting 24 to 72 hours. They are usually self-limiting once metabolic and other medical causative factors are diagnosed.

In delirium, impairment of perception is most disturbing with patients frequently experiencing vivid visual hallucinations and tactile disorganization. Patients might characteristically pick at sheets, see things in the room, respond in a hyperalert fashion to their environment, and require a great deal of support or even physical restraints at times to prevent them from injuring themselves.

Delirium constitutes an acute medical emergency and should be quickly evaluated. Evaluation of possible medication toxicity and concurrent acute illness, that is, infection, metabolic problems, and stroke, is necessary. Judicious use of antipsychotic medications can control potentially hazardous behavior. Benzodiazepenes are less desirable than antipsychotics such as haloperidol due to the potential for memory impairment from these medications.

MOOD DISORDERS

Mania, depression, and mood liability with associated anxiety or agitation are common with affective disorder. A number of medical illnesses are also associated with depression (Table 16-1). Often, elderly patients present without complaints of mood disturbance but with serious complains of weight loss, appetite disturbance, and insomnia. Although sleep changes with age are characterized by more frequent awakenings, patients with depression characteristically show marked negativity in the morning, and improve as the day progresses. Patients with sleep reversal often are depressed, characterized by insomnia at night and hypersomnolence during the day.

Table 16-1. *Illness Associated with Mood Disorder*

Endocrine disorders
Hyperthyroidism
Hypothyroidism
Addison's disease
Cushing's disease
Diabetes
Hypoparathyroidism
Hyperparathyroidism
Viral Infections
   Influenza
   Hepatitis
   Viral pneumonia
Collagen and vascular disease
   Systemic lupus
   Rheumatoid disorders
Cancer
   Carcinoma of the pancreas
   Occult carcinoma
CNS disorders
   Parkinson's disease
   Multi-Infarct Dementia
   Alzheimer's disease
   Normal pressure hydrocephalus

(continued)

Table 16.1. *(continued)*

Focal lesions of the nondominant lobe
Subarachnoid hemorrhage
Medication intoxication
    Benzodiazepines
    Beta blockers
Anemia
    Iron deficiency
    Megaloblastic

When changes like these are noted, intervention is critical, as depression represents one of the most treatable disorders in medicine. A wide selection of antidepressants exists today. Antidepressant medication requires 3 to 6 weeks at a therapeutic level to be effective. Older patients customarily tolerate smaller doses and are often started at lower doses, for example, desipramine hydrocholoride 25 mg per day, increasing to 75 mg over a 3-week period, depending on their tolerance and side effects such as dryness of mouth, constipation, and hypotension.[7]

Tricyclic antidepressants without active metabolites, such as desipramine and nortriptyline, are most efficacious in the elderly due to the lack of accumulation of excess amounts of active medications leading to potential toxicity. Patients who do not respond to tricyclic antidepressants often benefit from monamine oxidase inhibitors (MAOIs). These agents act by inhibiting activity of the microsomnal enzyme monamine oxidase (MAO), which intracellularly deaminates norepinephrine, serotonin, and dopamine to inactive metabolites, rendering them ineffective in normal mood function. A special diet restriction to prevent tyramine loading, which leads to a potentially severe hypertensive crisis, is necessary with MAOI antidepressants.

Patients who have good compliance and are able to follow diets without reckless use of medications are good candidates for, and often benefit from, MAOI antidepressants. Caution should be exercised in the use of MAOI medications with other drugs such as cold preparations and tricyclic antidepressants.

The most troublesome adverse effects of antidepressants in the elderly are anticholinergic, cardiovascular, and neurologic. Anticholinergic side effects include blurred vision, constipation, dry mouth, sinus tachycardia, urinary retention, increased or decreased sweating, confusion, and delirium. Cardiovascular side effects include postural hypotension, dizziness, hypertension, sinus tachycardia, premature atrial and ventricular beats. Arrhythmic effects include ECG changes such as ST segment depression and T-wave flattening, or in version and QRS prolongation, and pedal edema. Neurologic side effects include confusion, drowsiness, muscle tremors, twitches, restlessness, and in rare circumstances, seizures associated with overdose or preexisting seizure disorder. On rare occasions precipitation of a psychotic experience such as hallucinations, delusions, and activation of schizophrenic or manic psychosis can occur in patients who are predisposed. Allergic reactions such as rash can also occur.

In clinical practice these medications have a good margin of safety and are quite effective in 65 percent of depressed patients. Blood levels of antidepressants are readily available and should be utilized as a guide to treatment.

Psychotherapeutic intervention, both individually and with the family, is critical in the treatment of depression. Ongoing reassurance to the patient and ventilation of conflicts contributing to depression increase compliance, expedite recovery from the illness, and allow for careful monitoring of medication effects. Patients with no previous history of mood disorder are routinely maintained on antidepressant medication for a 6-month period. At this time medication is tapered and the need for further medication reassessed. Patients with a history of Bipolar Affective Disorder, or who have been resistant to improvement on antidepressants alone, are candidates for lithium carbonate. Other medications used in the treatment of depression, especially in patients with significant medical difficulties or with low energy, or who are intolerant of tricyclic antidepressants, include methylphenidate (Ritalin). There is some evidence that depressed patients with significant medical illness may benefit from methylphenidate. Side effects include anxiety, agitation, and tachycardia.

All depressed patients should be asked if they have a history of suicide attempts, and whether they currently have intention to commit suicide. The assumption that such a question gives the idea to the patient is completely without foundation. A high risk of suicide in indicated by the presence of a realistic suicide plan with the intention to carry it out. An elderly man with a history of social isolation, living alone, alcoholism, and a possible concurrent terminal illness is at great risk. Alcoholism especially heightens the risk. Although women attempt suicide more often than men, it appears that men are more successful in their suicide attempts. Women over age 65 demonstrate a decrease in both suicide attempts and completed suicides. Additional factors which increase the risk of suicide are prior attempts, family history of suicide, anniversary of a loss, the presence of serious medical illness (commonly seen in the elderly), hostility or absence of any strong feelings, withdrawal, remoteness from social supports, and refusal to accept help.

Intervention in regard to suicide attempts include acknowledgement of risk, placing the patient in a safe and supervised environment such as the hospital, continuing monitoring of the patient's mood state and intentions, as well as appropriate support of medication and intensive psychotherapy.

Pseudodementia, a state of mental flatness with difficulty in concentration and thinking, associated with depression, often goes undiagnosed. Patients with pseudodementia, unlike patients with dementia, often complain bitterly about memory deficit, as well as a lack of energy and an inability to carry out tasks. Their affect is flat, and they socially isolate or remove themselves from activities, like the patient with dementia without affective symptoms who appears interactive to his environment and rarely complains of memory deficit difficulties. The proper utilization of antidepressant medications can be extremely dramatic in the improvement of these patients.

PARANOID DISORDERS

Paranoid disorders in the elderly may be primary or secondary. Patients with dementia frequently develop a defensive guardedness and a need to explain through magical reasons their inability to remember events. The loss of keys and personal possessions frequently leads to paranoid rationalizations, which, as a result of ongoing stress or even an inherent biochemical link with the basic dementia, can lead to paranoid psychosis. Acute paranoid reactions are often associated with medical illness or reactions to medications. Sensory deprivation or sleep disturbance associated with concurrent medical illness, pain, or incontinence may also occur. Disturbances in milieu, such as frequent awakenings as a result of a sick roommate, may lead to a progressive exaggeration of paranoid symptoms or frank psychosis in some patients.[9]

Late onset schizophrenia or paraphrenia in elderly patients is characterized by paranoid ideation in the absence of a deterioration in personality such as is seen in schizophrenia. Characteristically, patients with a lifelong history of schizophrenia with onset in adolescence or early adulthood, in fact, show improvement with age. The onset of paranoid ideation, however, in the late fifties and sixties often heralds a syndrome of paranoid ideation with preservation of personality that is difficult to treat. These patients notoriously refuse to enter into treatment and often isolate themselves with elaborate preoccupations.[4]

Physical impairments, such as auditory and visual deficits, significantly increase vulnerability to paranoid disorders. Paranoid disorder in Bipolar Affective Disorder (manic-depressive illness) may be as high as 45 percent of patients with severe auditory handicaps, well above the usual expectations of paranoid symptoms in these patients (10%).[16] Careful screening of sensory functioning in elderly patients can often decrease difficulties with paranoid preoccupations. Maintenance on antipsychotic medications is also helpful. Injectable medications of a long-acting form of fluphenazine (Prolixin) or haloperidol (Haldol) can be of great assistance in these difficult, noncompliant patients.

Effective therapeutic utilization of the court with conservatorships may often assist these patients in getting necessary help and lessening the frustrations of the caregivers through appropriate legal channels. Environmental and personal changes alone are sufficient to ameliorate some symptoms in paranoid patients, although medications are mainly the first line of defense. Patients in rehabilitation settings or in long-term care settings often have a worsening of underlying paranoid ideation. Appropriate use of medications, support of others, positive environment, and reassurance, as well as assistance by staff members to whom the patient may have a special positive relationship, can lessen conflicts and difficulties.

Characterologic rigidity can also lead to paranoid reactions in patients undergoing rehabilitation. A case [paraphrased from 3] illustrating this follows:

An 80-year-old woman was admitted for convalescent hospital rehabilitative care following a hip replacement due to a fall. The patient had been living independently, having been widowed 10 years before. Her general level of daily skills and functioning including driving to friends' homes, playing bridge, and generally experiencing a positive level of functioning. As a result of her loss of ambulation and placement in a nursing home for rehabilitation, she developed an increasing level of anxiety manifested by a paranoid reaction to her environment. Being an autocratic and controlling person requiring an inordinate level of control of her environment premorbidly, the patient became hypercritical of everyone who attempted to assist her. Much of her anguish and fear in regard to her recent losses were projected toward her environment. She made frequent complaints about the staff and physicians, as well as the administrator. She was therefore transferred on two occasions to other facilities. When a psychiatric consultation was requested, the interview led to an initial marked defensiveness and anger at having to see someone for these problems. After the initial evaluation, however, it became quite obvious that the patient was open and willing to talk about her recent losses and fears in this regard. Low-dose antipsychotics were administered to control symptoms relative to fears that people were robbing her, and that her estate, in fact, was being taken away. On antipsychotics and psychotherapeutic interaction, with changes in the milieu that allowed her to have greater control of her environment, the remainder of her course in the skilled nursing facility led to a positive result.[3]

Illness was experienced in this woman through fears of death and loss of control. The potential pain, helplessness, and infirmity provoked a great deal of fear and anxiety. The other patient with a characterologic disorder who is under stress can demonstrate many of the mentioned symptoms.[10]

PERSONALITY DISORDERS

Patients with schizoid personality, characterized by social isolation and withdrawal, frequently do well in later life as they are often isolated and ignored by society. Patients with more paranoid characterologic features often become more problematic with age due to their drawing greater attention to themselves. Patients prone to hypochondriasis often worsen with age due to the ambivalence of their libidinal projection into physical illness and a preoccupation for others to be obsessed with their body and their generalized sense of helplessness. These patients are most benefited by focusing on their interpersonal needs in regard to feelings that they may have of loss, attachment, and love, rather than continuing to focus on their somatic preoccupations.

Patients with obsessive-compulsive personalities in which maintenance of order and control is often exaggerated and maladaptive are at greater risk of unresolved grief reactions and depressive illness. Efforts toward aiding these patients and expanding their general sense of mastery through occupational therapies, recreational therapies, and enhanced staff interaction through the possible use of medications for treatment of frank depression or anxiety are helpful.[14]

Patients with passive-aggressive and dependent personalities often are in a pathologic, ongoing relationship with a spouse or loved one. The loss of these supportive and sacrificing partners in the codependent relationship frequently leads to problems in the rehabilitation setting. Favorable approaches dealing with positive reinforcement for independent activities and an increasing sense of narcissistic awareness and well-being from their own assertiveness and interaction often greatly assists these patients.

OTHER TREATMENT OPTIONS

Psychotherapy is underutilized in the elderly, and staff involvement and support, as well as the use of the psychiatrist to assist in a greater understanding of the case and to promote psychotherapeutic intervention by staff, is extremely critical to motivation and rehabilitative factors in such patients.[14]

The utilization of community self-help groups, formal patient mutual support groups, is not yet fully developed but may be an important area of treatment over the next decade in elderly patients living in residential facilities.

Underutilization of family groups and support services in residential settings today represents a major problem. Families are critical to the recovery and enhanced well-being of the elderly as they are on every other level of interaction. Greater utilization of family support groups and education of families as to caretaker issues will further facilitate and enhance treatment outcome in this population.

SUMMARY

Screening for psychiatric illness in patients admitted to rehabilitation settings is imperative.[12] The awareness of a patient's mental capacity, premorbid and at time of treatment, allows greater understanding of rehabilitation potential and treatment strategies. Appropriate utilization of psychiatric consultation and a positive, optimistic attitude toward intervention for behavioral problems improves prognosis and shortens the length of stay for elderly patients.

REFERENCES

1. Albert, M. (1985). Assessment of cognitive function in the elderly. *Psychosomatics, 25,* 310.
2. American Psychiatric Association. (1987). *Diagnostic and statistical manual of mental disorders,* 3rd ed., rev. Washington, D.C.: American Psychiatric Association.
3. Borson, S., et al. (1987). Psychiatry in the nursing home. *Am. J. Psychiatry, 144,* 1412.
4. Bridge, P.T., and Wyatt, R.J. (1980). Paraphrenia: Paranoid states of late life. *J. Am. Geriatr. Soc., 28,* 1983.
5. Cohen, G.D. (1976). Mental health services and the elderly, needs and options. *Am. J. Psychiatry, 133,* 65.
6. Folstein, M.F., Folstein, S.E., and McHugh, P.R. (1975). Mini-mental state: A practical method for grading the cognitive state of patients for the clinician. *J. Psychiatr. Res., 12,* 189.
7. Lazarus, L.W., Davis, J.M., and Dysken, M.W. (1985). Geriatric depression: A guide to successful therapy. *Geriatrics, 40,* 43.
8. Mayo Clinic Health Letter, Nursing Homes. (1987). Rochester, MN. Mayo Clinic.
9. Miller, B.L., et al. (1986). Late-life paraphrenia: An organic delusional syndrome. *J. Clin. Psychiatry, 47,* 204.
10. Myers, B.S., Kalayam, B., and Meital, V. (1984). Late onset delusional depression: A distinct clinic entity? *J. Clin. Psychiatry, 35,* 347.
11. Ouslander, J.G., and Beck, J.C. (1982). Defining the health problems of the elderly. *Annu. Rev. Public Health, 3,* 55.
12. Robinson, R.G., Lepsey, J.R., and Price, T.R. (1985). Mood disorders in post stroke patients. In C.A. Shamoian (Ed.), *Treatment of affective disorders* (Chap. 6). Washington D.C.: American Psychiatric Press.
13. Rovner, B.W., et al. (1986). Prevalence of mental illness in a community nursing home. *Am. J. Psychiatry, 143,* 1446.

14. Salzman, C. (1982). A primer on geriatric psychopharmacology *Am. J. Psychiatry, 139,* 67.
15. Schamm, L.H., et al. (1987). The neurobehavioral cognitive status examination comparison with the cognitive capacity screening examination and the mini-mental status examination. *Ann. Intern. Med., 107,* 486.
16. Solomon, P., Leiderman, O.H., and Mendelson, J. (1987). Sensory deprivation: A review. *Am. J. Psychiatry, 114,* 357.
17. Steinman, L.A. (1979). Reactivated conflicts with aging parents. In P.K. Ragan (Ed.), *Aging parents* (pp. 126–143). Los Angeles: University of Southern California Press.
18. Stults, B.M. (1984). Preventive health care for the elderly (special issue on personal health maintenance). *West. J. Med., 141,* 832.
19. Zimer, J.G., Watson, N., and Treat, A. (1984). Behavioral problems among patients in skilled nursing facilities. *Am. J. Public Health, 74,* 1118.

CHAPTER 17

Substance Abuse in Older Persons with Disability: Assessment and Treatment

STEVEN D. HOPSON-WALKER

A discussion of substance abuse among older persons touches on two of the three great taboos in our society: sex, death, and drug abuse. This chapter deals with the effects of drug abuse, including alcohol, on older persons. In the lengthy history of substance abuse, aging is a rather recent topic. Fifteen years ago, the average age of alcoholics in treatment was between 35 and 50 years of age. Today the age range has expanded greatly, from 20 to 70 years of age. About 10 percent of older Americans, or about 3 million people, have a substance abuse problem. Men outnumber women at the rate of about 12 to one in alcohol abuse.[1] Prescription drug abuse may be higher in this population since 25 percent of all older Americans take prescription drugs. The primary abused substance for men is alcohol, while for women it is alcohol in combination with sedatives.[1]

A major issue in assessing substance abuse with the older population is that almost all substances remain in the system longer and create dysfunction more readily because of such changes in older persons as decreases in lean body mass and body water, while kidney and liver functions become less efficient.[1] What might be a small amount of diazepam (Valium) for a 24-year-old female may be a harmful, abusive, or addictive amount for a 74-year-old woman. The amount of drug necessary to cause misuse problems for the elderly is therefore much lower than for the younger abuser.[1] The lack of general knowledge of drug effects on older persons among many health professionals is a major problem in this area.

Research indicates that there are two types of alcohol abusers: an early onset group (prior to age 40) and a late onset group. The late onset group makes up about one-third of all abusers.[1] With this later group, the stresses of late life, including chronic illness, seems to increase the level of abuse.[16]

Substance abuse occurs when a person no longer uses the substance for comfort, but uses it to avoid physical or psychic discomfort. Commonly reported reasons for normal substance use are tension reduction, euphoria, or feelings of power and control. Often a person will use various substances to achieve each of these effects. However, when the person begins using substances to avoid physical craving, to deal with acquired increased tolerance, or out of psychologic desperation, they have gone from normal substance use to substance abuse or addiction. At this stage, there are personal and social problems that they also are trying to avoid by the substance abuse. That first drink in the morning now has an entirely different purpose—avoiding discomfort. A disability in late life can produce the physical and psychologic discomfort that increases the risk of substance abuse.

Alcoholism is defined as a progressive disease in which there is physical craving (usually after the first drink), behavioral and cognitive deficits, psychologic dependence, feelings of inadequacy, and significant interpersonal problems.[10] No longer can alcoholism be viewed as only a physical problem because the progressive deficits are clear in all areas of the alcoholic's life: physical, psychologic, and social.[7] The major social problems created by this disease are family and relationship disruptions, legal problems, occupational issues, and financial maladies. By the time the older person usually enters treatment, disruptions due to substance abuse can be documented in all areas if an extensive assessment is conducted.

DIAGNOSTIC ISSUES

UNDERDIAGNOSIS

With the older rehabilitee, we often do not think of possible substance abuse to account for decreased performance. We first look for psychosocial stressors in his or her life, a psychiatric disorder, or a major physical problem. Naively, these performance changes may even be attributed to the normal aging process. Only after every other diagnosis fails do we usually consider the possibility of substance abuse. Generally, professionals in the field have subscribed to the popular view that substance abuse disappears in old age due to maturation or burnout, even though current studies refute this.[4]

Substance abuse and alcoholism can be mistaken for many other diagnoses in older persons. In its later stages, substance abuse creates much confusion and can cause dementia. Many substances can create strong feelings of paranoia. Alcohol withdrawal often contains all of the symptoms of clinical depression or dysthymia; however, after 10 to 20 days of detoxification, it usually clears up. Many substances (cocaine and amphetamines) and alcohol withdrawal can create symptoms of anxiety which can be wrongly diagnosed as Generalized Anxiety Disorder. Substance abuse and withdrawal usually create physical problems, aches, and pains, so a somatoform disorder is often diagnosed. An adjustment disorder to the tasks of aging is often given without considering that the debilitation could be due to substance abuse. A case can be made that some substance abusers are borderline or dependent personalities, but these diagnoses are often given without further assessment of substance abuse issues. In short, we often apply a label to the older rehabilitee's clinical picture without analyzing the causes (often substance abuse) of this picture.

PHYSICAL ASSESSMENT OF SUBSTANCE ABUSE

A proper physical assessment for substance abuse should focus on epigastric distress, loss of appetite, liver dysfunction, kidney problems, neuritis, cognitive deficits, and nutritional deficiencies. Although the normal aging process creates a decrease in organ size and efficiency, substance abuse creates additional problems with all of these functions.

Many substances, when abused, create epigastric distress and a loss of appetite. When the substance is discontinued, the distress diminishes and the appetite returns. With alcohol abuse, cirrhosis may be present, creating a diminished ability to process most drugs and important vitamins and minerals.[16] There will particularly be a deficiency of B vitamins due to the liver dysfunction.

An evident decrease in the renal system's ability to filtrate and secrete waste products is often present. Water retention is often evident in alcohol abuse. In the final stages of some substance abuse, the person loses control over basic bodily functions.

Often with alcohol abuse, the extremities become numb and the person may even speak of "paralysis." Peripheral neuritis has been caused by basic malnutrition and other factors. Generally, the older abuser eats very little or eats a very unbalanced diet; therefore, he or she is often suffering from basic malnutrition.[16]

Finally, there will be numerous neurologic complaints: headaches, memory loss, and a lack of orientation.[8] In the last stages of abuse, more of the substance is needed (more often) to avoid headaches, which are actually signs of the progressive addiction syndrome. Abusers will complain of losing items and not being able to find their way to well-known places in their environment.[16] Overall, most major functions are disrupted by substance abuse, particularly in the later stages of abuse. The appearance is different from the normal aging process because the many functions tend to become impaired simultaneously instead of sequentially and in degrees beyond what normal aging would bring.

PSYCHOLOGIC ASSESSMENT OF SUBSTANCE ABUSE

Since substance abuse can present a problem in differential diagnosis, it is important to review the psychologic assessment tools currently available. Although projective tests can be used, objective personality and intellectual tests have been used more successfully to diagnose substance abuse.

On the Bender-Gestalt test, besides overall signs of organicity, the substance abuser usually draws "dog ears" and tremulous lines. On the Wechsler Adult Intelligence Scale (WAIS), there is usually a large amount of scatter between the subtests, with those tests measuring "old learning" being higher. The most common peaked profiles on the Minnesota Multiphasic Personality Inventory (MMPI) are 27 (depression and anxiety scales) and 49 (psychopathic deviancy and mania scales). One is usually diagnosed as "agitated depression" and the other as "antisocial personality type." Overall, these traditional tools only give us general assistance in diagnosing substance abuse.

The most complete method of assessment is an extensive life history interview, optionally with the family's assistance. Because abusers deny their problems, most questions need to be asked at least twice in different forms. Questions need to cover five areas: drinking history, physical problems, employment and financial history, family and relationship problems, and legal problems. Patterns should be noted and progressive deterioration should be observed. With employment, efforts should be made to acquire factual information about actual job titles and duties; the actual length of employment and the true reason for the job losses should be obtained from records and the family (after appropriate releases are signed). The number of relationships and separations should be noted as possible indicators of previous abuse problems.

Often, in a lengthy substance-abusing relationship, there may have been many separations that are not spoken about. Parent-child resentments and animosities should be recorded. With regard to the legal history, both alcohol- and nonalcohol-related problems should be asked about; besides citations for driving while under the influence and public drunkenness, multiple divorces, child support issues, repossessions, and assaults should be looked at closely.

Several methods can be used to overcome the typical denial in order to obtain an accurate history.[9] One can administer a questionnaire within the first 7 days of treatment and then again 2 weeks later. Questions can be raised about the discrepancies. Another appropriate method is to have family members fill out the same questionnaire and discuss the discrepancies immediately in a family therapy session. In either case, the effects of substance abuse emerge very quickly and the diagnosis becomes clear.

If traditional testing is not useful and the life history analysis is suspect, then there is one more method of assessment to obtain the proper diagnosis. A drug-free environment can be created in a hospital setting for 3 to 7 days. The person can be taken off all mind-altering substances whether they are addictive substances or not. Other medications that have sedating or antidepressant side effects should also be discontinued, if possible.

The person should then be observed for the following changes: If the person is a substance abuser, the previously observed depression, paranoia, and confusion will decrease. Physical complaints will increase due to the withdrawal process, and intellectual skills may improve (memory, old learning, and new learning). Often, anxiety, anger, and guilt will increase during the first 3 days and possibly reappear on a 30-day cycle.[13] These symptoms are a part of the withdrawal-recovery process, which is also a grieving process. In short, many traits that seem diagnostically significant will dissipate after 3 to 7 days in a drug-free environment.

PSYCHOLOGIC DYNAMICS

Substance abusers often exhibit a characteristic pattern of cognitive-behavioral traits. First, the abuser's guilt and anxiety about his or her life is projected onto the environment, including the family members, employers, and others, who are seen to be the cause for all of the person's problems and catastrophes. Second, it is very important for the abuser to be in control of the family agenda, that is, power is an important issue to them; therefore, they manipulate others, socially and emotionally, to get their needs met. Abusers also tend to focus solely on their own needs without considering others. They tend to think that their needs "should" or "must" be met "right now," that is, they tend to be demanding. They also seem to be very suspicious of others due to a lack of confidence and security. This suspicious thinking is a particularly salient characteristic in the later stages of abuse. Another cognitive characteristic is that they tend to have "one-channel" thinking or "tunnel vision." There is only one solution that they adhere to for many different problems, and they will stubbornly maintain this solution in the face of contrary facts. Finally, as Yochelson and Samenow demonstrated, their cognitive processes tend to be "fragmented"; they are unaware that their current statements contradict a statement made minutes earlier.[15] They will often adamantly deny a contradiction and then state another one.

These cognitive patterns create interpersonal characteristics typical of abusers. They are constantly demanding immediate gratification; there is no waiting for long-term solutions or progress toward a goal. They often have many rationalizations to explain their needs, but usually the "need" is based on prior poor planning and problem solving. When others (friends, family members, etc.) look beyond the adult facade, what really is observed is a "temper tantrum" thrown by a "terrible" 2-year-old. The tantrum is dressed in adult language to cover childlike emotional needs.

Substance abusers do have the ability to present themselves in a positive image when it serves their needs, but within a short period, they can be behaving in an antisocial or a negative manner toward others.[14] It is often a mistake to accept the "new leaf" without looking under it; both the gregarious, friendly person and the negative ogre are both faces of abuse—neither should be assumed to have changed while substances are being abused.

The substance abuser also tends to be irresponsible. They cannot be trusted to follow through or to be punctual. In other words, their actions seldom follow their words. Due to this inconsistency, feeling statements should not be believed either; the current feeling can change in an instant depending on the personality of level of abuse. The most predictable statement about them is that they will be unpredictable.

Their problem-solving methods are often very inflexible. They refuse to listen to alternative solutions. They are very fearful of losing control, and new solutions mean new demands are placed on them with the possibility of failure. Along with this, the cornerstone of the substance abuser's personality is denial: denial of substance abuse, denial of problems, denial of caring, and denial of other solutions.[9] "I have no problem, what is wrong with you?" is the common statement heard by friends, family members, and professionals. Until this characteristic pattern is dealt with, no other changes can be expected.

FAMILY DYNAMICS

The families of substance abusers also exhibit some common behaviors.[2,11] Basically, they become the dysfunctional family type that is sometimes called the "old business" family, that is, there are many unresolved conflicts.[12] Most discussions evolve into arguments about past resentments. Such families have great difficulty focusing on the "here and now." Every family member seems to have an investment in not making changes. Everyone has to "win" the argument, when ultimately the substance abuser is always the loser. The families are usually enmeshed, chaotic, and highly emotional. Most past feelings are unresolved, so the result is that every family topic is an explosive minefield.

Another analysis that can be done is to observe and do a check list on the family dynamics. After one or two sessions with the substance abuse family, this check list can easily be done. First, the family members should be observed for being very enmeshed and overly involved in one another's lives. However, one member may have disengaged from the family. Second, such families are neither rigid nor flexible, but are very chaotic in their adaptation patterns; there are many "fires" (emergency problems) with no focus, and the roles and family rules are very confused. Third, their communication is highly emotional and random. Family members frequently make comments from "left field." All discussions are highly charged and frequently lead back to the past. All rational explanations are very superficial and seem to crumble under close questioning. This is a highly dysfunctional family that has learned to argue in a very destructive fashion. It is an old business family: old fears, old resentments, old guilts, old roles, and old games. This family is highly invested in not changing. Except for the one who has disengaged (at times), no one in the family is able to discontinue the destructive process. In conclusion, once a check list of the family's cohesion, adaptability, communication, and old business is completed, the substance abuse dynamics should be clear.

DIFFERENCES WITH OLDER SUBSTANCE ABUSERS

Given the characteristics noted here, there are some variations and differences with older persons. Due to more years of abuse and practice, older abusers often seem more stubborn and more demanding. Also, they often use physical problems as part of their denial or refusal to participate in treatment, claiming not to feel well. Although they often do have some physical limitations, good medical care, family support, and therapeutic guidance usually can overcome these obstacles.

As can be imagined, the older person's family problems, after years of abuse, are much more enmeshed and deeply rooted. The abuser may target one family member as the focus of resentment, and this creates problems for the entire family. It is, therefore, even more important with these families that all members begin to deal with their problems in therapy and Alanon.

As aging advances, substance abuse occurs more quickly and debilitates functioning more readily. In other words, the older person who begins abusing substances later in life usually becomes addicted in a shorter time.[1] This creates more denial on the family's part because the family members have not previously experienced the "abusive" behavior—only the "aging" behavior. In the majority of the cases of older abusers, there have been past indicators of problems, but there is also often a longer history of appropriate functioning in the family and at work. This can present a confusing picture to the therapist and to the family.

With regard to differences in therapy with older abusers, the increased brain damage (such as the Wernicke-Korsakoff syndrome) often makes them less able to function in the usual verbal therapies. The detoxification process can be longer than the traditional 72 hours, and once they enter treatment, the program schedules need to go at a slower pace. This means that they could benefit from a longer stay in either outpatient or inpatient treatment. Older persons adjust quickly to group modes of therapy and these can be very effective.

BASIC GOALS IN THERAPY

PROCESS GOALS

In treating the older substance abuser, family involvement is imperative.[5] Even though process goals may not be discussed with the patient, they need to be clear to the therapist in order to give a direction to the therapeutic endeavor. These goals are the most important ones that assist in restructuring the destructive process of abuse and addiction. Whatever the individual and family dynamics in the past, the overall goal is to discontinue the past patterns and teach new, more productive methods of problem solving and communication.

The first family process goal is to increase *cohesion* so that the family can work together on the substance abuse problem. This goals works against two existing counterproductive forces: disengagement and enmeshment. Most substance abuse families are highly enmeshed and one or more members may have disengaged. The goal is to teach the family members how to work together without taking over one another's roles or responsibilities. This goal also means reincorporating the disengaged into the family system. This will change the old interactions and produce new ones, while decreasing the common family enabling process. Due to the many years of abuse, the most problem solving requires a concerted effort by the entire family.

The second process goal is to, through time, increase the substance abuser's, and the family's *adaptability* to change. The withdrawal and recovery processes bring new problems to a family system that has usually been very chaotic up until now. They seldom have focused on the actual problem and seldom have produced lasting solutions. Consequently, there has usually been continual stressors and a sense of constant failure. This chaos often, at first, changes to a rigidity in solution formulation, but this is a necessary step in reaching the ultimate goals of flexibility in the face of change. Many of the concepts in Alcoholics Anonymous are helpful in changing the family's developed rigidity: "one day at a time," "easy does it," etc.

The final process goal is to increase the family's *communication* so that it is more open and rational. Generally, the substance abuse has created a family pattern of random and highly emotional interactions. Many small, innocuous conversations end in explosive, emotional arguments. Everyone is fighting a battle without knowing the cause. Seemingly rational arguments, when confronted, quickly unravel; there is no focus or resolution in the communication. Most interactions create pain, sadness, and anger. This process goal usually cannot be reached without the assistance of a third party (a therapist), who consistently creates an atmosphere of openness and clear, communicative analysis.

In summary, the general process goals of any therapeutic encounter with an old substance abuser and the family are to increase family cohension, family adaptability, and clear communication.

CONTENT GOALS

When dealing with substance abuse, the most appropriate model of content goals is a problem-solving model.[6] The therapeutic encounter must be consistent, concrete, and to the point. Ethereal discussions of life change benefit this person very little and ultimately lead to increased anger and the termination of therapy.

There are six basic content goals:

1. Reduction of resistance and denial
2. Clarification of the basic problem: abuse
3. Clarification of previous poor solutions
4. Clarification of family goals.
5. Clarification of current problem-solving skills
6. Expansion of family resources

The first step is necessary to help the family cope with the older person's denial about his or her substance abuse. It may take numerous therapeutic sessions to deal with this. Until the person (and the family) admits to the abuse problem, no further goals can be discussed or clarified. The therapist needs to assist the family in being honest and assertive with the abuser. Once the denial subsides, continued clarification of the basic abuse problem will be needed. In other words, the family and abuser often easily lose sight of the never-ending potential for abuse as the person progresses in treatment. If denial cannot be overcome, therapy should be discontinued.

The next content goal is to clarify the family's previous attempts to deal with the abuse problem. The common patterns include avoidance, blaming, enmeshment, disengagement, enabling, and emotional blackmail. What also becomes evident is that the common solutions have become a major problem themselves. It will take much time to have the family see this and to unlearn these interactive solutions and to learn new ones.

The next content goal is to clarify the goals of each family member. Again, these should be as concise and clear as possible. They should be goals that can lead to specific behavioral changes. Each member is required to state at least one goal. Besides the termination of substance abuse, the goals usually center around relationship changes. Other concerns are often about medical, legal, or financial problems. Once these goals are stated, new solutions to them are sought. What are the current family resources: emotional, financial, physical? If the family can focus on their resources with the help of a third party in a rational and open manner, they usually find that they can derive new alternative solutions.

However, there are many times when the old patterns and current solutions are not adequate. The therapist must help the family deal with the addiction and its attendant problems by developing new resources. A necessary adjunct to therapy is always Alcoholics Anonymous (AA) or Alanon. These organizations provide all family members support and direction. Basic behavioral contracts for all members, rehearsals, and periodic emergency conferences are necessary in developing new problem-solving skills for the family. Natural reinforcers (loss of support, money, or health) are usually available to be used by the family in changing the abuser's behavior. The specific methods used to fulfill these six content goals are discussed at length below.

PSYCHOTHERAPY ISSUES

Before specific treatment methods are discussed, a brief overview of psychotherapy parameters is needed so that the different guidelines for treating the older substance abusers can be understood. Psychotherapeutic issues, domains, and types are not completely distinct but are each on a continuum that assists us in observing the overall picture more clearly. There are four basic continua which are listed in Fig. 17-1.

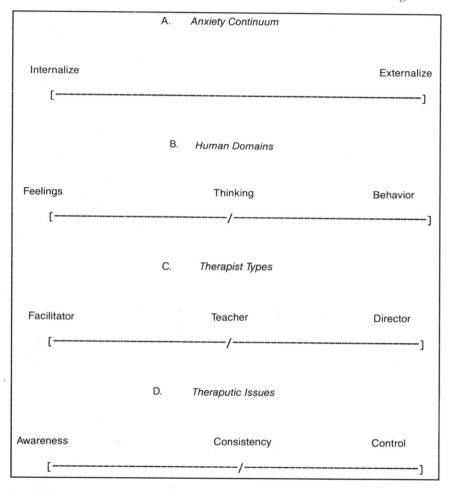

Fig. 17-1. Parameters of psychotherapy.

Differences between diagnostic categories can be stated by utilizing an anxiety (stress) continuum that describes how stress is handled.[3] Substance abusers predominantly externalize their anxiety and blame others. There are three areas of human domain: feeling, thinking, and behavior. Abusers notably deny their feelings and have distorted thinking. The initial goal is to create behavioral changes and then to focus on thinking and feeling changes. Of the three basic therapist types, the facilitator, the teacher, and the director, the director is the type that is necessary in confronting abuse problems. This type of therapist usually requires behavioral consistency and clear examples of progress and change; a continual lack of progress usually means the termination of therapy. Finally, there are three therapeutic issues required for effective therapeutic experiences: awareness, consistency, and control. In dealing with abusers, the major issue is that of maintaining control of the therapeutic situation by utilizing the group or the family. By starting therapy on the right side of the continuum and dealing directly with abuse, the chances of a successful intervention are increased.

KEY AGENTS OF CHANGE

The specific agents of change which work with geriatric substance abusers should be divided into three phases of treatment: the initial phase, the action phase, and the maintenance (or follow-up) phase. The action phase is the longest and most central phase of treatment; it is generally what is described as the therapeutic process. However, without proper initial and maintenance phases, the action phase is usually not effective.

Initial Phase

During this phase, the goal of therapy is to obtain the abuser's full commitment to therapy and behavioral involvement. The first key agent of change is the involvement of other people, that is, family, friends, professionals, or recovering abusers. A group of significant others is generally better at breaking through the abuser's denial and resistance. Individual therapy or intervention is usually not as effective at this point. Many family members and professionals may have tried to help this person before. A group of family members or prior abusers can be much more clear and consistent about the patient's abuse and the multiple problems it has created. Also, the group is necessary to promote behavioral consistency and more adaptive problem solving.

Another important agent of change in family or group therapy during this phase is a clear commitment from all concerned individuals. Every family member must be committed to the therapeutic process; every group member must agree to help this person. Without a clear commitment to spend the needed time and energy on the abuse problem, there will be no consistency, and the enabling behavior of the dissenting party will always disrupt future therapeutic efforts. If no family or group commitment is given, the therapeutic process may have to be terminated at this point.

The third key agent of change during this phase is the confrontation of resistance. The therapist must encourage the family or group not to participate in the denial and resistance, but to quickly point it out. Resistance takes many forms: denial of abuse, denial of relationship problems, denial of financial problems, denial of the need for help, etc. In short, anything that disrupts that therapeutic process of recovery can be viewed as resistance—even what appears to be a "good, logical" argument. Confronting the resistance maintains therapeutic control of a potentially volatile situation.

Action Phase

During the action phase, the therapist should concentrate on the client's abuse problems and other actual problems created by the substance abuse and the problems which may have started the abuse: medical, legal, family, and financial problems. This is the time to educate the abuser and the family about addiction, so that their fear and guilt will subside. Due to the withdrawal process, the abuser's feelings may change on a daily basis and his or her cognitive functions are still impaired. Physical and psychologic withdrawal may continue for several months; therefore, the proper focus is to plan on problem solving and behavioral change for a lengthy period.

Another agent of change in this phase is the creation of cognitive dissonance between the abuser's past behavior and his or her current feelings not to abuse again. If the abuser is not drinking and is helping others, dissonance is created between the past and current lifestyles. Among family members, this dissonance causes a change from their past perceptions of the patient and their typical interactive process. What they would normally do, they cannot, and what they find difficult to do, they must: confront denial, state facts, be honest, be assertive, and be consistent.

The next principle is that the therapist must seldom trust the words of the client and must continually request behavioral demonstrations of stated internal changes or insights. This promotes both therapeutic consistency and control. Since the abuser externalizes anxiety, he or she needs to learn to deal with it in a constructive manner. Therefore, placing demands and difficult tasks before abusers and requiring them to deal with the tasks in group, without reverting to old patterns, is a helpful procedure to promote recovery.

The therapist, with abusers and their families, must continually set boundaries and be concrete and factual. Goals should be clear, simple, and concise. Alternatives should be limited to those that are possible within the family resources: seven AA meetings may not be possible that week if transportation resources are limited. In other words, the therapist must guard the abuser and the group (family) against both pessimism and undue optimism at this stage of recovery. The therapist should encourage them to work with and follow through on one problem at a time. There should be specific family or group contracts for action with specified reinforcements and consequences.

Maintenance Phase

Once the intensive phase of treatment is completed (usually 30 days to 6 months), there are several key factors in continued treatment success. First, the therapist should "hope for the best but expect the worst." In dealing with substance abusers, relapse is the rule and should be expected. By setting appropriate expectations, the therapist is less likely to blame the client for a relapse and will have a better chance for honest appraisals or success. When dealing with families, all members are required to work on recovery and follow through; each member should be confronted with failures to be consistent—no one gets "off the hook." Abuse requires continued therapeutic vigilance at all times.

If resistance re-emerges and all interventions have failed, paradoxical intention might be used. For example, the therapist might say, "I guess this situation is hopeless; we might as well let her have another drink." This usually restates the actual danger, and the family will begin mobilizing itself again. The family or group should be taught that emergency meetings are also a key to dealing with the many crises of recovery. Extra therapy sessions may be required. The critical point of the maintenance phase is that the recovering family or group system discovers that it is always stronger than any one person, including the therapist. The family system in many respects becomes used to providing the treatment and the individual therapist helps the family to help the abuser.

REFERENCES

1. Atkinson, R., and Kofoed, L. (1983). Alcohol and drug abuse in old age: A clinical perspective. *Subst. Alcohol Actions Misuse, 3,* 353.

2. Cicirelli, V.G. (1983). Adult children and their elderly parents. In T.H. Brubaker (Ed.), *Family relationships in later life* (pp. 31–46). Beverly Hills, CA: Sage Publications.
3. Cutter, F. Problem solving roles as alcohol treatment. Presented to Western Psychological Association, April 1975.
4. Drew, L.R. (1968). Alcoholism as a self-limiting disease. *Q. J. Stud. Alcohol.* 29, 956.
5. Herr, J.J., and Weabland, J.H. (1979). *Counseling elders and their families.* New York: Springer.
6. Hirshowitz, R.G. (1973). Crisis theory: A formulation. *Psychiatr. Ann., 3.*
7. Jellinik, E.M. (1960). *The disease concept of alcoholism.* New Haven, CT: Hillhouse Press.
8. Jellinek, E.M. (1952). Phases of alcohol addiction. *Q. J. Stud. Alcohol., 13,* 673.
9. Kellerman, J.L. (1980). *Alcoholism, A merry-go-round named denial.* Center City, MN: Hazeldon Foundation.
10. Milam, J., and Ketcham, K. (1981). *Under the influence.* Seattle: Madonna Publishers.
11. Peters, T. (1987). *Thriving on chaos.* New York: Knopf.
12. Silver, R. *Reaching out to the alcoholic and the family.* Center City, MN: Hazeldon Foundation.
13. Solberg, R.J. (1980). *The dry-drunk syndrome.* Center City, MN: Hazeldon Foundation.
14. Steiner, C. *The game alcoholics play.*
15. Yochelson, S., and Samenow, S.E. (1976). *The Criminal personality.* New York: Aronson.
16. Zimberg, S. (1983). Alcohol problems in the elderly. *J. Psychiatr. Treatment Eval., 5,* 515-528.

CHAPTER 18

Motivational Dynamics in Geriatric Rehabilitation: Toward a Therapeutic Model

BRYAN KEMP

Motivation is one of the most important factors that affects rehabilitation and adaptation to disability and chronic disease, yet it is also one of the most enigmatic processes. It has been described by Fishman[5] as the "single most important problem facing the rehabilitation worker," a statement subscribed to by other authors as well.[19,20,24] Despite its importance, motivation remains something like the weather: everyone talks about it but no one does anything about it.

Motivation has great relevance for geriatrics, where health problems and social losses often present obstacles to effective functioning. The capacity to overcome adversity, to improve function, and to continue to be involved in life has a lot to do with motivation. The importance of motivation can be seen in such diverse behaviors as complying with subbested health procedures, expending effort during rehabilitation, participating in social activities, and even as an aspect of depression. Proper understanding of motivation by professionals can have an enormous impact on the well-being of older persons who have a disability.

Part of the problem in understanding motivation has been a lack of models or theories that could be used clinically. To be useful, a model must be simple enough to be understood, yet complex enough to encompass multiple aspects of behavior. Barry and Malinowsky[2] reviewed the literature on motivation for rehabilitation in 1965 but found few practical approaches which the clinician could use. Lane and Barry[10] noticed a decline in interest in theories of motivation among professionals in rehabilitation because, in part, the results of most research held little practical value.

The purposes of this chapter are (1) to present a model of motivation that is both utilitarian and understandable, (2) to discuss the impact that disability and rehabilitation has on motivation (and vice versa), (3) to discuss age differences in motivation, and (4) to recommend approaches to assessing and improving motivation.

As Weiner[23] points out, a theory or model of motivation must meet several critiera to be useful. First, a model of motivation must be concerned not only with behavior, but with the thoughts and feelings of the person as well, for, as we will see, these are also motivated phenomena. Second, a model of motivation must take a subjective viewpoint of the person, for it is ultimately the person's perceptions and experiences of the world that are most important in understanding his or her motivation. Third, a single model of motivation must be able to explain both normal and abnormal behavior.

The word motivation itself comes from the Latin *movere*, meaning "to move." Like all movement, motivation has two interrelated dimensions. The first is the direction of movement. In physical reality the direction of an object is described as a vector. In psychologic reality the direction of behavior is described by the choices and decisions people make. One problem that motivation theories must be therefore able to answer is why a person chooses to do a certain thing (or not to do it), to have a certain thought, or to feel a particular way. The other dimension of movement is the force of the action. In the physical realm, force is how much energy is moving the object. In the psychologic realm this is analogous to effort, intensity, or persistence. All motivation theories must also be able to account for why behavior persists (even in the face of major obstacles), why it isn't initiated (no effort), and why it attenuates. Thus, motivation includes both the directional and the effortfulness aspects of overt acts, thinking, and feeling.

THEORIES OF MOTIVATION

Two ways to characterize previous theories are to note whether they employ a single-factor approach or a multifactorial approach to motivation and whether they attribute motivation to some internal attribute of the person or regard it as something modifiable by the environment.

Single-factor approaches stress a single motive as the important determinant of behavior at any given time. This factor might be a sexual or aggressive motive,[7] any one of a number of drives,[8] or any one of a number of needs.[12] Each of these is similar in that they tend to see the measurement of motivation as akin to using a yardstick. In these theories, different people have various "amounts" of the motive which account for their behavior, while other factors, such as learning or social customs, help to account for individual differences in the display of the motive. Even Maslow's "need hierarchy" is a variant of this because it prioritizes which single motive is operating at the time. Such theories adhere to an idea that motivation exists along a univariate dimension, people simply having "more" or "less" of the given motive (e.g., a need for security, affiliation, aggression, approval, etc.).

Multifactor theories stress the interplay of several forces and processes. Atkinson and Feather's theory of achievement motivation,[1] although it stresses a single need (achievement), nevertheless acknowledges that several processes go into its development and expression. McDaniel described a useful approach for rehabilitation when he suggested that motivation is a *product* of the utility or value of an objective and the probability of a successful outcome relative to the costs or risks of the effort needed.[13] The model presented below is a multifactor theory. It stresses four determining factors in motivation and it applies this model to a wide range of behavior.

A MODEL OF MOTIVATION

The present formulation draws on the earlier efforts of McDaniel,[13] Atkinson and Feather,[1] Miller, Galanter, and Pribham,[15] and those in the phenomenology movement, such as Weiner.[23] In the current model, motivation is the result of the interplay of four variables, all of which interact dynamically (they change, depending on each other). This model has been described earlier for its relevance to rehabilitation.[9]

The basic unit of motivation (M) is called a "motive system." It is expressed as a simple equation:

$$M_{\substack{\text{direction} \\ \text{effort}}} = \frac{W \times B \times R}{C}$$

Where W stands for wants, B for beliefs, R for rewards, and C for costs.

A person's *wants* includes the person's desires, wishes, needs, and goals. For most purposes wants can be understood in terms of what people want to get for themselves (or, in some cases, not get) and what they want to do (or not do). A person's goals are one of the key features in initiating behavior and are strongly related to behavior and outcomes. To a great extent, people get what they want. A person who wants to get better after an illness will have a more favorable outcome than a person who doesn't want to get better. It is important to determine what a person wants from rehabilitation, why he or she wants it, how life would change if he or she got it, and how that goal developed. Generally speaking, the more specific the goal, the more likely a person is to achieve it. Mento, Steele, and Karrem[14] reviewed over 100 studies which clearly demonstrate this. These studies also clearly demonstrate that goals of moderate difficulty are more likely to be achieved compared to goals of greater or lesser difficulty.

Examples of what a person may want from rehabilitation include an improvement in activities of daily living (ADLs), reduction in pain, and better overall function. Sometimes health care interventions and rehabilitation are not successful because the practitioner does not really understand what the person wants (and sometimes the patient or client doesn't either). An older person may not take medicine as prescribed because he or she wants the physician to pay special interest in his or her problems. Knowledge of what the person wants promotes more complete understanding of motivation.

Beliefs are expressed in terms of expectations, assumptions, understanding, or perceptions. All beliefs reflect the person's subjective view. They may or may not correspond to what others believe. They may or may not even seem logical, but they are the cognitive component of the person's motivation and, most importantly, they are what the person acts upon. At least three areas of belief are important in order to fully comprehend a person's motivation. These are beliefs about (1) the situation and/or task the person is facing; (2) the future as the person sees it, and (3) the person himself or herself. As a person appraises the dimensions of a situation or task, he or she begins to formulate ideas about how well he or she can cope with it. If a task looks too difficult, the person will believe it cannot be done. If the future looks long and hopeful, the person will feel optimistic and energetic. If the future looks bleak, the person will not show much effort. If people have a strong belief in their own capabilities, they will try harder. If people have a low appraisal of their capabilities, they will give up more easily. Beliefs and wants interact with each other. For example, if a person has only a moderate belief that he or she can accomplish something, yet greatly wants it, more effort will be put forth than if he or she had the same belief but only weakly desired the outcome. If a person sees a situation as aversive, he or she will want to leave it.

Rewards include reinforcement, benefit, outcome, and payoff. Behavior which does not result in some form of reward is not continued. Rewards generally fall into three classes. They include events which (1) bring pleasure through the senses (e.g., a good meal, a hug, a visually pleasing environment), (2) produce a sense of success (e.g., a job well done, achieving a goal, receiving praise), or (3) produce a sense of meaning or purpose (such as one's role in life or usefulness). Behavior may be *initiated* based on a person's desires and beliefs, but in order to be *maintained*, there must be sufficient rewards.

Costs include risk, price, and any negative consequences to effort. Costs act in ratio to the above three variables. In its simplest form, motivation is the dynamic balance between the three variables in the numerator and the one variable in the denominator. There are also three groups of costs. The first are physical costs. These include such things as time, physical effort, pain, and even money. For example, it takes both time and effort to maintain a regular exercise program. Second are psychologic costs. These often include emotions evoked by engaging in certain behavior, especially the emotions of fear or guilt. Another common psychologic cost is threat to self-image. We tend not to do things that are too inconsistent with our view of ourselves. If we see ourself as shy, we aren't inclined to give a speech before a group. Finally, costs may be social, especially the feedback of peers, family members, and the public in general. If others do not approve of our behavior or some other aspect of us, we pay the price of their rejection.

A great deal of behavior can be understood by looking at it in this dynamic manner. In its simplest form, if the product of the three numerator variables is greater than the denominator, the person is "motivated". If the denominator is greater, the person is "unmotivated". More behavior can be understood, however, if we also realize that no motive system (the four-variable complex) stands alone. Instead, every motive system must be viewed in relationship to at least one other. For example, the motive to engage in daily exercise is best understood if we also view it in relationship to the motive not to exercise. This is extremely important because the content of each of the four variables is usually quite different for each motive system; the total behavior, therefore, cannot be understood by only looking at half the equation.

Our final formulation of motivation, then, looks like the following:

$$\text{Ultimate M} = \frac{M_1 = \dfrac{W_1 \times B_1 \times R_1}{C_1}}{M_2 = \dfrac{W_2 \times B_2 \times R_2}{C_2}}$$

Where M_1 is the motive system to do one thing and M_2 is the motive system to either not do M_1 or to do something entirely different (an M_3, M_4, or M_5, etc.).

STUDIES OF MOTIVATION, REHABILITATION AND AGING

Rosillo and Fagel[18] found that improvement in rehabilitation tasks correlated well with the patient's *own* appraisal of his or her potential for recovery but not very well with others' appraisals. This points out the importance of taking the subjective viewpoint as more critical in understanding motivation than the staff's appraisal.

Stoedefalke[21] reports that more frequent feedback (reinforcement) for older persons in rehabilitation can help to improve their performance and feelings of success. Thus older persons can improve in physical therapy but sometimes modifications have to be made to provide feedback more often. Rabin, Froman, Trotter, and Kraft (cited in Fordyce[6]) described an older man with a stroke who was referred to improve his performance in physical therapy. A close analysis of the therapy process revealed that the therapist would not give feedback until several components of the walking sequence were completed, rather than complimenting him on achieving any single component. The older man was becoming discouraged at his lack of progress and he was showing less "motivation." They concluded that he was not receiving reinforcement (feedback of success) often enough. A modification of the feedback procedures dramatically improved performance. Improvement followed when reinforcement was linked exactly to the target behavior. Without such corrective analysis, the older person may have ended up being seen as having a problem with motivation or the therapist may have concluded that older persons don't have much rehabilitation potential. Older persons are known to learn differently than younger persons and to benefit from breaking complex tasks (such as walking) into simpler components and immediately reinforcing each component.

MacCartney, Benson, and Brewin[11] were interested in why ADLs were not carried out in a sample of persons (some old) who suffered from chronic illness even though adequate ability was present. They had patients will out specialized questionnaires to explain their lack of performance. Over 50 percent indicated that it just wasn't important to them (they saw no rewards in it), 30 percent said it took too long, and 20 percent said it was too risky to be independent in these activities because it would upset an established family pattern. Thus, different factors may account for the same behavior in different people.

Other authors[16] showed that older persons with chronic illness have low initial aspirations with regard to their ability to perform various tasks. As situations in which they succeeded or failed occurred, their aspirations changed to more closely reflect their abilities. However, Prohaska, Pontiam, and Teitleman[17] found that older persons may have different beliefs about their abilities than do younger persons. When persons of both ages were given an unsolvable problem, younger subjects ascribed their failure to not trying hard enough. Older subjects, on the other hand, ascribed their failure to inability. Thus, on future trials younger subjects would try harder and older subjects would give up. This is extremely important because it illustrates that what people believe regarding their successes and failures highly influences their subsequent behavior. If the cause of failure is seen as an immutable characteristic of the person, then little effort in the future can be expected. If, on the other hand, failure is seen as caused by a changeable factor, then increased effort may result.

Eisdorfer[4] found that the performance of older persons in a difficult learning task increased significantly when their anxiety was reduced. Older persons may have higher anxiety in rehabilitation situations because they fear failure or looking bad to the therapist. If anxiety is high enough, then the behavior becomes redirected toward simply reducing the anxiety and not toward mastering the task.

Weinberg[22] found that subjects set their own goals for task achievement even if they were directed to adopt the investigator's goals. Mento, Steel, and Karren[14] found that the best performance at difficult tasks, as many rehabilitation tasks are, occurs when the person sets a very specific goal. If the person simply tries to "do better," then performance is not improved as much. Kemp and Vash[9] found that among persons disabled with a spinal cord injury the presence of specific goals for the future was strongly related to overall adjustment to the disability. Thus, what a person wants and how specific and realistic these goals are helps to determine overall performance.

THE EFFECT OF DISABILITY, REHABILITATION, AND AGING ON MOTIVATION

Disability, the rehabilitation procedure, or aging itself can have important effects on various components of motivation. Most people certainly do not want to have a disability. It has not been one of their life goals. Yet, when faced with a disability, people have to decide sooner or later what they want from that point forward. Some people don't want to be disabled so strongly that their goals may initially be directed only toward trying to remove it, such as by denying its existence, trying to find a miracle cure, or going from doctor to doctor. Some people (a minority) don't want to live anymore because of the extreme personal pain they feel in their lives. Often the person displays negative comments, suicidal thoughts, depressed affect, and limited behavior because they have something they don't want and it's been forced upon them. Therefore, behavior early after a disability can partially be seen as driven by a desire to reduce the personal pain. During the process of rehabilitation there has to be a shift toward wanting to improve functioning, in other words, to improve what the person can do. Individuals who can state goals, desires, and wishes for the future that are not limited to restoring bodily functions that have been permanently lost are likely to be better rehabilitation candidates.

Beliefs pay a very large role in motivation after a disability. What a person believes about being disabled, what he or she believes the consequences and implications are for the future, and how the procedures of the rehabilitation task are viewed are major determinants of motivation. A person who views rehabilitation procedures as too difficult or too painful will not engage in them readily. A person who believes that his or her future is over will show little motivation because in this person's scheme of things it isn't logical, and people do follow their own, personal logic. If older persons believe that rehabilitation is only for younger persons (or if their physicians believe it), then they won't ask for it. If policy makers believe that older persons can't benefit from rehabilitation, then there won't be many provisions made for it. If the disabled person has lost belief in himself or herself (has little confidence), then there will be few attempts to engage in difficult tasks. If the person with a disability believes nothing can ever be done to improve things, then there are likely to be depressive feelings and little effort.

One real difference between younger and older persons in rehabilitation is that the older person has a foreshortened future. Younger persons can more easily look forward, 10 or more years if necessary, to improved circumstances. The future may be perceived as being very foreshortened by some older persons, leading to a response (rightly or wrongly) of giving up. Obviously, it becomes of paramount importance to assess the belief system of every person in rehabilitation who is disabled in order to understand that person's motivation and to correct illogical or incorrect beliefs.

Having a disability, participating in rehabilitation procedures, and, to an extent, being older are frequently not very rewarding experiences. In fact, these conditions need to be looked at as possibly being very punishing circumstances. Some authorities[6] suggest viewing rehabilitation in a punishment paradigm. The onset of a disability is associated with a major and sudden reduction in the usual reinforcers (by definition, punishment). Reductions in sources of pleasure, success (such as in doing daily activities), or meaning drastically affect the person's behavior and outlook. Thus, reductions in rewards begin to affect the person's beliefs, and may lead to fixed beliefs that things will never get better. Too often, little attention is given to what rewards will be present at home to help maintain the behavior after discharge from a hospital. While in the hospital, therapists, physicians, nurses and others reward independent behavior. But at home, is someone going to reward the opposite behavior? Older persons have objectively lower physical abilities than younger persons. If adjustments are not made in rehabilitation to compensate (such as physical therapy procedures), then the older person will not receive as much reinforcement as the younger person. If the older person has lessened self-confidence, views the task as difficult to begin with, and also receives less reinforcement because he can do less, then there are apt to be problems with motivation.

Disability, rehabilitation, and aging often extract high costs from a person for performing even daily living tasks. The onset of a disability has many aversive aspects, including physical pain, social rejection, sometimes a diminished sense of self-worth, and the requirement to participate in procedures which, once easy, are now difficult. Such aversive conditions may cause behavior to be redirected from improvement-oriented activities to behavior directed toward reducing the aversive conditions. Thus a person may be late to treatments, not want to participate at all, or spend excessive time fantasizing about how things used to be.

In summary, once motivation is seen to be multiply determined and once each of the component variables is carefully examined in the context of disability, rehabilitation procedures, and the effects of aging, the person's effort in rehabilitation can be more clearly analyzed and interventions can be more systematically developed.

RECOMMENDATIONS FOR ASSESSING AND IMPROVING MOTIVATION

Using this model, motivation can be improved by following both general and specific guidelines.

GENERAL POINTS

On a general level, four principles are important:

1. Motivation must be considered within a dynamic framework wherein at least four variables are operating at once and where at least two motive systems are present. Further, the ultimate out-

come is determined by the patient's subjective viewpoint on all of them.

2. Motivational "problems" seldom arise unless there is more than one person involved. Many times health professionals want patients to improve so that the professional will feel that he or she is doing a good job, being successful, and making a difference. This phenomenon is quite common in treating older patients, especially if staff members feel pessimistic or somewhat helpless, or have unrecognized emotional involvement with the patient. It is therefore important to determine whether there really is a problem with the patient or whether it exists with someone else.

3. Each person usually has a particular component that is the most critical in preventing better motivation. The features that are key to understanding motivation vary from person to person, even under the same circumstances. For one person, it may be their beliefs that are least conducive to motivation; for another, the absence of appropriate rewards; for still another a cost that others do not yet perceive. However, if each factor is thoroughly explored, the key feature will emerge.

4. There should always be an attempt to understand the alternative motive systems operating. Behavior is controlled by multiple factors and often contradictory motives. Full understanding requires an examination of both.

SPECIFIC STEPS

Proper intervention for the patient who appears to be poorly motivated requires careful assessment and thoughtful treatment.

1. The therapist or other professional should explore what the patient wants and why he or she wants it. If the patient's wants appear to be unusual (e.g., if the patient with a stroke wants to play volleyball), the therapist should find out why. This can be done by asking what would be different if the patient's wishes were fulfilled. The patient should be assisted in establishing attainable goals. If there seems to be a "problem" with motivation, especially in initiating a behavior, the patient may not want the right thing from the rehabilitation process.

2. The therapist should explore the patient's beliefs about the situation, self, and future, listening for key words that reflect faulty beliefs, expectations, or assumptions. Frequently, maladaptive beliefs are irrational and are sustained by faulty thinking habits and

distorted logic.[3] If these faulty beliefs can be identified, they usually are amenable to change through clarifying the logic and pointing out the flaws in thinking. For example, persons who never get angry because they think they shouldn't could be counseled to determine why they think this way and assured that angry feelings are sometimes normal.

3. The practitioner should establish abundant rewards in rehabilitation by finding out what is important to the patient, relating health procedures and practices to it, and making sure that rewards are frequent and closely linked to the desired behavior. It is also important to determine which rewards will sustain the behavior once the patient is home and to try to improve their frequency. Rewards may be operating in the home environment which sustain the undesired behavior. These should be identified so that they can be reduced.

4. The therapist should reduce undesired costs. This can be done by encouraging the patient to orally express emotional factors (e.g., fear, guilt, worry) associated with the task. The patient's self-image in relation to the task must also be considered. Is it difficult to incorporate the patient's previous self-concept into what is being asked of him or her? The patient should be told what to expect in terms of physical costs (e.g., physical therapy). The therapist should make sure there are not hidden costs perceived by the patient that is untrue. For example, if improvements are attained in rehabilitation, will it cost the attention of others? In that case the costs may be too great. Motivation is understandable, it is important, and it is dynamic. It can be improved and, as a result, an older person's rehabilitation efforts can be more successful.

REFERENCES

1. Atkinson, J., and Feather, N. (1966). *A theory of achievement motivation.* New York: Wiley.
2. Barry, J.R., and Malinowsky, M.R. (1965). *Client motivation for rehabilitation: A review.* Rehabilitation Research Monograph Series, No. 1. Gainsville, FL: University of Florida.
3. Beck, A.T. (1976). *Cognitive theory and the emotional disorders.* New York: International University Press.
4. Eisdorfer, L. (1968). Arousal and performance: Experiments in verbal learning and a tentative theory. In G.A. Talland (Ed.), *Human aging and behavior* (pp. 107–121). New York: Academic Press.
5. Fishman, S. (1962). Amputation. In J. Garrett and E. Levine (Eds.), *Psychological practices with the physically disabled* (pp. 362–381). New York: Columbia University Press.

6. Fordyce, W. (1970). Behavioral methods in rehabilitation. In W.S. Neff (Ed.), *Rehabilitation psychology.* Washington D.C.: American Psychological Association.

7. Freud, S. (1926). *The problem of anxiety.* New York: Norton.

8. Hull, C. (1943). *Principles of behavior.* New York: Appleton-Century-Crofts.

9. Kemp, B.J., and Vash, C.L. (1971). Productivity after injury in a sample of spinal cord injured persons: A pilot study. *J. Chronic Dis., 24,* 51.

10. Lane, J.M., and Barry, J.R. (1971). Recent research on client motivation. *Rehabil. Res. Pract. Rev., 13,* 53.

11. MacCartney, B., Benson, J., and Brewin, C.R. (1986). Motivation and problem appraisal in long-term psychiatric patients. *Psychol. Med., 16,* 431.

12. Maslow, A.H. (1970). *Motivation and personality, rev. ed.* New York: Harper & Row.

13. McDaniel, J. (1976). *Physical disability and human behavior.* New York: Pergamon Press.

14. Mento, A., Steele, R.P., and Karren, R.J. (1987). A metaanalytic study of the effects of goal setting on task performance: 1966–1984. *Organ. Behav. Hum. Decis. Process, 39,* 52.

15. Miller, G., Galanter, E., and Pribham, K. (1960). *Plans and the structure of behavior.* New York: Hold, Rinehart & Winston.

16. Nadler, I.M., et al. (1985). Level of aspiration and performance of chronic psychiatric patients on a simple motor task. *Percept. Mot. Skills, 60,* 767.

17. Prohaska, T., Pontiam, I.A., and Teitleman, J. (1984). Age differences in attributions to causality: Implications for intellection assessment. *Exp. Aging Res., 10,* 111.

18. Rosillo, R.A., and Fagel, M.L. (1970). Correlation of psychologic variables and progress in physical therapy: I. Degree of disability and denial of illness. *Arch. Phys. Med. Rehabil., 51,* 227.

19. Staats, A. (1960). A case in a strategy for the extension of learning principles to problems of human behavior. In L. Krasner and L. Ullman (Eds.), *Research in behavior modification* (pp. 278–291). New York: Holt, Rinehart & Winston.

20. Steger, H.G. (1976). Understanding the psychologic factors in rehabilitation. *Geriatrics, 31,* 68.

21. Stoedefalke, K.G. (1985). Motivating and sustaining the older adult in an exercise program. *Top. Geriatr. Rehabil., 1,* 78.

22. Weinberg, R., Bruya, L., and Jackson, A. (1985). The effects of goal proximity and goal specificity on endurance performance. *J. Soc. Psychol., 7,* 296.

23. Weiner, B. (1986). *An attributional theory of motivation and emotion.* New York: Springer-Verlag.

24. Williams, T.F. (Ed.) (1984). *Rehabilitation in the aging.* New York: Raven Press.

CHAPTER 19

Assessment and Treatment of Disabled Families in Geriatric Rehabilitation

MARK D. CORGIAT

Families with dysfunctional dynamics pose a special problem for geriatric rehabilitation professionals. These families are often exquisitely vulnerable to the stresses involved in caring for an ill or disabled older member. They often have difficulty accepting new information, training, reassurance, or support. Dysfunctional families also find it difficult to make consistent commitments to support a disabled older member.[38] Their unsatisfying interactions with staff and the patient often impede or prevent effective treatment.[20,26]

Recognizing dysfunction in the family can be critical to the success of the rehabilitation program. This is particularly true in rehabilitation of older persons. Disabled older persons are likely to receive most of their informal care and support from their families. Elaine Brody concludes that 80 to 90 percent of medically related and personal care services, instrumental activities of daily living (IADLs), and transportation services are provided to the elderly by their families.[2] Family members, usually adult children, are also most likely to bridge the expanding needs of the older person and formal health care organizations.[32] And family support has been associated with delaying institutionalization of the disabled elderly.[2,12]

Strong relationships between successful geriatric rehabilitation efforts and the family's ability to provide care and support have been noted by several authors. Loeble and Eisdorfer[21] consider "proper preparation of family members" (p. 54) a necessary element in rehabilitation of the elderly. Levenson and Beller[20] state that "inadequate family functioning . . . would impede optimal rehabilitation if not ameliorated" (p. 366). Miller, Berstein, and Sharkey[23] suggest that successful rehabilitation programs for the elderly can only be maintained if family relationships are understood and managed. And Versluys[37] notes that "rehabilitation failure, when there is no other observable reason, may be the result of disordered family dynamics" (p. 59).

The purpose of this chapter is to present a paradigmatic approach to understanding the relationships among family dynamics, problem-solving strategies, and impaired coping abilities found in some families with disabled older members. Family paradigms provide a structure for organizing and understanding the similarities and differences among families at all stages of the family life cycle. Three such paradigms are identified as dysfunctional problem-solving strategies that are often used by these families. Suggestions are given to assist the practitioner in identifying family paradigms and problem-solving strategies.

CRITICAL ISSUES IN LATE-LIFE FAMILIES

Families in late life have a number of unique characteristics. Many families are multigenerational, often including three, four, or five generations. The existence and number of generations in a family are important because the family influences, and is influenced by, the various generations.[36] For many families multigenerations create a collection of people upon whom older family members can rely. For others, the adult child generation may be experiencing difficulty at the same time the older generation is in need of assistance and therefore may not be available to provide support.[3] In any case, the multigenerational aspects of a family are important considerations for health care providers.

Late-life families are also unique with respect to their lengthy family histories. Such families have a large reservoir of experience and well-developed communication and coping patterns. However, a long family history is not necessarily a positive attribute.[3] There may be residual tension from unresolved earlier life conflicts, well-entrenched maladaptive patterns of communication, or a long history of failed coping experiences. Whether positive or negative, the existence of a long family history is important. As Brubaker and Brubaker[4] note, the way that family members have previously dealt with stress is likely to predict the way in which the family will handle current and future stresses.

Older families are also characterized by significant transitional life events that are important and potentially stressful for all family members. Retiring from employment, coping with the death of an older family member, and experiencing chronic illness or disability are life events that frequently occur in late life.[19] Each of these events typically involves many family members as willing or unwilling participants in family change.

Retirement has been associated with decreases in feelings of self-esteem and self-worth, although successful negotiations of this change are the rule.[19] Retirement also brings about changes in scheduling and socialization patterns. With more available free time, grandparents may become more involved with grandchildren and other family members. Conversely, they may become withdrawn and isolated if they fail to adapt to the loss of employment-related socialization opportunities. Decreasing finances can also change postretirement consumption patterns, rendering some older family members reliant on their adult children for financial assistance.

Coping with the death of a spouse or parent is another transitional life event that typically involves all family members in the normal process of bereavement. It can also transform parent-child relationships. The surviving parent may turn to children in place of the spouse, calling upon them as confidants or helpers.[19] Previously dormant sibling rivalries can also escalate in the absence of parental intervention. In most cases the family is central to the process of adapting to the death of an older family member.

Perhaps the most difficult adjustment for late-life families is that related to coping with chronic illness that causes disability of an older family member. These families may need to confront multiple problems in physical caregiving, emotional upsets, and decisions about legal matters, financial matters, and institutionalization.[18] The family must often fact conflicting demands. They must balance their own needs against the responsibility of responding appropriately to the increasing needs of the ill or disabled older member. This balancing act is frequently performed for one or more sets of parents or grandparents at the same time adult children are confronting their own developmental changes. The balance is often precarious.

Most families are able to provide ongoing care for an older ill or disabled member despite the associated stresses and uncertainties. The family is able to successfully balance individual needs against the family's ability to respond to the needs of the ill or disabled older member.[38] Such families tend to have a stable premorbid adjustment that has helped them mobilize resources to deal with previous crises.[31] They have well-defined family roles. They have the ability to adapt to change.

There is closeness and affection among family members. While such families may become temporarily overwhelmed, they typically respond by achieving new levels of adaptation.

For less stable families, the strain involved in caring for an ill or disabled older member can have profound effects on family functioning. When the family is strained by having to cope with a disabled older member in conjunction with having its own unfulfilled needs or insufficient resources, it may cease to be a willing source of support. Feelings of guilt arising from inabilities to meet filial responsibilities may precipitate additional problems in other family members.[33] Growing tensions may lead the family to unresolved conflicts about issues of dependency, role transitions, and continuity. The potential for family conflicts can become amplified as the balance of independence and dependence needs of the older person shifts.[7] And inevitable role transitions resulting in new expectations may reactivate old conflicts causing more confusion and chaos in the family.[34]

Dysfunctional family dynamics often render less stable families unable to utilize information and assistance provided by rehabilitation professionals. They are unable to understand and transmit accurate and explicit information.[27] Their rigid role definitions interfere with family adjustment to illness and disability.[8] Conversely, they may be chaotic and continually unstable, leaving no one in charge of family decision making.[25] As a result, interventions by rehabilitation team members are often debated, poorly followed, or simply ignored. Yet these families often demand repeated and continued intervention by health care professionals.[31]

While some families may exhibit their dysfunctional processes through conflicts with the health care system, others develop pervasive internal problems. Disparate and strong needs of the patient and family bring them into serious conflict.[22] The disabled older member is seen as a burden and source of chronic stress. The family's responses often lead to overprotection, neglect, encouragement of dependence, and punitive action toward the patient. Similarly, the disabled family member may respond with denial, avoidance of treatment, and a succession of inappropriate demands. In some cases, the family's ability to adapt is so impaired that permanent disruption occurs.[31]

FAMILIES, PARADIGMS, AND PROBLEM SOLVING

Family paradigms represent the family's commitment to a set of priorities concerning fundamental human issues. They form a set of well-defined beliefs concerning each member and the interactions among members. Family paradigms provide the tacit rules which govern family relationships. They construct the perceptual context in which family interactions and behaviors take place. The family paradigm exemplifies each family's characteristic mode of perceiving itself and its interactions with the social world.[28,29] It is a central and remarkably stable feature of a family.[9]

Family paradigms do more than define family priorities, they also represent the family's set of strategies for solving problems.[11] Every family develops its unique styles and strategies for dealing with the basic problems associated with family life.[9,15,30] Each must work out ways of resolving the problems associated with day-to-day living. Every family must address the large issues of birth and death, growing up and growing old, that mark longer family histories. All must define and maintain boundaries. All families must deal with such fundamental dualities as individual versus group interests and change versus stability. They must provide security while allowing freedom for individual growth. Each must also be firm enough to endure, yet flexible enough to adapt. In doing so, families operate as though guided by a "family paradigm;" a model of what the family is, can be, or should be.[9]

When confronted with problems, families do whatever they do best. Each family, guided by its own paradigm, applies its version of problem solving.[9] When this doesn't work, the family tries harder. Defined paradigmatically, families try harder by doing more of the same. As a result, family problem-solving strategies tend to develop semi-autonomous lives of their own to which people in the system become habituated. Consequently the repertoire of strategies becomes limited as family members repetitively apply the same solution to different problems without regard to its appropriateness.[13] For many families this means meeting the challenges of daily life with an unchanging repertoire of well-established approaches. The tendency to repeatedly apply the same problem-solving strategies for different problems leads many families into difficult situations. According to Bolin,[1] new problems often result from the very behaviors that were intended to resolve the problem initially. In other words, the original problem is met with an attempted solution that intensifies the original difficulty and so on. In time the "solution" to the problem becomes more of a problem than the problem itself.[39]

A classic example of the solution becoming the problem is offered by Herr and Weakland.[14] They discuss the case of a widowed woman living alone who was coping well until her daughter decided that "something has to be done with mother." The problem did not reside with the mother; she was already coping adequately. Rather the problem was created by the family's belief that "there is a problem with mother." The more the family tried to solve the problem, the more problems they created. They moved mother into the son's home where she fell over unfamiliar furniture and broke her hip. She argued with family members constantly, stated that she hated living in her son's home, became depressed, and told them that she wished she were dead. The family responded to mother's threat of suicide by moving her to another child's home. When asked about this tactic the family responded that they could not let her live alone because she was depressed. The mother's depression was actually the result of being forced to live with her children. This family is caught in a vicious cycle of creating more problems by applying the same type of solution over and over. Herr and Weakland[14] suggest that most problems encountered when counseling late-life families are "problems created and perpetuated by inappropriate solutions" (p. 102).

The paradigmatic view of family disablement is based on this tendency of families to perpetuate problem-solving strategies. While the most likely response to any challenge is for a family to respond in a manner consistent with its paradigm and organization, disabled families carry a mandate of their paradigms to incapacitating extremes.[9] Even when coping mechanisms fail, disabled families do not try new strategies. According to Constantine[9] they may "initiate a search for solutions, or seek advice, or run around in circles, or give up, but whatever they do it will come from their existing repertoire, and will, at least at first, consist of variations on established family themes" (p. 199). For this reason, as families of different types become overstressed they are prone to distinct modes of failure.

PARADIGMS AND FAMILY TYPES

Although family paradigms cannot be directly observed, all families can be understood in terms of paradigms. Family paradigms are templates for patterns of behavior that, by their redundancy, become recognizable as characteristic of a family's way of dealing with life. Kantor and Lehr's research suggests that fundamentally different types of families can be distinguished by such patterns.[15] Through direct observation they defined three basic family paradigms: closed, open, and random families. Similar findings have been described through clinical observation[22,28,29] and theoretical argument.[9,24,25] Overall, the findings suggest that these three paradigms embody real and important differences in the way families organize and operate. Closed, open, and random families, guided by different paradigms, differ in the way they solve problems. Each is especially good at different tasks. And their divergent goals and methods makes each family prone to different types of difficulties.

Closed, open, and random families operate on a continuum ranging from functionally adequate "enabled" families on the one hand to "disabled" ones on the other. Enabled families are those that successfully balance the needs and interests of the family against those of individual members. Such families tend to resemble one another regardless of their paradigmatic commitments. Conversely, disabled families characteristically manifest extreme expressions of their paradigms. As a result they are typically more distinct.

THE CLOSED FAMILY

The primary focus of the closed family is one of stability, security, and belonging. The conventional traditional family is well representative of the closed family paradigm.[9] Such families are homeostatic, stressing maintenance of normal established family patterns. Since continuity and uniformity are given priority, the family unit tends to be seen as more important than the individual. In a conflict of needs and interests the family comes first over individual members.

Closed families also have a paradigmatic commitment to control information and regulate dissemination. Consequently, communication tends to be channeled and restricted. As a result, family members have many secrets which they will not share with one another or the outside world. According to Kantor and Lehr,[15] "Locked doors, careful scrutiny of strangers in the neighborhood, parental control over media, supervised excursions, and unlisted telephones" (p. 120) are characteristic of closed families.

When confronted with problems the closed family tends to rely on tradition and loyalty to solve them. The more difficult the problem, the stronger will be the attempts to control and pull the family into line. If the problem is not solved, the family will become more isolated from the world, more intensely connected internally, and more rigid, and they will become increasingly dysfunctional.

The disabled closed family is characterized by dogmatism and conformity. The family is protected from the outside world, which is seen as chaotic and threatening. The more closed the system, the more dedicated to stability, the more likely it is to block or deny any information that challenges the family paradigm. In such a family there is little room for subjectivity, and even less tolerance for diverse viewpoints. The disabled closed family is aptly described by Kantor and Lehr as "sealed off from the world."[15]

Dysfunctional closed families commonly have one "identified patient." The identified patient is used to sustain the family process. An older disabled parent might function as the center of a middle-aged daughter's life, keeping her busy with appointments, medication, and cleaning. Thus the daughter will have neither the time nor energy to deal with hidden issues threatening the stability of her marriage. The daughter's need to use her mother's disability to avoid facing other issues can handicap her mother. Interventions to increase her mother's functioning will likely be perceived by this family as potentially threatening challenges from the outside world.

THE RANDOM FAMILY

The random family is best conceptualized as the antithesis of the closed family.[9] While the closed family values stability and continuity, the random family values change. Such families are morphogenic, promoting continual change by opting for novelty and variety rather than stable continuity. Since novelty and variety are given priority, individual interests tend to be seen as more important than whole family concerns.

Communication in the random family is often incomplete and chaotic, with information being easily lost or ignored in the rapid pace of continual change. However, new information from both family members and others is highly valued as a source of variety. In fact, the emphasis on individuality tends to foster territoriality about ideas and competition among family members for new input.

When confronted with problems, the random family relies on spontaneity and creative individuality. In the face of chronic stress or repeated crises the family can become locked in a highly competitive fight for survival, with "everyone out for themselves." Any difficult decision will readily be terminated without having to reach a solution since truth in the random family is necessarily subjective. As family members work with increasing independence to find solutions, the family process can become more chaotic and uncoordinated. The search for individual solutions leads toward greater separateness and more chaos as the family becomes increasingly dysfunctional. The disabled random family's emphasis on individuality above all else frequently renders them unable to function in a coordinated way. The needs and interests of individual members are lost in the quest for independence and self-gratification. The relationship between the individual and the family becomes one of fierce independence, and at times counterdependence. Truth in the family is always relative, subjective, and determined by the individual, not the family as a group. Consequently the family is often unable to define and address problems whose solutions require consensual family participation. Since the family favors the individual over the family unit, as paradigmatic mandates are carried to extremes, the family tends to be sacrificed for individual interests.

The disabled random family will likely view proposed interventions requiring family cooperation as a threat to individuality. The drive for individual autonomy will prevent members from consensually responding to the needs and interests of others. Frequent bickering and spontaneous outbursts of angry hostile arguing are likely to characterize family meetings. The older disabled member will find little emotional or instrumental support as all family members vie for limited resources. Family members in need are typically unable to compel the attention and support of others in the family and eventually become viewed as a burden.

THE OPEN FAMILY

The core image of the open family is that of adaptability and participation. The needs of the individual and the group are equally important to the open family and adaptability to the interests of both is the family's core goal. Although open families emphasize flexibility and change, they do not value change as an end in itself. Rather, change is valued insofar as it is goal-directed and improves the family's effectiveness in meeting those goals.

Successful integration of individual and family needs requires effective communication. The open family considers the sharing of feelings, thoughts, and ideas as essential to effective family functioning. Consequently they tend not to censure information or regulate communication either within the family or in extrafamilial interactions. Unlike the closed family, open families perceive the environment as a masterable source of information useful for problem solving.

When confronted with problems the open family will persistently try to hammer out a consensual solution. Family members will gather more information and try harder to communicate. When faced with an insolvable problem they will inundate themselves with information and immerse themselves in discussion. This infinite loop of more information and more communication serves only to heighten the already excessive ambiguity. They will frequently open themselves to outside influences which may disenfranchise members or make them dependent on outside influences. A confusion between "insiders" and "outsiders" and of roles and priorities frequently occurs.[15] Family members will continue to communicate but may eventually withdraw emotionally.

This disabled open family is distinct in its "continuing, seemingly endless, intensely emotional negotiations without resolution, characterized by high levels of ambivalence and confusion" (p. 317).[9] These families are dominated by the belief that it is always possible to solve problems in a manner that will meet the needs of all. Members are expected to disclose fully to one another and to participate in all family discussions. Disabled open families are typically nontraditional and lack leadership, discipline, and clear family rules.

Dysfunctional open families will have difficulty meeting the emotional and instrumental needs of an older disabled member. The constantly shifting rules and endless negotiations render the family unable to move beyond exploring possible approaches and solutions. Such families tend to have long histories of unresolved problems and incomplete projects. The needs of an older member can easily become another pending project as family members search for a consensual solution to providing care without upsetting the balance between individual and family interests.

It should be clear that no single paradigm has a clear and universal advantage in all circumstances. Closed families may function very well during periods of little change, but be less well adapted to periods of rapid flux. While they typically achieve stability and security, they tend to sacrifice a measure of individualism. Conversely, random and open families are effective promoters of individuality, but are likely to be less effective at achieving group identity and consensual decision making.

ASSESSMENT AND TREATMENT

Much has been written about assisting normal families that are temporarily overwhelmed by the needs of an older disabled family member.[18,40] Health care professionals can often assist these families by providing needed information, training, reassurance, or emotional and instrumental support. Kaplan and Mearig[17] promote informal problem solving as an effective approach to helping families. Zarit and Zarit[40] propose interventions consisting of providing information, assisting with management of behavioral problems, and providing emotional support. Brummel-Smith[5] suggests using the family conference as a vehicle for a three-step intervention strategy. The first two steps are directed toward increasing family knowledge and promoting family problem solving through the exchange of information between rehabilitation professionals and family members. The last step is to identify those families that continue to struggle with caregiving despite being provided information, training, and specific suggestions.

Less has been written about assisting disabled families confronting the challenges of providing care and support to an older disabled family member. While providing information, training, reassurance, and support are effective interventions with well-functioning families experiencing a crisis, they are often not effective with disabled families.

Appropriate intervention for the disabled family starts with careful assessment of the family's interactional and problem-solving styles. Understanding the family as a process rather than a moment is essential for effective family intervention. A thorough assessment includes an understanding of the family's problems as well as its strengths and assets. In short, the purpose of the evaluation is to develop a clear and comprehensive picture of how a particular family is working in its present context.

Of particular importance in assessing the family is the identification of the family's paradigm and problem-solving style. As noted above, paradigms provide a way of organizing and making sense of the similarities and differences among families. As such they are related not only to the kinds of problems a family is likely to experience, but also to the probability of success associated with various approaches and techniques of therapy. Clinical assessment that differentially identifies disabled family types is important since treatment goals and approaches related to each can differ substantially.

Observable manifestations of family paradigms can be found in all aspects of routine family functioning. Thus, observation of the family during early stages of contact with the rehabilitation team can assist in differentiating family styles. Observations for the purpose of identifying the family's paradigmatic commitments should focus on interactional aspects of family funtioning. For example, how skilled are family members at listening to one another? Are they willing to listen to one another? How do family members demonstrate positive feelings toward one another? Are family members able to be honest with one another about factual things? Can family members admit problems to one another? Can people say what they want to other family members? How does the family share responsibility? How does the family negotiate? How does the family make decisions? Are members able to compromise? Are family interactions fraught with double messages, blaming, bribes, threats, defiance, inappropriate jokes, put-downs, sarcastic comments, or speaking for others? Are there hidden agendas, secrets, myths, taboos, or power struggles? Does the family have any fun together? Does the family allow for individual differences?

A family's orientation toward internal opposition and disagreement is one of the best distinguishing features of the family's paradigm. For example, the closed family expresses its paradigmatic commitment to continuity by striving to control and eliminate disagreement. If attempts at control fail, the disabled closed family may use scapegoating to isolate the opposer, thereby diminishing his or her influence. The random family, with a paradigmatic commitment to oppose control, tends to foster internal disagreement as a form of individualism. However, its commitment to individualism at the expense of family unity also renders it unable to use dissension as a resource for promoting family interests. By contrast, the open family values and includes disagreement to the extent that it is goal-directed and improves the family's effectiveness as a unit.

Problem-solving styles are another valuable clinical marker for differentiating family paradigms. Therapist-directed decision-making tasks, such as card sorting[4,28] or spending imaginary money, will generally produce a sample of family behaviors useful for identifying family problem-solving styles. Closed families often approach such tasks by applying tried and true techniques to arrive at a quick single decision. The authority figure within the family typically leads, with minimal discussion, to that solution which is "best for the family." The more disabled the family, the more limited their repertoire of problem-solving techniques and the more established their hierarchical approach to authority. In contrast, the disabled random family will use creativity to generate many alternatives, but more often be unable to arrive at a consensual solution. The open family will likely be best at merging novel and proven methods in its attempts to solve tasks. However, the disabled open family's paradigmatic commitment to solving problems in a manner that fully balances individual and family interests will frequently render it unable to solve the easiest of tasks.

Ideally, paradigmatic family assessment should culminate in the development of a map of the family's structure and basic organization. The "family system map" provides one means of graphically representing the family system.[9] Family system maps organize and systematize data into visual metaphors of the complex relationships found within the family. Unlike structural family diagrams which emphasize linear analytic analyses, the family system map facilitates a merging of analytic and intuitive thinking. As such it provides greater flexibility in describing boundaries and relationships within the family. Correctly done, a family system map gives the therapist access to the same type of unarticulated information that is revealed through family sculpture.[10]

Figure 19-1 depicts a system map of an extended family living in the same household. The family consisted of the grandmother, Dorothy, her daughter Iris, her son-in-law Jim, and her granddaughter Cathy. Dorothy and Cathy were initially seen during a home visit requested by a family friend. Iris was notably absent during the home visit. Dorothy was found to be severely depressed and desiring to live independently. By her report she had been depressed for several months. Subsequent evaluation at a rehabilitation outpatient clinic revealed that Dorothy was indeed able to live independently. A medical history revealed that Dorothy had suffered a small stroke approximately 1½ years prior to the home visit. At the time of her stroke the treating physician had recommended that she live with her daughter for 6 to 8 weeks. At the time of the home visit she had been living with her daughter for over a year.

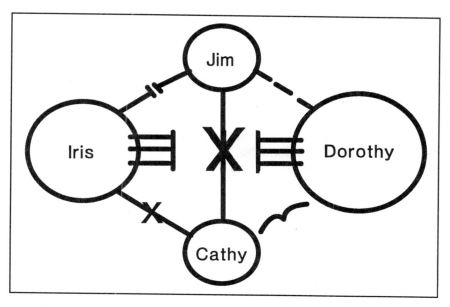

Fig. 19-1. Map of an extended family system depicting conflicted (⊣ ⊢), overinvolved (≡), disconnected (—✗—), covert (− − −), and allied (⌒⌒) family relationships.

During family meetings with the therapist Iris maintained that the physician had determined that her mother needed to reside with her for an indefinite period of time. Other family members did not challenge this assertion. In fact, no one was considering the possibility of Dorothy again living independently. Family meetings were characterized by supervicial complaints from Dorothy and quick meaningless solutions offered by Iris. Jim, who was typically detached from family discussions, would occasionally support a weakened version of Dorothy's complaints and observations. He rarely supported his wife's point of view. Cathy was a silent observer who shared supportive smiles with her grandmother.

As the family system map suggests, this was a disabled closed family with very strong boundaries between the family and the outside environment. A manifestation of this could be seen in the family's unwillingness to bring Dorothy's mental state to the attention of health care providers. The map also depicts family relationships that were dominated by a conflicted overinvolvement between Dorothy and Iris (≡). Jim, who was detached from his daughter, shared a covert supportive relationship with Dorothy (− − −). This covert relationship was useful to fuel the conflict in his relationship with his wife Iris (⊣ ⊢). Cathy had an alliance with her grandmother (∼∼), but remained disconnected and uninvolved with her parents.

The principle use of a family system map is in planning interventions.[9,10] The map allows the therapist to target specific family problems and plan interventions tailored to the family's paradigmatic expressions.

Consider the family mapped as above. Appropriate rehabilitation goals would clearly have included assisting Dorothy's move back to independent living status. However, the conflicted enmeshment between Dorothy and her daughter dominated all family functioning. In terms of the map, that conflict filled the family space, and subordinated all other family relationships; it had become the focal point of nearly all family interactions. As such Dorothy was functioning as the scapegoat, maintaining a balance in the family by allowing the others to ignore all other interactional problems that threatened family stability. Consistent with their closed paradigm the family was using Dorothy to meet its paradigmatic mandate to maintain family stability and continuity. Providing this family with information regarding Dorothy's need to live independently or offering support and reassurance would have been ineffective interventions because the family's paradigmatic commitments would dictate that Dorothy's individual needs be secondary to the family's interest in homeostasis.

Alternatively, a family conference was used to target the conflict between Dorothy and Iris. It was noted to the family that it seemed to be dominated by the anger and resentment between these two. Such an approach brought the conflict into the open, established interactional issues as acceptable topics for discussion within the context of therapy, and reframed the conflict as a family concern. The family's discussions were therefore not focused on Dorothy's needs, but rather the family's current sense of frustration and stress. The famiy eventually decided that moving Dorothy back to her own house would be the best way to reduce the stress that was affecting all family members.

Knowing that a family is guided by paradigmatic commitments is not enough to form a prescription for a treatment strategy. Rather, the paradigmatic perspective highlights certain issues that are more or less relevant in one type of family versus another. In conjunction with a family systems map, the paradigmatic approach helps identify potentially important issues and directions for working with a given class of family.

Similarly, paradigmatic assessment provides direction for adapting therapeutic tasks to individual family interests. For example, if the family system is closed, problem-solving sessions may be used to promote communication among family members. Alternatively, the therapist may use direct paradoxical prescription, taking advantage of the closed family's tendency to see the therapist as an authority figure. Therapist modeling of acceptance of disagreement may help to increase the closed family's tolerance for diverse viewpoints. It is important to remember that the closed paradigm represents a commitment to resist change. Although family change may be necessary to re-enable a closed family, appeals to try something new will likely not precipitate it. And direct pressure will probably foster resistance. The morphostatic tendencies of the closed family render it more responsive to paradoxical techniques that tend to use the family's resistance to its own advantage.

Therapists can gain access to a random family by mirroring its random approach and participating in its informal style.[9] Random regimens typically respond to therapeutic techniques based on play. Interventions that generate family involvement and cooperation within the context of recreation tend to be most effective. For example, individual family drawings, family sculpture, role playing, and expressive techniques are among the best interventions to use with random families. Proposing such activities in a manner requiring increasing levels of family cooperation will help the random family learn to function as a coordinated unit.

Open families are unique in that they explicitly examine their process and structure.[9] Unlike closed families, they characteristically define manifest problems in terms of relationship difficulties, which leads the family to endless disabling negotiations without resolution. However, the family's tendency toward excessive discussion can be exploited to its advantage. The therapist can intervene in this process by placing a temporary ban on family talk about process and relationships. Instead, family conversation can be directed toward the pragmatic aspects of the manifest problem. For example, the open family might define the chief complaint related to caring for a disabled older member in terms of relationship problems between siblings. Rather than accept this definition, the therapist could suggest that the family members temporarily put aside discussions about how they are feeling about one another in order to solve some of their pressing practical needs. In this way the family's capacity for problem solving can begin to be redirected. Reframing the manifest problem can often be followed by contracting with the family to perform specific care-providing tasks between therapy sessions. Such an approach will help decrease the family's tendency to discuss matters excessively. It will also appeal to the open family's commitment to efficacy and pragmatism.

The overall paradigmatic intervention strategy should be one that moves the disabled family in a direction opposite to its paradigmatic tendency for exaggeration.[9] The therapeutic purpose is to move the family to a less extreme and more enabled version of itself. In all cases the therapist must be aware of the family's style in order to select interventions that will reinforce paradigmatic tendencies on the one hand or counter them on the other.

SUMMARY

Recognizing dysfunctional dynamics in the family that is caring for a disabled older member can be critical to the success of a rehabilitation program. Family paradigms provide a means of organizing and understanding family dynamics. They also provide a structure for recognizing patterns of behavior characteristic of an individual family's problem-solving approaches and typical modes of failure. Identification of a family's paradigm will help clinical practitioners match approaches and techniques to differing family paradigmatic commitments, thereby increasing the probability of successful intervention.

REFERENCES

1. Bodin, A.M. (1981). The interactional view: Family therapy approaches of the mental research institute. In A. Gurman and D. Kniskern (Eds), *Handbook of family therapy*. New York: Brunner/Mazel.
2. Brody, E., Poulshock, S.W., and Masciocchi, C.F. (1978). The family caring unit: A major consideration in the long-term support system. *Gerontologist, 18*, 556.
3. Brubaker, T.H. (1983). Introduction. In T.H. Brubaker (Ed.), *Family relationships in later life*. Beverly Hills, CA: Sage.
4. Brubaker, T.H., and Brubaker, E. (1981). Adult child and elderly parent household: Issues in stress for theory and practice. *Alternative Lifestyles, 4*, 242.
5. Brummel-Smith, K. (1988). Family science and geriatric rehabilitation. *Top. Geriatr. Rehabil.* (in press).
6. Buckley, W. (1967). *Sociology's modern systems theory*. Englewood Cliffs, NJ: Prentice-Hall.
7. Cantor, M.H. (1980). The informal support system: Its relevance in the lives of the elderly. In E.F. Borgatta and McCluskey (Eds.), *Aging and society*. Beverly Hills, CA: Sage.
8. Carpenter, J.O. (1974). Changing roles and disagreements in families with disabled husbands. *Arch. Phys. Med. Rehabil., 55*, 272.
9. Constantine, L.L. (1986). *Family paradigms: The practice of theory in family therapy*. New York: Guilford Press.
10. Constantine, L.L. (1978). Family sculpture and relationship mapping techniques. *J. Marriage Fam. Counsel., 4*, 13.
11. Costell, R., et al. (1981). The family meets the hospital: Predicting the family's perception of the treatment program from its problem solving style. *Arch. Gen. Psychiatry, 38*, 569.

12. Ede, D.R., and Rich, J.A. (1983). *Psychological distress in aging: A family management model.* Rockville, MD: Aspen Systems.
13. Ferrsira, A.B. (1963). Family myth and homeostasis. *Arch. Gen. Psychiatry, 9,* 457.
14. Herr, J.J., and Weakland (1979). *Counseling elders and their families: Practical techniques for applied gerontology.* New York: Springer.
15. Kantor, D., and Lehr, W. (1975). *Inside the family: Toward a theory of family process.* San Francisco: Jossey-Bass.
16. Kaplan, D., et al. (1977). Family mediation of stress. In R.H. Moos (Ed), *Coping with physical illness.* New York: Plenum.
17. Kaplan, D., and Mearig, J.S. (1977). A community support system for a family coping with chronic illness. *Rehabil. Lit., 38,* 79.
18. Kemp, B. (1986). Psychosocial and mental health issues in rehabilitation of older persons. In S.J. Brody and G.E. Ruff (Eds), *Aging and rehabilitation: Advances in the state of the art* (pp.   –   ). New York: Springer.
19. Kuypers, J.A., and Bengston, V.L. (1983). Toward competence in the older family. In T.H. Brubaker (Ed), *Family relationships in late life.* Beverly Hills, CA: Sage.
20. Levenson, A.J., and Beller, S.A. (1984). Optimal assessment in geriatric rehabilitation. In D.W. Krueger (Ed), *Rehabilitation psychology: A comprehensive textbook.* Rockville, MD: Aspen Systems.
21. Loeble, J.P., and Eisdorfer, C. (1984). Psychological and psychiatric factors in rehabilitation of the elderly. In T.F. Williams (Ed), *Rehabilitation in aging.* New York: Raven Press.
22. Minuchin, S. (1974). *Families and family therapy.* Cambridge, MA: Harvard University Press.
23. Miller, M.B., Bernstein, H., and Sharkey, H. (1975). Family extrusion of the aged patient: Family homeostasis and sexual conflict. *Gerontologist,* Aug., 291.
24. Olson, H.O., et al. (1983). *Families: What makes them work.* Beverly Hills, CA.: Sage.
25. Olson, D.E., Sprenkle, D.H., and Russel, C.S. (1979). The circumplex model of marital and family systems: Cohesion and adaptability dimensions, family types and clinical applications. *Fam. Process, 18,* 3.
26. Peck, B.B. (1974). Physical medicine and family dynamics: The dialectics of rehabilitation. *Fam. Process, 13,* 469.
27. Pentecost, R.L., Zwerenz, B., and Manuel, J.W. (1976). Intrafamily identity and home dialysis success. *Nephron, 17,* 88.
28. Reiss, D. (1981). *The family's construction of reality.* Cambridge, MA: Harvard University Press.
29. Reiss, D. (1982). The working family: A researcher's view of health in the household. *Am. J. Psychiatry, 139,* 1412.
30. Reiss, D. (1971). Varieties of consensual experience: Relating family interaction to individual thinking. *Fam. Process, 10,* 1.
31. Rustad, L.C. (1984). Family adjustment to chronic illness and disability in mid-life. In M. Eissnberg, L. Satkin, and M. Jansen (Eds.), *Chronic illness and disability through the life span.* New York: Springer.
32. Shanas, E. (1979). The family as a social support system in old age. *Gerontologist, 19,* 169.

33. Silverstone, B. (1979). Issues for the middle generation: Responsibility adjustment, and growth. In Ragan P. (Ed), *Aging parents.* Los Angeles: University of Southern California Press.

34. Steinman, L. (1979). Reactivated conflicts of aging parents. In P. Ragan (Ed), *Aging parents.* Los Angeles: University of Southern California Press.

35. Strain, J.J. (1978). *Psychological interventions in medical practices.* New York: Appleton-Century-Crofts.

36. Troll, L.E., and Bengston, V.L. (1979). Generations in the family. In W. Burr et al. (Eds.), *Contemporary theories about the family.* New York: MacMillan.

37. Versluys, H.P. (1980). Physical rehabilitation and family dynamics. *Rehabil. Lit., 41,* 58.

38. Watzlawick, P., Beavin, J.H., and Jackson, D.C. (1976). *Pragmatics of human communication: A study of interactional patterns, pathologies, and paradoxes.* New York: Norton.

39. Weakland, J.H., et al. (1974). Brief therapy: Focused problem resolution. *Fam. Process, 13,* 141.

40. Zarit, S.H., and Zarit, J.M. (1984). Psychological approaches to families of the elderly. In M. Eisenberg, L. Sutkin, and M. Janssn (Eds.), *Chronic illness and disability through the life span.* New York: Springer.

PART IV

Organizing Rehabilitation Programs

CHAPTER 20

Rehabilitation in Acute Care Settings
LAWRENCE S. MILLER

Rehabilitation physicians have always maintained a concern for the functional problems of patients of all ages. The rehabilitation approach has traditionally involved a team of health professionals to assist each patient in achieving his or her highest level of functional independence. The rehabilitation team typically works in a multidisciplinary fashion with each member, including the physician, aware of the strengths and expertise of the other team members. The rehabilitation team not only works with medical and physical problems but assesses emotional and cognitive functioning, psychosocial status, family resources, and other community resources. This comprehensive approach should not be restricted to a relatively few individuals but should be available for all patients treated in the medical community. Rehabilitation units of acute care community hospitals have usually included a large number of geriatric patients with stroke, arthritis, amputation, hip fracture, etc. Unfortunately, there are not enough rehabilitation units in acute hospitals to provide the necessary opportunities for all who could benefit.

During the last two decades, physicians in family medicine and internal medicine who have been concerned about issues such as dementia, falls, and pharmacologic interactions in the elderly person provided an impetus for development of geriatric specialization. As the field of geriatrics expands it will need to offer the comprehensive services of rehabilitation to all the geriatric population. If the primary care physician becomes as familiar with the comprehensive approach to the patient as the rehabilitation physician, there will be ultimate benefit for the older population. This chapter examines the role a geriatric rehabilitation unit can play in an acute care hospital, contrasts this with a general rehabilitation unit, and reviews the kinds of patients most appropriate for a geriatric program in an acute care hospital.

REHABILITATION UNIT: REGULAR OR GERIATRICS?

What are the differences between a stroke or arthritis rehabilitation unit in the community hospital compared to an age-defined geriatric rehabilitation unit? If approached solely on the basis of outcomes this is a difficult question to answer. Without sound research data (of which there are few), there is little ability to adequately evaluate the differences in rehabilitation care. Rehabilitation units that follow appropriate procedural guidelines and effectively document progress and outcomes will certainly meet the minimal criteria for certification by the various local and national agencies. However, by only reviewing individual patient charts, it is difficult, if not impossible, to determine whether or not a change in organization toward an age-defined unit might have resulted in substantial improvements in patient function. For example, many years ago a home health agency nurse mentioned that patients discharged from one rehabilitation unit consistently made better adjustment at home than patients discharged from other rehabilitation units. The more successful rehabilitation unit devoted much effort in discharge planning, including identifying community resources, close follow-up care, examining the home environment, extensive patient family education, etc. However, this additional effort did not appear evident in the medical record in comparison to the other facilities.

In another example, a demented patient, bedridden and incontinent for several months in a nursing home, was admitted to a general rehabilitation center for a 1-week evaluation with the opinion that there was no potential for improvement. The record showed that the patient was seen by an internist, physiatrist, physical therapists, and rehabilitation nurses who determined that the patient was severely demented, would not eat, would not cooperate, and therefore should be discharged. The patient's son, a physician, did not have a "good feeling" about the rehabilitation program and arranged for his father to go to another center, a geriatric rehabilitation center. On admission it was determined that the patient did not have Alzheimer's dementia but rather Multi-Infarct Dementia, severe depression, prostatic hypertrophy, and, in fact, a hip fracture sustained in a fall at the nursing home 3 months previous, leading to an inability to walk. Following hip replacement, prostate surgery, and antidepressant treatment, the patient showed dramatic progress and improved to a supervised level of ambulation, independence in activities of daily living (ADLs) (including feeding), and continence of bladder. He still remained too unsafe and confused for board and care living but was able to return to an intermediate care facility as an active person. Even after retrospective review of the medical chart from the first rehabilitation center, there was no indication of less than adequate care.

What factors, then, differentiate between a regular rehabilitation unit and a "geriatric" rehabilitation unit? Mostly, it is the advanced education, special training, and personal concern of the entire rehabilitation team, especially the physician, for geriatric patients. It is the day-to-day consideration of geriatric problems that makes the geriatric rehabilitation unit special. The careful assessment of cognitive problems, medical stability, pharmacologic issues, psychiatric features, etc., give the geriatric patient the special consideration that ultimately will result in maximally improved functional recovery and quality of life. And it is these differences which result in the person living independently or partially assisted versus incapable and maximally assisted.

One study appears to document the effectiveness of a specific geriatric rehabilitation unit.[3] This study was performed at Highland View, a rehabilitation and chronic disease hospital in Cleveland. This study demonstrated that development of a specific geriatric rehabilitation program within the hospital resulted in improved care and a higher percentage of patients returning home. The program specifically selected staff who had knowledge, interest, and sensitivities to geriatric management.

A recent study[1] evaluated the effect of the diagnosis-related group (DRG) on outcomes following hip fractures. The length of hospital stay dropped from 16.6 days pre-DRG to 10.3 days post-DRG. In this study, there did not appear to be any rehabilitation hospital referrals. The number of persons with hip fracture who were referred to nursing homes increased dramatically, from 21 to 48 percent; moreover, 200 percent more patients remained institutionalized 6 months after discharge compared to the pre-DRG period. Unfortunately, the Health Care Financing Administration and the California Professional Review Organization have developed policies which effectively limit rehabilitation centers from admitting hip fractures. Many rehabilitation centers will not even consider taking a hip fracture patient. Obviously, the clear results of these policies is to sentence more older persons to spend the rest of their lives in nursing homes at great expense to their families and to the Medicaid system. This trend must be reversed by increasing geriatric rehabilitation opportunities, not restricting them.

The concept of rehabilitation is recognized as being important for the training of geriatric specialists. The American Geriatric Society guidelines for geriatric fellowships place "emphasis . . . on a much greater awareness and familiarity with physical medicine and rehabilitation."[2] In the past, it was found, however, that geriatric fellows at University of California, Los Angeles, did not benefit from rehabilitation rotations with rehabilitation residents on a general rehabilitation unit. After trying a number of different general rehabilitation programs, a rehabilitation center with a specific geriatric focus was chosen. The geriatric fellows have since uniformly found this rotation to be stimulating and highly beneficial to their practice in the field of geriatric medicine. The fellows are primarily involved in a one-to-one preceptor relationship with the rehabilitation physician. Specific training is provided in the unique aspects of neuromusculoskeletal examination of older persons. Preexisting medical and functional conditions are discussed in relation to the current illness and disability. Concerns relating to cognitive impairment, medical problems, pharmacology, etc., are carefully evaluated. The geriatric fellows learn what to expect from a comprehensive geriatric rehabilitation program.

CHOOSING STAFF FOR GERIATRIC REHABILITATION UNITS

With the advent of Medicare in the 1960s through the 1970s, the belief was that geriatric physical therapists (PTs) would abound, that PTs would have contracts with several nursing homes, provide care to meet all the therapy needs, and still bill Medicare at a rate high enough to live in the nicest neighborhoods. Notwithstanding this, the facts showed that the majority of patients in nursing homes still did not receive adequate therapy. (and most PTs did not become rich). The point is that taking care of old people in and of itself does not make one a qualified geriatric health care provider.

Physical therapists presently receive at least a bachelor's degree from college and have special training in many areas of basic sciences and the neuromusculoskeletal system. Many PTs also have master's degrees and there is a push for a master's to be required for all registered therapists in the future. The most lucrative positions for PTs remain nursing home contracting and private practice, which includes musculoskeletal treatment and sports medicine. Hospital-based PTs are involved primarily in orthopedic management but also take care of the rehabilitation needs of acute care patients. They may subspecialize in the treatment of arthritis, hand injury, head injury, spinal cord injury, pediatrics, etc. Within the rehabilitation hospital, PTs treating the disorders of general rehabilitation patients such as stroke or hip fracture consider "geriatrics" to be the least stimulating of all rotations.

Several years ago my institution conducted a study on older stroke patients which involved measuring the rate of improvement in mobility on a functional assessment scale. We then evaluated average rates of improvement obtained by each individual PT both in physical therapy and on ADLs for occupational therapy. We were able to identify a few PTs who achieved rates of improvement above the mean by at least one standard deviation. These PTs were already recognized by their clinical performance but in addition had the attributes necessary for success in treating geriatric patients. The majority of other PTs' scores stayed within the mean and standard deviation.

The PTs treating the geriatric patient recognized that adjustments in treatment must be made for differences in motivation, and ability for exercise will often be much less than with a young adult. They also recognized that improvement is often slower due to coexisting conditions, such as arthritis or cardiopulmonary problems, so they adjusted their expectations accordingly. Older persons may fatigue easily and have increased discomfort with even small amounts of exercise. Therapists learned to perform a careful physical assessment to determine the degree of musculoskeletal abnormalities and to check with physicians about the degree of cardiac and pulmonary function. They need to help the patients achieve goals for improvement and, as much as possible, work within the individual patient's level of comfort.

Physical therapists should also recogize that many geriatric patients had once been active citizens, even if they presently are inactive and retired, and thus not to devalue the patient. Often, the common use of first names by PTs will annoy the patient and therefore the therapist should determine initially how the patient wishes to be addressed. The PTs should continually review the objectives of the treatment plan and identify reasonable short-term and long-term goals for the patient. There should be frequent communication with the physician when there are areas that are interfering with anticipated recovery, that is, fatigue, depression, shortness of breath, impaired balance, etc. This information brought to the attention of the physician may focus his or her attention on a problem that may not have been considered previously. There are no specific techniques or "high tech" equipment specifically needed for the geriatric patient. The best advice for the management of geriatric patients for any health professional is to follow this simple concept: "Treat with concern and respect."

The *occupational therapist* (OT) also has a college degree and may have a master's degree. The OT's involvement relates more to functional skills, particularly skills involving the upper extremities. In geriatric management, the OT is involved not only in ADL training but also in evaluating and helping the patient in the performance of normal household activities and community activities. They often will provide help in developing hobbies and projects that will be of long-term benefit and pleasure. Again, the OT should be aware of the issues of geriatric management discussed previously. Since OTs are working more with judgment and cognition, they are in a position to help the patient in orientation and cognitive training. They are able to make proper judgments as to the patient's ability for problem solving and safety. The OT who would be successful with geriatric patients must also be aware of the older person's individual and specific needs. For instance, geriatric patients often will have impaired vision from cataracts and require a work area with indirect lighting. In fact, one OT stated that many geriatric patients really did not care to watch television, read, or play cards. Their most enjoyable leisure activities included listening to music and having someone read to them from the newspaper. It is not surprising that this OT achieved outstanding results with her geriatric patients.

A *speech pathologist* can play an important part in the rehabilitation team even in those patients not having primary impairments of communication. Speech therapists have a master's level of training in their field. Speech pathologists may work primarily with school districts, with children, or only with voice problems. In the rehabilitation team, speech therapists work with stroke patients who have aphasia and dysarthria, swallowing problems, or cognitive dysfunction. Speech therapists play an important role in cognitive training and reorientation programs for those patients who have Multi-Infarct Dementia or Alzheimer's. They provide a daily structured program that helps reorient and focus these patients in their activities. They advise family members in caring for cognitively impaired patients.

The importance of a *neuropsychologist* is well-known to geriatricians. However, a neuropsychologist with background in rehabilitation provides additional benefit. There is opportunity to discuss specific methods of intervention among the rehabilitation staff members so that they can more effectively work with the patient with cognitive impairments.

The role of the *rehabilitation psychologist* is also of vital importance. Dealing with depression and adjustment to functional impairment is as important to the geriatric patient as to the patient of any age with a functional impairment. The psychologist involved in the geriatric unit needs to be able to identify the degrees of cognitive impairment, often with the help of the neuropsychologist and other team members, and to be able to provide the appropriate supportive management that will be of benefit. If direct counseling and supportive sessions are not deemed to be of benefit in selected cases then the psychologist may supervise a behavioral management approach with team members.

The *rehabilitation nurse* has had experience and training in dealing with nursing issues related to varying disabilities including strokes, spinal cord injuries, etc. Many rehabilitation nurses have taken a comprehensive examination and have become a certified rehabilitation registered nurse. The rehabilitation nurses perform not only nursing duties but are able to assess the functional abilities of the patients. They become involved in appropriate training for ADLs, transfers, and bowel and bladder management, including carefully monitored timed voiding programs and catheterizations. It was not long ago when bladder training consisted of clamping the catheter and only male nurses were allowed to catheterize a male patient. Rehabilitation nurses involved in a geriatric program must in addition have the knowledge, skills, and attitudes that the nurses on geriatric evaluation units posses. These are discussed elsewhere in this book.

Finally, one must consider the role of the *physician-director* of a geriatric rehabilitation unit. A well-training physiatrist, knowledgeable in inpatient rehabilitation management, in conjunction with a geriatric specialist, could successfully direct a geriatric rehabilitation unit.

A *physiatrist* has training in the various specialties of neurology, orthopedics, and rheumatology, and is able to identify many factors contributing to the physical impairment and functional deficits in the elderly patient. However, physiatrists generally do not have much training in internal medicine and are not exposed to "geriatric training."[4] It is often said that physiatrists were probably the first specialty that developed a team approach for geriatric patients with major functional impairments. Nevertheless, their focus did not relate to many of the unique problems of geriatrics, including prevention of falls, evaluation of dementia, incontinence, depression, or pharmacologic management.

There have been questions raised as to whether *geriatricians* by themselves could manage a rehabilitation unit. Certainly geriatricians should possess the skills necessary to manage a team approach and are aware of medical management and functional problems in the geriatric patient. However, they do not have appropriate training in neuromusculoskeletal assessment nor do they typically learn therapy options available in the management of functional impairment. The following case may clarify the benefits of physiatric management:

A 76-year-old woman was admitted to the acute hospital because of progressive inability to walk and frequent falling. She was evaluated by an internist, rheumatologist, general physician, neurologist, and orthopedic surgeon. The initial impression was spinal stenosis, lumbar radiculopathy, herniated disc. However, magnetic resonance imaging (MRI) scans, myelograms, and other tests did not disclose a surgically correctable lesion. EMG findings showed mild nerve conduction slowing. The patient demonstrated weakness of the lower extremities. Ironically, she was referred to the rehabilitation center for two reasons. First, the "skilled" rehabilitation unit attached to the hospital refused to admit her since she did not appear to have any "rehab potential." However, this patient only had Medicare with no extra funds to pay a deposit at the skilled rehabilitation facility or at any convalescent facility. These issues were not disclosed to the rehabilitation center on referral, only that this patient developed some type of spinal cord degenerative condition with neuropathy that might benefit from rehabilitation.

On evaluation at the rehabilitation center, the physiatrist noted definite wakness of the left quadriceps but also a severely arthritic, unstable left knee. (Arthritis of the knees had been mentioned by various physicians at the other hospital but did not appear to them to be of major consequence.) The physiatrist determined that a knee replacement would allow this patient to achieve mobility. The orthopedic consultant was reluctant to perform surgery because of the patient's obesity and weakness. After much pleading, the orthopedist was convinced that without a knee replacement the patient would be sent to a nursing home for the rest of her life, most likely bedridden because of her obesity and inability to transfer without maximal assist. Even if the surgery was not successful she could be in no worse position. The patient tolerated the surgery well, regained strength in the left knee, became independent and ambulatory with a walker, and was able to return home with appropriate resources to assist her.

This case illustrates the problems with functional impairment in the elderly. Problems are often of a multisystem nature that are not readily identified by individual or even multiple specialists. The physiatrists is able to evaluate the effect of multisystem involvement and often can urge other specialists to provide the type of management that leads to improved function.

REFERRAL TO A GERIATRIC REHABILITATION UNIT

What is an appropriate referral to a geriatric rehabilitation unit (GRU)? Ideally, a GRU will provide all of the resources available at a geriatric evaluation unit (GEU) plus the rehabilitation evaluation and management of the physical impairments. A regular rehabilitation unit, for an impaired functioning geriatric patient without a specific diagnosis such as stroke, would generally not provide comprehensive geriatric management. In fact, the general rehabilitation unit would probably not accept that type of patient, stating that the "patient did not meet Medicare guidelines." A physician should consider referral to a GRU for a patient who, after repeated outpatient evaluations, continues to have difficulties with function, or does not improve following attempted management with outpatient or home therapy. Hospitalized geriatric patients recovering from an acute illness such as congestive heart failure, pneumonia, or addominal surgery, and who, after a reasonable period of recovery and medical treatment, still appear quite unsteady and unable to manage effectively at home, would also be appropriate referrals.

One must consider whether the assistance available at home is sufficient to allow the patient to improve in functional ability in the home setting. The other consideration must be, if nursing home care is planned, will the patient have potential to improve, given the limited physician management, nursing management, and therapy available at the nursing home setting? Before referring the geriatric patient to a nursing home, the physician should ask, "Am I giving this patient a life sentence to institutional care without the possibility of parole?" The patient first is entitled to a comprehensive geriatric rehabilitation assessment. Not only is this necessary for humanitarian reasons but it will reduce the costs of long-term nursing home care.

The following case illustrates the concept of the lack of awareness by the medical profession for geriatric rehabilitation management:

A 74-year-old man had a 1-year history of progressive difficulty with ambulation and back pain. His family physician of many years had prescribed large doses of amobarbital sodium–secobarbital sodium (Tuinal) at night along with large doses of aspirin–oxycodone hydrochloride and (Percodan) meperidine hydrochloride (Demerol) for pain complaints. Because of progressive pain and weakness he was referred to a neurosurgeon, was diagnosed as having lumbar spinal stenosis, and underwent a decompressive laminectomy. While in the hospital he was evaluated by an internist, cardiologist, and the neurosurgeon. Following surgery, the patient was discharged home. After 3 months at home the patient was confused, lethargic, could barely walk the 10 ft. to the bathroom, and would fall frequently. He needed total physical care, was often incontinent of bladder, and became essentially nonfunctional. Al physicians involved in his care were aware of the local rehabilitation center and regularly referred "appropriate" patients for rehabilitation care. Retrospectively, the physicians on his case said they did not consider medical or rehabilitation management for this patient since they felt he had severe psychologic problems, cognitive problems, refused to stop drinking, and displayed a complete lack of motivation. They assumed that nothing more could be offered the patient from a medical point of view.

A friend of the family, a dentist, had involvement with a geriatric rehabilitation program and was aware of the excellent results obtained with complex geriatric rehabilitation assessment. The decision to admit the patient to rehabilitation was risky. The patient could not be admitted to an acute medical bed since he did not have a diagnosis under DRG. Because the patient was cognitively impaired, had behavioral problems, and was entirely unmotivated with no specific outcome goals on admission, he did not meet guidelines for rehabilitation care under

Medicare. Nevertheless, this patient had become severely disabled over a 1-year period and deserved a comprehensive evaluation. After a careful assessment, findings included severe hypothyroidism with inadequate thyroid replacement, a daily medication regimen, including alprazolam (Xanax), 5 mg; amobarbital sodium–secobarbital sodium, 400 mg; and aspirin–oxycodone hydrochloride, 8 to 12 tablets, was administered. The back and lower extremities were stiff and weak from prolonged bed rest and immobilization. He was ataxic, confused, and disoriented. He had also developed further behavioral problems that appeared to be related to alcohol withdrawal.

The patient remained in the geriatric rehabilitation unit for 3 weeks. He was taken off all sedating medications and was placed on doxepin hydrochloride (Sinequan) for depression and acetaminophen (Tylenol) for pain. He was given appropriate thyroid replacement. He received intensive therapy (physical, occupational, speech, and psychologic). At the time of discharge the patient was alert and oriented, cognitively intact, and was able to ambulate, slightly unsteadily but without assistive devices. It was recommended to all his physicians at discharge that he not be given any further sedatives or narcotic medications. On 6-month follow-up the patient had maintained his independent level of function and had returned to his family business part-time.

This patient was referred only because one person was aware of the care available at a geriatric rehabilitation unit. A second point that needs to be made is that the Medicare regulations are established in such a way as to almost prohibit comprehensive assessment and management of a chronically functionally impaired elderly patient.

SUMMARY

Geriatric rehabilitation is an important aspect of geriatric care. This chapter points out what constitutes a geriatric rehabilitation unit and stresses the need for increasing the awareness of geriatric rehabilitation. A description of the services and type of professionals involved is reviewed. One should consider rehabilitation assessment for any geriatric patient who has functional difficulties that have not been successfully managed despite visits to various specialists. Before World War II, there were major rehabilitation centers for poliomyelitis, but stroke patients went to nursing homes, spinal cord–injured patients died, and head-injured patients went to mental institutions. Presently, there are no polio centers, but there are federally funded spinal cord rehabilitation centers, and an explosion of head injury programs (the number one venture capital investment in health care today!). It is time to provide rehabilitation for the functionally impaired elderly as well.

REFERENCES

1. Fitzgerald, S.F., et al. (1987). Changing patterns of hip fracture care before and after implementation of the prospective payment system. *JAMA, 258,* 218.
2. Guidelines for fellowship training programs. (1987). *J. Am. Geriatr. Soc., 35,* 792.
3. Lefton, E., Bonstelle, S., and Frengley, J.D. (1983). Success with an inpatient geriatric unit; A controlled study of outcome and follow-up. *J. Am. Geriatr. Soc., 31,* 149.
4. Redfern, J.B. (1984). Geriatric rehabilitation. In A.P.Ruskin (Ed.), *Current therapy in physiatry* (pp. 90–99). Philadelphia: Saunders.

CHAPTER 21

Rehabilitation in Private Practice
CATHERINE E. BANNERMAN

The primary care physician has several roles in the rehabilitation of the elderly. The first is to recognize the need for and initiate rehabilitation. This requires both an accurate assessment of disability, and familiarity with the various settings and resources available for rehabilitation. The second is to manage medical problems during rehabilitation. Finally, as perhaps the only member of the rehabilitation team who has continued follow-up with the patient, the primary care physician must ensure that gains established are maintained, and that progress continues after discharge.

ASSESSMENT AND REFERRAL FOR REHABILITATION

In the elderly, the degree of disability caused by a problem is often more significant than the particular underlying medical diagnosis. For example, a person with diabetes, hypertension, and coronary artery disease may function very well and be more active than someone with an osteoarthritic hip or knee pain which limits his or her mobility. In many cases, improving a patient's ability to function is more important than curing the disease. In geriatrics, the physician's goal is not only to treat illness but to maintain a patient's function within the context of his or her disease. Assessing the need for rehabilitation thus becomes part of routine, ongoing medical care, and a rehabilitation approach is adopted for acute medical problems.

There is an obvious need for rehabilitation following an acute event which results in abrupt loss of function such as stroke or hip fracture. The need may be just as great, but less obvious, for patients hospitalized with acute medical problems such as pneumonia, which can cause a more insidious loss of function due to bed rest. Persistent physical disability following hospitalization for acute medical illness has been well described.[7] Decline in function in the elderly can also occur gradually in the community, leading to incapacity just as devastating as that caused by an acute event.

The primary care physician must be able to recognize the need for rehabilitation and refer appropriately in all three situations. This is most difficult in the case of gradual functional decline occurring in the home. But it is as important to intervene in this situation as in the acute case, before the patient loses the ability to remain independent in the community. Assessment of gradual decline requires being aware of a patient's functional capacity as well as his or her medical diagnoses. The ability to climb stairs, get in and out of a bathtub or car, dress oneself, or cook a meal may be as important as monitoring blood pressure.

The traditional "review of symptoms,"[1] which is part of a complete history and physical examination, does not really assess a patient's functional capacity. After a detailed series of questions about cardiac, respiratory, and musculoskeletal problems, it still may not be clear how far or fast a patient can walk and whether help is needed for the activities of daily living (ADLs) such as dressing or writing a check. Even the physical examination, unless done in great detail, may not reveal the true picture of a patient's functional state. It is therefore important to develop and maintain a relatively formal functional assessment of elderly patients, to monitor over time. The Katz Index of Independence in Activities of Daily Living Scale[3] is an example of a brief, easily administered scale which rates the ability to perform ADLs. Such a questionnaire, in combination with specific maneuvers on physical examination to test strength and mobility,[5] provides a good functional assessment which can be performed in an office setting.

The answer to functional decline may not always be rehabilitation, but recognizing a significant change is the first step toward improving function. Joint replacement may be required to alleviate immobility caused by painful osteoarthritis of the hips or knees. But fear of falling can also cause functional decline from self-imposed immobility with resultant muscle weakness, general deconditioning, and even flexion contractures. In this case, gait training to restore confidence and muscle strength is the intervention which will allay further deterioration. Depression can also cause diminished mobility, weakness, and loss of functional capacity. Treatment of the depression is important, but physical therapy to improve joint range of motion and general muscle strength may be as important to maintain function.

In all cases, recognizing functional decline is crucial in preventing loss of independence, as the key to maintaining function in the elderly is early intervention.

Having recognized the need to improve a patient's function either after an acute medical event or due to gradual deterioration, the physician must be aware of the resources available to do this in order to refer appropriately. The many possible rehabilitation settings include acute and convalescent hospitals, inpatient rehabilitation centers, in-home rehabilitation, and outpatient therapy. The choice of settings depends on many factors including the cause and degree of disability, the amount of community and family support available, and the patient's financial resources. Due to increasing pressure to discharge patients quickly after acute hospitalization, rehabilitation which might previously have taken place in the hospital must be done in the community. This places a growing burden on the community-based primary care physician and family for organizing and participating in rehabilitation.

MEDICAL MANAGEMENT DURING REHABILITATION

The actual involvement of the primary care physician depends on the setting of rehabilitation. In an inpatient unit where medical care is provided by the rehabilitation team, the primary care physician may function as an adjunct member of the team, available for consultation and liaison with the family. Other settings, such as convalescent hospitals, in-home rehabilitation, and outpatient therapy, require more active involvement by the primary physician. This means that first, the physician must have a good understanding of the role of the other persons involved in rehabilitation. Second, the physician must anticipate and manage the medical problems that may arise. Finally, the physician must maintain contact with the patient's family and support system.

Rehabilitation of the elderly is best accomplished by a multidisciplinary team with the consistent reinforcement and cooperation of all involved. This may be a "core team" consisting of physical or occupational therapist, nurse, physician, and social worker, or may involve many more disciplines depending on the setting and the patient's needs. In order to function effectively as part of such a team, the physician must be familiar with the basic procedures and terminology of the other members.

Although it is basic to rehabilitation, the exact role of the occupational therapist or physical therapist is not usually taught in medical school. And during residency training, the scope of the social worker beyond that of discharge planner, and the roles of the various therapists, are usually gleaned through observation rather than by specific instruction. Disciplines such as speech therapy, recreation therapy, and art therapy remain somewhat mysterious, and like occupational therapy, physical therapy, and social service, may not be used optimally because of inappropriate or complete lack of physician referral.

Therapists need to know about a patient's underlying medical problems, and the physician should be familiar with basic procedures and techniques of therapy.

An example of the working relationship needed in rehabilitation is seen in the case of stroke care. Speech and gait training following a stroke are coordinated with the efforts of a social worker or the family to provide an appropriate physical environment after discharge. Similarly, there is little point in gait training unless the symptoms of angina which occur with exertion are assessed and controlled. In this case, the physical therapist and physician must coordinate their efforts.

Rehabilitation is not a static state. It is an active process with physical and functional changes occurring. In the elderly, this is often reflected by changes in medical status with new medical problems arising, exacerbation of old problems, and almost inevitably, a change in medication requirements. This group tends to have several coexistent medical diagnoses, which may all be "stable" in a familiar environment with a predictable activity level and steady number and dose of medications. These problems can quickly become active with the significant stresses imposed by a rehabilitation program, which often involves a great increase over prior activity levels and a complete change of diet and environment.

There are also medical problems which arise as a direct result of the primary disability which is usually the immobility imposed by a stroke, hip fracture, or severe medical illness. These "secondary disabilities" include pressure sores, flexion contractures, and venous thrombosis. In addition, bed rest has a devastating effect on overall muscle strength and bone density,[4,6] particularly in the elderly who have less reserve than younger patients. Depression is another secondary disability which can be just as harmful to the progress of rehabilitation if not recognized and treated.

The best approach to all these secondary disabilities is preventive. Particularly in the acute medical setting, the primary care physician must be able to anticipate these problems in order to initiate appropriate preventive measures.

The common types of acute medical problems which occur during rehabilitation include exacerbation of cardiovascular disease and musculoskeletal pain due to increased activity. Gastrointestinal problems such as duodenal ulcer disease, gastritis, and constipation may develop due to pain medication, nonsteroidal antiinflammatory drugs, and dietary changes. Bladder infections are common complications, particularly with instrumentation involved in the investigation of incontinence or in bladder training. In inpatients, anxiety and insomnia are caused by the unfamiliar environment and change in routine. Since a change in symptoms does not necessarily mean new disease, the primary care physician who is aware of a patient's previous medical history is best able to put new symptoms in context and avoid unnecessary investigations which are costly, time-consuming, and interrupt rehabilitation.

In both inpatients and outpatients, medication requirements change throughout the course of rehabilitation and must be reviewed on a regular basis. For example, antihypertensive requirements may diminish with bed rest during acute illness, increase with more activity, then diminish again as exercise tolerance improves. Angina and cardiac arrhythmias may be exacerbated by vigorous therapy, and cardiac medications must be adjusted appropriately. Pain medication is more likely to be needed in the early stages of rehabilitation with extra effort and stress placed on muscles and joints by mobilization exercises, gait training, and endurance activities. As rehabilitation progresses, antiinflammatory or other pain medications originally given on a routine basis can be given prn (as required), then gradually eliminated. Insulin requirements may decrese dramatically, particularly in inpatients, reflecting a higher-than-usual amount of activity and a more carefully regulated diet. Hypnotics may be needed as a patient first settles into an unfamiliar, busy ward environment, but should not be continued routinely.

In an inpatient setting, "medication rounds" is an effective way of reviewing medications, both routine and prn, with nurses and other team members. This format has been successfully used in the Rancho Los Amigos Medical Center Geriatric Inpatient Rehabilitation Unit in Downey, California, where, as a teaching site, both family medicine residents and pharmacy students also participate. A retrospective study[2] showed that prior to initiating medication rounds, the total number of drugs per patient increased by 3 percent from admission to discharge. With the advent of formalized medication rounds, the total number of drugs decreased by 35 percent from admission to discharge. Medications most often affected were antihypertensives and analgesics. Given the high incidence of adverse drug reactions in the elderly, it is certainly worthwhile to minimize the total number and doses of medications. Taking the time to formally review medications seems to be a successful way of doing this.

In private practice, where this format for rounds is not feasible, regular brief review of the medication book is useful, particularly to keep track of the dosing frequency of prn medications. For outpatients, a separate medication list in the chart is helpful.

FOLLOW-UP AFTER REHABILITATION

Having passed through an acute illness and rehabilitation, the patient and family must then cope with reassimilation into the community with whatever disability the patient may be left with. If not discharged home, but to a board and care or nursing home, the patient must adapt to a new, and significantly different, environment. As probably the only member of the rehabilitation team who will continue to follow the patient after discharge, there are several ways in which the physician can help the patient and family through this difficult transition.

No matter how much progress has been made, the patient may experience anxiety and disappointment on discharge, particularly from an inpatient program. This letdown occurs as patients that were able to remain hopeful and anticipate further progress while in rehabilitation face the permanence of their disability as they perceive the end of rehabilitation. The disappointment is more acute if they are discharged to a less independent setting than the one they had been living in. The physician can help in this situation by explaining the origin of these feelings to the patient and family, by reassuring the patient, and by encouraging the family to be more supportive. It may be important for the physician to actually demonstrate the patient's ability to the family in order to encourage the family's support. When appropriate the physician should also reassure the patient and family that progress is likely to continue after discharge.

Whether or not the primary care physician has been involved in the patient's rehabilitation, it is important that the patient's functional status on discharge be noted in some detail. Small improvements in ambulation, strength, or bladder training may be very significant in terms of a patient's functional ability. The physician must have a baseline in order to monitor progress with appropriate feedback to the patient and family.

With the growing proportion of elderly in the population and the emphasis toward shorter hospitalization for acute medical problems, primary care physicians need to incorporate a rehabilitation approach into the management of medical problems. This means that from the onset of treating a patient, the goal is to restore function, not simply cure disease. The aim of rehabilitation is to allow the patient to function as independently as possible in the community. As more rehabilitation takes place in the home and outpatient settings, community-based physicians will inevitably become more involved in all stages of their patient's rehabilitation.

REFERENCES

1. Degowan, E.L., and Degowan, R.L. (1976). *Bedside diagnostic examination* (pp. 24–26). New York; Macmillan.
2. Gelalich, K., Williams, B., and Bannerman, C. Effect of medication rounds in geriatric rehabilitation unit. (Submitted for publication.)
3. Katz, S., et al. (1963). Studies of illness in the aged. *JAMA, 185,* 94.
4. Kottke, F.J. (1966). The effects of limitation of activity upon the human body. *JAMA, 196,* 825.
5. Mobility Assessment Scale. University of Southern California Division of Geriatrics at Rancho Los Amigos Medical Center Geriatric Assessment Clinic, Downey, California.
6. Treharne, R.W. (1981). Review of Wolff's law and its proposed means of operation. *Orthop. Rev., 10,* 35.
7. Warshaw, G.A., et al. (1982). Functional disability in the hospitalized elderly. *JAMA, 248,* 847.

CHAPTER 22

Geriatric Rehabilitation in the Long-Term Care Institutional Setting

DAN OSTERWEIL

A discussion of rehabilitation for the elderly in the long-term care institutional setting is a challenge because the available literature on rehabilitation focuses more on the acute care hospital and the rehabilitation center environments. In the minds of many, nursing homes are portrayed as sites of final disposition when all other alternatives have been exhausted and not sites for rehabilitation. Admission to a skilled nursing facility (SNF) is often identified as a bad outcome. An SNF is in fact a viable and appropriate alternative to the acute rehabilitation center. The basic principles of geriatric rehabilitation described by previous authors are equally valid in the long-term care institutional setting (Table 22-1), although some modification may be necessary.

As a geriatrician, it is important to adopt Howard Rusk's philosophy as it relates to stroke victims: "Every stroke patient should have a trial at rehabilitation, because there are no reliable indicators during the acute phase as to which patients will do well and which will not." This approach is equally pertinent to all geriatric disabilities. In most cases the outcome is unknown and the intensity and extent of rehabilitation effort and expected goals must be individualized. The cost-effectiveness

Table 22-1. *Basic Principles of Rehabilitation*

Treatment of the underlying disease
Prevention of a secondary disability
Treatment of primary disabilities
Realistic goals
Emphasis on functional independence
Enhancement of residual function
Provision of adaptive tools
Altering the environment
Team approach
Attention to motivation and other psychological factors (of both patients and caregivers)

of rehabilitation in adults has traditionally been measured by functional independence and an income-generating life. In geriatrics, cost-benefit ratios cannot be assessed in that way. Attention has been focused instead on functional outcomes that save cost in the long run and on quality-of-life issues. Among adult stroke survivors, for example, following short-term rehabilitation, 30 percent lived more than 11 years while 70 percent lived 3 to 7 years.[3] Short-term rehabilitation that leads to independent living is considered less expensive than permanent institutionalization. A rehabilitation effort leading to restored self-care skills of an institutionalized or homebound older person is cost-effective. Caring for this patient is less costly than caring for a "total care" nursing home resident. Improving the quality of life following rehabilitation is difficult to measure and therefore rarely reported as an outcome. Nevertheless, it should also be considered a target goal.

DEFINITION OF REHABILITATION

Many definitions have been used to describe rehabilitation. The most common is, "The restoration of previous level of function and/or maximizing the level of function to self-sufficiency or to gainful employment at his highest attainable skill." While this is generally true for adults with single–organ system involvement, it may be more complex for geriatric patients. The complexity stems from coexisting morbidity due to multiple chronic diseases, and sensory, cognitive, and affective impairments.

Geriatric rehabilitation has been defined to include several groups, including elderly persons who are not obviously ill but whose physical fitness is impaired; restoration of chronically ill persons without obvious visible signs of disability (*e.g.*, those with cardiac and pulmonary disease); and restoration of obviously disabled persons (e.g., those with hemiplegia, arthritis, fractures, amputations, and neuromuscular disease).[4,6] An appropriate operational definition of rehabilitation for the geriatric population in the long-term care setting might be: the process of delivering the minimal services which maintain the present or highest possible level of function. Rehabilitation potential in the geriatric population differs from prognosis in the sense that we do not always consider cure as our goal, but rather maintenance of function. The following discussion focuses on the role of the long-term care institution as a rehabilitation center, in addition to its customary role as a custodial center.

REHABILITATION IN AN INSTITUTIONAL LONG-TERM CARE SETTING

Conceptually, we can divide the target population into two categories: (1) individuals who are admitted to a long-term care facility for a specific purpose and are expected to go back to independent living; and (2) individuals who reside in congregate living facilities or nursing homes who have multiple medical problems that may contribute to disability, and which therefore have an impact on the quality of life, as well as caregiver burden. The first category includes (a) elderly persons with hip fractures with prolonged course of recovery. According to Medicare guidelines, a diagnosis of hip fracture without an associated disability in activities of daily living (ADLs) is usually denied a chance for a rehabilitation program within an acute rehabilitation center; (b) stroke victims who require a multidisciplinary team effort and who are unable to comply with 3 hours of a rehabilitation program per day; (c) patients who are eligible for a rehabilitation center, but suffer from depression. Lack of compliance due to depression may disqualify an older person from a program in a rehabilitation center. Even if accepted, it may be difficult to document any progress. (d) a special subgroup are elderly persons with an acute event such as stroke or fracture with a preexisting dementia syndrome. Dementia limits ability to successfully comply with a rehabilitation program within strict guidelines and time constraints.

The second category consists of elderly persons that suffer from multiple irreversible disabilities, and that are residing in a long-term care institutional setting. These persons may suffer from dementing disorders, urinary incontinence, agitative behavior, mobility problems, insomnia, depression, malnutrition, or hearing and visual impairments. This category constitutes 90 percent of the SNF-dwelling elderly, while the first category makes up 10 percent of the nursing home population.

Elderly persons from the first category are admitted to an SNF for a specific reason and have a good chance of returning to independent living. Therefore, the focus of rehabilitation is restoration of instrumental ADLs (IADLs) and ADLs. The second group is more likely to stay in a long-term care setting. For them, independence in ADLs and prevention of a secondary disability should be the focus.

The long-term care setting has some advantages over an acute hospital rehabilitation center for geriatric patients. The pace is slower, lasting months versus weeks. The focus is on the *individual*, with little or no concern as to how fast one progresses. Since those patients are 10 percent of the SNF population and are often cognitively more functional, they may get special attention by staff. The transfer back to independent living is more gradual and therefore may be less stressful.

ASSESSMENT OF REHABILITATION POTENTIAL

Searching for rehabilitation potential is not synonymous with looking for a cure, but rather the potential for reducing the amount of assistance provided while maintaining the highest possible level of function. The following factors play a role in determining rehabilitation potential: demographics, clinical, and cognitive and psychologic.

Demographic Factors

There is a debate in the literature regarding the effect of age on rehabilitation potential. Early reports summarized the experience in nursing homes and county boarding homes but were limited to short-term outcomes. They found younger hemiparetics to improve to a greater extent than older patients. Cain[5] and Reynolds, Abramson, and Young[14] stated that overall rehabilitation potential decreased with increasing age. Others have found no correlation between age and remaining physical disability.[1]

In other studies, age has not emerged as a significant prognostic factor.[2] Anderson, Bourestom, Queensburg, and Hildyard[2] found older people to be slower in making gains by the time of discharge, but 3 months after discharge older patients had done as well as younger patients. Reports showed high mortality in the first year poststroke; especially in the old-old (>80 years of age), which translates to a poor prognosis.[8] Others found rehabilitation to be specifically effective for patients over 85.[12]

Site of Residence. There is no consensus as to the role residence plays in determining rehabilitation potential. Some feel that residents of long-term care institutions have little or no potential, whereas others have shown improvement in more than 50 percent of stroke patients who resided in nursing homes prior to the stroke.[9,14] The site of residence is indeed a negative prognostic factor if the patient resides in a nursing home due to poor socioeconomic status rather than due to his or her disability and medical condition.

Socioeconomic and educational status emerge as significant factors in determining rehabilitation potential in stroke patients.[2,10] Family support with good financial resources is an important factor in determining rehabilitation outcome.

Clinical Factors

Studies have shown that those who had a shorter delay from onset of the acute event to the beginning of rehabilitation training were discharged earlier from the hospital. This may have to do with having fewer complications to overcome such as depression, contractures, and poor motivation, as well as the timing per se. Starting rehabilitation training early may help avoid developing undesirable patterns of motion that later would have to be unlearned. It is generally accepted that an interval of more than 30 days from an acute event to start of rehabilitation adversely affects outcome. The degree of neurologic deficit does not emerge as a predictor of rehabilitation outcome in stroke. The degree of functional impairment and behavioral problems have emerged as significant factors. Patients with very little neurologic recovery may function independently in certain key tasks such as ambulation. To walk, one needs greater amounts of muscle strength than are needed in fine motor control. On the other hand, even when muscle strength is good in the hands and wrist, the person may be impaired when there is not sufficient return of sensation or motor control.

Both excessive flaccidity and excessive spasticity for an extended period of time are poor prognostic signs. Sensory deficits on the involved side seem to have a greater effect on function.[16] This has also been associated with shorter hospital stays.[17] More recently, somatosensory evoked potentials have been used to predict the degree of motor recovery. Additionally, visual field defects have an adverse effect on rehabilitation potential, both in learning self-care activities and mobility. Some patients recognize their visual field deficits early and begin to learn how to compensate while other patients are unable to adjust to a persisting visual field defect.

There have been a large number of reports contrasting damage of the right hemisphere with that of the left hemisphere, with the focus on unilateral involvement of the brain. However, when brain damage is deep and involves the commissures and/or corpus callosum, the professional should be aware that the effects may be bilateral. It is generally well understood that damage to the left hemisphere affects language, aphasic naming, and time concepts, whereas damage to the right hemisphere affects performance, spatial orientation, stereognosis, and neglect of the more paretic limb.

Finally, severity of the condition is a factor in professional decision making about rehabilitation. Elderly persons who have conditions with greater severity may receive less rehabilitation than persons whose conditions are mild.[1] In a study of stroke patients in a rehabilitation hospital, it was found that the severity of disability following stroke was a more important factor than age in determining rehabilitation potential. Table 22-2 summarizes other factors that adversely affect rehabilitation potential. Table 22-3 summarizes factors that increase the length of stay.

Table 22-2. *Factors Adversely Affecting Outcome*

Severe weakness on admission
Perceptual/cognitive dysfunction
Homonymous hemianopia
Poor motivation
Multiple neurologic deficits
Interval from onset to admission >30 days
Inability to walk at time of discharge
Persistent urinary and/or fecal incontinence

Table 22-3. *Factors That Increase Length of Stay*

Weakness on admission
Homonymous hemianopia
Perceptual dysfunction
Hemisensory deficits
Multiple neurologic deficits
Slow functional recovery

Psychologic Factors

Family support and resources are strong predictors of rehabilitation potential. Patients with good support tend to do better irrespective of the primary cause of the disability. Psychologic factors that adversely affect rehabilitation are behavioral aberrations. Agitation, abusiveness, and wandering in dementia patients are identified as a disability and are a target for the rehabilitation program. Oversedation is another factor that adversely affects rehabilitation potential and needs to be carefully watched for. Cognitive dysfunction and poor motivation even with intact cognition are barriers to successful rehabilitation.

Site of Rehabilitation. The overall trend in the literature favors rehabilitation centers. Most data are derived from comparisons with rehabilitation on acute medical or surgical wards. One can learn from those studies that stroke rehabilitation could help 80 percent of those patients who are now referred to nursing homes for poststroke care. Empiric data documenting the benefits of an SNF as a site of intensive rehabilitation are limited. For appropriate patients there are, however, multiple resources available in the SNF. Registered physical therapists on site with a team of restorative aides are available in many SNFs. They can conduct gait training and muscle strengthening exercises. Occupational therapists, speech therapists, and even respiratory therapists are also available and these services are reimbursable through private and governmental insurance programs. In most SNFs the social worker is the resource person for psychologic support. In addition, psychiatrists and clinical psychologists are available on a fee-per-service basis. In the last 5 years a trend has started, mainly in not-for-profit and Veterans Administration nursing homes, to hire full-time medical directors trained in internal medicine and geriatrics who can be leaders of the rehabilitation team. Although the trend is there, a comprehensive geriatric rehabilitation program is not yet available in most mainstream community skilled nursing homes. However, the essential elements almost always exist.

In considering an SNF as the preferred site for rehabilitation for geriatric patients, one needs to take into account the barriers to acute rehabilitation centers. The following cases exemplify these barriers.

CASE 1
Mr. A.T., a 97–year–old divorced male, suffered a stroke with aphasia. He also had multiple associated medical problems. Functionally he had poor vision and was dependent on supervision and minimal assistance for his ADLs. He resided alone in a retirement hotel prior to the acute event. He was admitted to an SNF for gait and ADL training, as well as daily speech therapy. Following the program he became ambulatory with a walker and improved his communication skills.

CASE 2
Mrs. L.C., a 92-year-old female with Paget's disease, osteoporosis, and a fracture of the hip, was admitted for gait training. The main associated problem was persistent pain. The SNF program consisted of adequate pain management and physical therapy. After 9 weeks she was able to reach her goal of ambulation with a walker. Ultimately she returned to a board and care facility.

CASE 3

Mrs. M.P., an 87-year-old white female with dementia, who lived in a board and care facility, fell and fractured her left hip. Recovering from her acute fracture, it became obvious that she was unable to follow simple commands. She had also become incontinent. Evaluation showed bladder dysfunction, which was diagnosed as an atonic neurogenic bladder with high postvoid residuals and overflow incontinence. She was then managed using intermittent catheterizations.

CASE 4

Mrs. S.K., a 92-year-old vigorous woman, suffered multiple strokes leaving her with aphasia, dysphasia, and significant flexion contractures. She required two-person assistance for transfers and tube feeding. The plan of care consisted of preventing pressure sores and maintaining adequate nutrition via the percutaneous gastrostomy tube. Her family provided continued support and asked to declare her "no code." Eighteen months after the stroke and prolonged bed rest she developed a spontaneous hip fracture while turning in bed and was put in traction. Due to decreased mobility in bed, she developed a sacral pressure sore. A difficult problem at this point was pain due to the fracture requiring continuous attention. The plan update at this time included immobilization of the affected lower extremity, skin pressure reduction, and pain management. Her rehabilitation program was limited to pain control and treatment of the pressure sore, which eventually healed completely.

In all of these patients, there was limited rehabilitation potential, and most would not have been accepted for admission to an acute rehabilitation center. However, interventions designed to enhance function or reduce caregiver burden were valuable.

Case 1 had good potential with provision of speech and physical therapy and relocation to a congregate or assisted living arrangement. Case 2 had an excellent potential to go to a lower level of care, provided that a walker was allowed and pain was controlled. Case 3 had a poor rehabilitation potential for independent functioning since it was unrealistic to expect withdrawal of assistance with ADLs, and intermittent catheterizations would be required. Case 4 had the poorest rehabilitation potential of all, but had some limited chronic rehabilitation goals such as pain control, skin care, and nutritional support.

PSYCHOGERIATRIC REHABILITATION PROGRAM IN LONG-TERM CARE

The mental health needs of residents of nursing homes are underscored by the fact that almost 90 percent experience behavioral problems such as agitation, abusiveness, or wandering.[7,15] In a study of a Utah nursing home, some residents were so heavily sedated that they had to be awakened for meals. There is often a low expectation for the maintenance of activity, and in some instances lower activity levels may be encouraged to maintain order. Various researchers have addressed behavior management programs for targeted problems including dressing, bathing, personal hygiene, eating, continence, ambulation, activity participation, social skills, agitation, prevention of self-injury, and disruptive behaviors such as screaming and verbal abusiveness. Recently special care units in long-term care institutions have been developed. The goal of these units is to foster maintenance of function in those with a dementing disorder which otherwise is usually associated with progressive functional deterioration. By using a specially designed environment and providing special activities the units compensate for intellectual and functional deficits. Their success is judged by lack of deterioration rather than by improvement of function. Several programs were described in the recent literature.[13] Special training for health care workers on such units is required. There have been some reports of improvements in care and enhancement of function when team members receive additional training.

Project ADAPT targeted consultation focused on improving motivation and physical rehabilitation skills of nursing home staff. Emphasis was on individual treatment plans outlining the responsibilities of the client and staff members for the ensuing 3 months. Outcome evaluation consisting of measuring deterioration in the client's functioning. Preliminary data showed improvement in behavior, continence, and ambulation. The overall impression was that the program was successful in establishing positive behaviors of both clients and staff.[11]

SUMMARY

The role of the long-term care institution as a rehabilitation site for a selected geriatric population has been described. There are different target goals in this type of rehabilitation program, as well as special limitations. Even when services are available, the provision of rehabilitation programs in the long-term care institution may be limited by the third-party payers. Limited but important functional gains enhance the client's quality of life and may lead to less caregiver burden. Such interventions should be reimbursable. The long-term care community will do itself a favor by changing its public image from a site of custodial care to a rehabilitation center in the true meaning of the word.

REFERENCES

1. Adler, M.K., Brown, C.C., and Acton, P. (1980). Stroke rehabilitation: Is age a determinant? *J. Am. Geriatr. Soc.*, 28, 499.

2. Anderson, T.P., et al. (1974). Predictive factors in stroke rehabilitation. *Arch. Phys. Med. Rehabil. 55*, 545.
3. Anderson, T.P., et al. (1978). Stroke rehabilitation: Evaluation of its quality by assessing patient outcomes. *Arch. Phys. Med. Rehabil., 50*, 170.
4. Brody, S.J., and Ruff, G.E. (1986). *Aging and rehabilitation: Advances in the state of the art.* New York: Springer.
5. Cain, L.S. (1969). Determining the factors that affect rehabilitation. *Jo. Am. Geriatr. Soc., 17*, 595.
6. Dasco, M.N. (1953). Clinical programs in geriatric rehabilitation. *Geriatrics, 8*, 179.
7. Goldman, H.H., Fader, J., and Scanlou, W. (1986). Chronic mental patients in nursing homes: Re-examining data from the national nursing home survey. *Hosp. Community Psychiatry, 37*, 269.
8. Henely, S., et al. (1985). Who goes home? Predictive factors in stroke recovery. *Jo. Neurol. Neurosurg. Psychiatry, 48*, 1.
9. Kelman, H.R. (1962). An experiment in the rehabilitation of nursing home patients. *Public Health Rep., 77*, 356.
10. Lehman, J.F., et al. (1975). Stroke rehabilitation outcome and prediction. *Arch. Phys. Med. Rehabil., 56*, 383.
11. Mallya, A., and Fitz, D. (1987). A psychogeriatic rehabilitation program in long term care facilities *Gerontologist, 27*, 747.
12. Parry, F. (1982). Physical rehabilitation of the old, old patient. *J. Am. Geriatr. Soc., 31*, 482.
13. Petchers, M.S., Roy, A.W., and Brickner, A. (1987). A post-hospital nursing home rehabilitation program. *Gerontologist, 27*, 752.
14. Reynolds, F.W., Abramson, M., and Young, A. The rehabilitation potential of patients in chronic disease institutions. *J. Chronic. Dis., 10*, 152.
15. Schmidt, L.J., et al. (1977). The mentally ill in nursing homes: new back wards in the community. *Arch. Gen. Psychiatry, 34*, 687.
16. Stern, P.H., et al. (1970). Effects of facilitation exercise techniques in stroke rehabilitation. *Arch. Phys. Med. Rehabil.*, Sept., 526.
17. Van Buskirk, C., and Webster, D. (1955). Prognostic value of sensory defect in rehabilitation of hemiplegics. *Neurology, 5*, 407.

CHAPTER 23

In-Home Geriatric Rehabilitation

JOSEPH M. KEENAN

In-home geriatric rehabilitation has evolved from the convergence of three major developments in health care. The fields of home care, geriatric medicine, and rehabilitation medicine have all experienced considerable growth within the past decade. Though none of these are new disciplines, current societal needs have brought about an increased interest in and emphasis on these fields. As a result, new medical expertise and technology has developed in each of these disciplines. A discussion of a few highlights of the current medical and societal trends will be useful in understanding the background and rationale for in-home geriatric rehabilitation.

The well-known demographic changes that have accompanied the dramatic increase in life expectancy in this country have focused unprecedented attention on the health care needs of the elderly.[16] Older persons, as a group, are recognized as an increasingly powerful social, political, and economic force in our society.[9] These changes have had a dramatic effect on the health care industry, which is constantly positioning for market share, and on policymakers, who must plan resource allocations for projected health needs. Traditional health care of the elderly, which often has been biased by ageism, fatalism, and nihilism,[11] is now being reexamined in the light of new knowledge and research in geriatric medicine and gerontology.

Geriatric training has received new emphasis in both medical and allied health fields. The boards of family practice and internal medicine have developed postgraduate certification of added qualification in geriatrics.[6] The health care industry, health educators, providers, and planners, are all actively responding to the challenge of meeting the burgeoning health care needs of this country's older citizens.

Home care offers a unique and appropriate response to many of the health care needs of the elderly. Long-term care in the home is often more affordable[3] and offers the additional benefits of the support of family, friends, and the familiar environment of the home. The expressed preference of the elderly overwhelmingly favors maintenance of independent living in their own homes, if appropriate supports are available.[7] There has been a dramatic increase in the availability of experienced home care personnel along with increased application of technology to the delivery of home care.[10] Thus, care in the home is available and appropriate for many acute and long-term conditions. Reimbursement issues still pose a major problem to the provision of home care. Legislation and policy changes are needed for improvement in this area.

Rehabilitation medicine has experienced phenomenal growth and development in the past several decades. It has evolved from a post–World War II model of physical restitution of war casualties focusing primarily on the return of physical function and employability of the individual, to a much broader therapeutic scope and philosophy. Modern rehabilitation takes a holistic approach, embracing the psychologic, social, and physical functioning of the individual, and includes environmental manipulation to enhance function and well-being. Geriatric rehabilitation, in particular, includes attention to the function and well-being of the family, and informal support systems to enhance its caregiving role and avoid burnout or injury. Douglas Fenderson, in his paper "Aging, Disability, and Therapeutic Optimism," eloquently chronicles the legislative actions and scientific and technologic advances which have brought about the modern philosophy and practice of rehabilitation.[11] Statistically, older persons have a much higher incidence of chronic disability than other subsegments of our population. It is precisely this quality of the "therapeutic optimism" of modern rehabilitation that is needed to counteract the therapeutic impediments of negative biases. Geriatric rehabilitation is well suited to the home setting, where both assessment and intervention can be accomplished in the individual's actual living environment with family and friends involved as needed.

In summary, it can be appreciated that developments in these three areas of health care have come to a logical and natural confluence in the rehabilitation of elderly in the home setting. For the remainder of this chapter, we will suggest a definition of in-home geriatric rehabilitation and discuss rationale, specific applications, and limitations for the same. Finally, we discuss the application of a team approach to home rehabilitation of the elderly.

DEFINITION AND RATIONALE FOR HOME REHABILITATION OF THE ELDERLY

The definition of home rehabilitation of the elderly in this discussion is broad and simple—intervention which enhances the function or well-being of the individual and caregiver in the home setting. It assumes that the intervention is holistic and has been derived from a comprehensive assessment of the patient, the home, and the caregiving support system. Comprehensive assessment is essential in rehabilitation. It allows us to develop benchmarks for measuring progress and to appreciate the interplay of function with various physical, environmental, and social systems. Experts in geriatric assessment stress validity concerns in the development of assessment instruments.[15] That is, does the assessment instrument, indeed, measure what it is supposed to? Nothing can enhance validity of assessment more than the actual measurement of function in the physical and social environment of the home.

The rationale for geriatric rehabilitation goes beyond the traditional vocational rehabilitation model of restoration of physical function and employability. Geriatric rehabilitation is often targeted at restoring and maintaining autonomy, self-esteem, and independent living. Successful rehabilitation may enhance function, may only slow the inexorable decline of function associated with chronic or terminal disease, or may provide a caregiver with the understanding, skills, and respite to deal with the declining patient.

Scientific research and modern technology as applied to the development of orthotics, prosthetics, and assistive devices have made a tremendous contribution to the quality of life in older persons. The typical decline of sensory function in old age—vision, hearing, balance—are major contributors to the loss of independence among the elderly. Modern rehabilitation has taken the concepts of personal prosthetics and expanded them to include the entire living space of the home, the so-called prosthetic environment. Ramps, widened doorways, lowered countertops, better lighting, elevators, grab bars, a transfer bench, lever doorknobs, and faucet handles are just a few examples of environmental adjustments that can mean the difference between independent living and institutional care of the elderly.[4] There is also application of new high-tech monitoring systems, using computerized biotelemetry to manage care of the elderly in the home. There are sophisticated tracking devices to monitor a person's activity within or out of the home, telephone hookups for monitoring various parameters of health such as blood sugar, home dialysis, or cardiac rhythm, and medical alert systems for a patient in distress.[12]

The cost of maintaining older people in their own homes is usually less than corresponding institutional care.[11] These costs may vary regionally but the cost-benefit trade-offs tend to favor the home setting for care of the less disabled, less dependent patient.[16] Correspondingly, the institutional setting may be more cost-effective for patients with higher levels of disability or dependency (see Fig. 23-1). The rationale for in-home rehabilitation is to try to maintain the patient in the lower range of disability or dependency or, at the very least, to slow the decrement of function so that institutionalization can be delayed.

Finally, one obvious rationale for home rehabilitation of a person of any age is the maintenance of care in a familiar setting with the intact support system of family and friends available to participate in the rehabilitation. Patients who have any degree of cognitive decline benefit from rehabilitation in familiar surroundings with familiar people in attendance. With institutional rehabilitation the older person's loss of autonomy lowers self-esteem and provokes the fear of permanent dependence.[1] These problems will aggravate the demotivation and depression frequently associated with severe illness in the elderly. At home the older person has the supportive relationships of friends and family. Self-esteem can be enhanced with meaningful involvement in simple household tasks, such as watering the plants or feeding a pet.[22] These considerations may seem trivial but they can be critical elements in sustaining the motivation for rehabilitation after serious illness.

APPLICATIONS FOR HOME REHABILITATION

An older person's recovery from a serious illness, such as a myocardial infarction, hip fracture, or stroke, often presents a major rehabilitative challenge. Pressures of the prospective payment system may force discharge from the hospital before the patient is sufficiently recovered to participate in an active rehabilitation program. This means there is a significant risk for intervening problems and loss of rehabilitation potential. Early discharge for an elderly person may result in any of a number of potential complications—skin problems, nutritional problems, deconditioning, contractures, etc., in addition to the morbidity

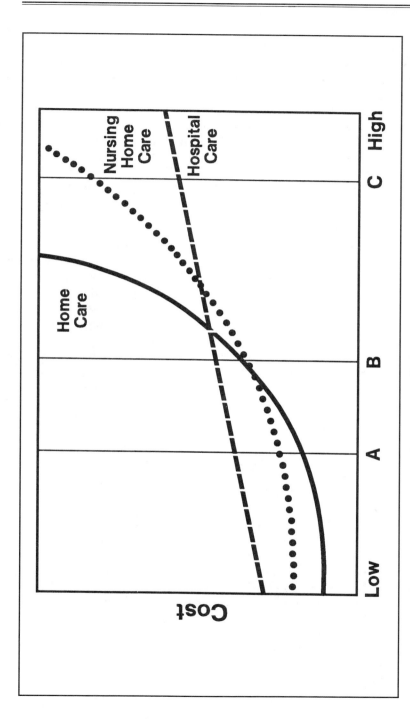

Fig. 23-1. Level of disability or dependence. A. Home care is most cost-effective. B. Above this point institutional care is most cost-effective. C. Acuity or instability of problems make hospital care most cost-effective. (Adapted from Drummond, M.F. [1980]. *Principles of economic appraisal in health care* [p. 100]. New York: Oxford University Press.)

associated with the original illness. All of these may prejudice the potential for rehabilitation and can even allow the goblins of ageism, fatalism, and nihilism to insidiously creep into decision making. Figure 23-2 depicts typical patterns of recovery from serious illness. Active rehabilitation can be managed either in the home setting or through an outpatient rehabilitation unit. The outpatient unit is often better equipped and staffed to handle active rehabilitation and, if transportation is not a difficulty, the added stimulation of dressing and going out of the home each day may even be therapeutic.

Another point at which home intervention may be appropriate in the recovery from major illness is at the termination of active outpatient rehabilitation. This is especially true if there has been incomplete return of function such as residual paresis following a severe stroke. The patient may experience a sense of abandonment and even be prone to late onset depression.[23] A follow-up maintenance rehabilitation program in the home helps preserve morale and functional gains. This maintenance therapy, as well as the early posthospital discharge home therapy, may not be reimbursed by Medicare. However, these are relatively low-tech interventions and can be managed in large part by a motivated patient with family support.

Home assessment and rehabilitation is also appropriate for the older patient with long-term health problems who begins to show an accelerated decline in function (see Fig. 23-3). Home assessment may be quite revealing. Simple environmental modifications or an adjustment in medical management may lead to a recovery of previous functional independence. Another common scenario is to discover on home assessment a truly worsening chronic process that is irreversible. Appropriate home interventions can slow the decline of function or provide support to caregivers, thus delaying, if not preventing, nursing home placement. Studies suggest that a significant proportion of those patients institutionalized for long-term care can, in fact, be managed at home if appropriate family support and home care programs are available.[19] Unfortunately, reimbursement for such home rehabilitation and maintenance programs are limited to a few demonstration projects and channeling programs.[16,17] Programs which can both conserve resources and maintain the dignity and autonomy of older persons in their own homes will become more fully appreciated as we encounter the increasing long-term care needs of older Americans.

There have been many individualized home rehabilitation and therapy programs developed for specific conditions and disease processes. These programs are often developed around a specific intervention, such as home dialysis, oxygen therapy, or parenteral nutrition. But they include comprehensive assessment of the needs of the patient and the

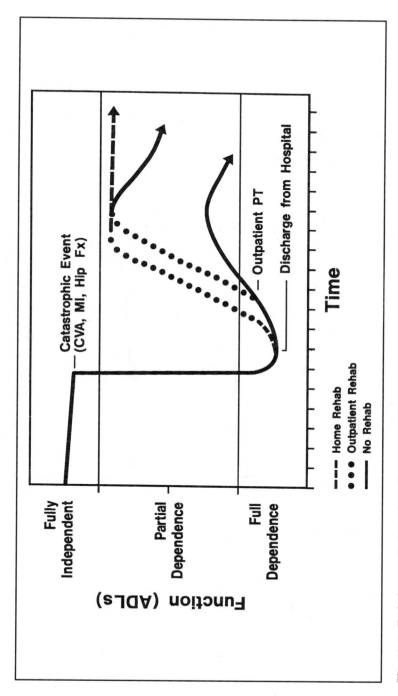

Fig. 23-2. Early home rehabilitation after catastrophic illness can preserve functional potential and prevent delays in outpatient rehabilitation. Home rehabilitation following outpatient therapy can help maintain functional gains. CVA = cerebrovascular accident; MI = myocardial infarction; Hip Fx = hip fracture; ADLs = activities of daily living; PT = physical therapy.

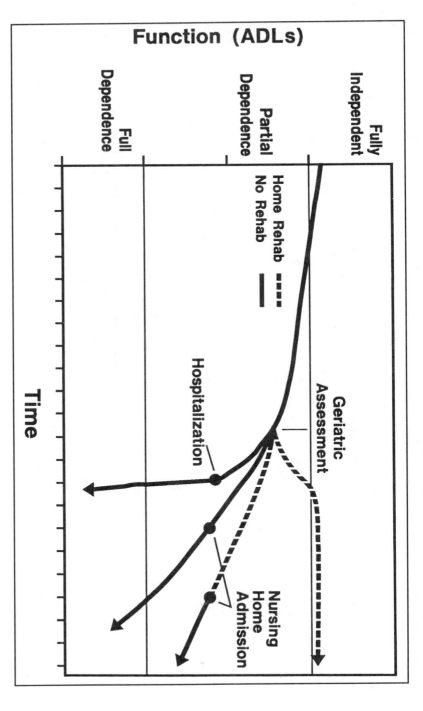

Fig. 23-3. Home rehabilitation following geriatric assessment in chronic illness can forestall functional decline and may even reestablish functional independence. ADLs = activities of daily living.

caregiver in the development of the total program. For example, home pulmonary rehabilitation includes patient and caregiver instruction in appropriate breathing and respiratory physiology, supplemental oxygen therapy, and medical management of the underlying pathologic process. In addition, the patient receives instruction in appropriate nutrition, hydration, and conditioning exercise. Environmental modifications are recommended to enhance the safety and efficient layout of the home. Results of a pulmonary rehabilitation program reported by Hodgkin, Asmus, and Connors indicated improved survival, improved function and activities of daily living (ADLs); and decreased psychosocial difficulties.[13] Perhaps the most striking finding in this study was a dramatic decrease in days of hospitalization required per year. An average hospitalization of 18 days per year prior to the pulmonary rehabilitation program was decreased to 6 days per year after 1 year of therapy. This represents an obvious economic benefit but, more importantly, a striking improvement in quality of life.

Despite tremendous cost savings for many of these programs, they are still not predictably reimbursed by Medicare or third-party payers. However, support for changes in these policies seems to be growing. In the 1988 United States legislative session, a bill which proposed expanded coverage for home care services, the Pepper-Roybal bill, (cosponsored by Representative Claude Pepper), demonstrated broad support among lawmakers but was narrowly defeated.

One exception to the problems of reimbursement for home care is hospice care. Home hospice expenses are covered if the program is certified by Medicare. Hospice is not often thought of as a rehabilitative process yet many of the same basic home rehabilitation concepts and interventions are used to support the well-being of the patient and caregiver and to decrease suffering. Thus, rehabilitative concepts and interventions can be applicable in successful dying, as well as successful living.

LIMITATIONS

Uncertain or unavailable reimbursement represents the greatest obstacle and limitation to the use of home geriatric rehabilitation.[8] The frequency of Medicare retrospective denials of payment for care, the strict interpretation of "homebound," and the lack of coverage for supportive or maintenance rehabilitation have all severely limited the appropriate use of these services. These restrictions are less a problem in the prepaid health care programs for the elderly, which often take advantage of the home care alternatives to institutional care.[21] There are also increasing numbers of older persons who are willing and able to pay for these services on a private basis.

Another potential limitation to home-based programs is the stability of the underlying medical illness or process. If appropriate management of the patient requires skilled personnel and extensive technology for around-the-clock monitoring or special back-up teams for potential emergencies, then home management is not safe or practical. Even if the appropriate personnel and equipment could be assembled in the home, the cost-benefit trade-offs become prohibitive, as was shown in Figure 23-1. There is considerable experience with the management of complex and serious illnesses in the home.[12] However, this is typically after the patient is stabilized and appropriate safety precautions have been established. Home rehabilitation programs also can offer the opportunity for earlier discharge after hospital stabilization of a medical process, with the continued subacute care in the home setting (post–myocardial infarction, post–cerebrovascular accident, postoperative parenteral therapy, etc.).

Geriatric home rehabilitation may be limited by the patient's or caregiver's acceptance of such a program.[18] These attitudes may be complicated by fear of abandonment, anxiety over caregiving responsibilities, or lack of conviction that such programs will be worthwhile or cost-effective. Providers must always be concerned about a possible underlying depression when there is apparent lack of motivation in an otherwise appropriate candidate for home rehabilitation. Such a situation can also raise legal and ethical issues if it appears that guardians or caregivers are not appropriately concerned about the needs or best interests of the patient. It is always the patient's prerogative to refuse a rehabilitative intervention; it is the provider's obligation to convey realistic expectations in a spirit of therapeutic optimism.

Finally, the extent and sophistication of special support services may limit the rehabilitation program that can be provided in the home setting. Most metropolitan areas have easy access to a full array of professional and technological services; however, smaller cities and rural areas are frequently deficient in both. Any physician or home care agency involved in the care of the elderly should work with hospitals and other providers to develop a full complement of services to support home programs. Many hospitals are finding it economically beneficial to be involved in the full spectrum of services available for the care of the elderly, from home care programs through supported living environments to skilled nursing, rehabilitation, and acute care facilities.[20] They are natural allies to those providers who wish to make better services and programs available in the home setting.

Some home programs, such as pulmonary rehabilitation, are dependent on a critical number of clients needed to support the infrastructure required for such services. If a particular patient would be greatly benefited by a home program that is not available locally, it may be appropriate for the patient to relocate in the community where the service is available. Similarly, if the patient lives in a remote or potentially inaccessible area, it is not advisable to establish home programs, such as ventilator-dependent care or parenteral therapy, that are critically dependent on professional support staff. Even a natural hazard, such as a snowstorm, could jeopardize the safety of such home care and that patient should also be advised to relocate closer to support services.

TEAM APPROACH TO HOME REHABILITATION

No single discipline has sufficient expertise for optimal home assessment and intervention. Thus, most successful home care programs use a team approach with a designated team member who functions as care manager. The care manager is responsible for the timely and appropriate consultation with the various professionals involved in the home care program. If a group of home care providers share the care of a number of patients in common, it may be expeditious for them to conduct periodic team meetings to discuss, adjust, and plan care. The weekly team meeting for some geriatric or home care programs will review the care of 25 to 30 patients in the course of a 90-minute conference, making it an efficient use of time for the professionals involved. Better interdisciplinary communication is the main benefit of such a meeting, but it also provides opportunities for some joint problem solving and decision making. The team meeting is also an ideal place to role-model interdisciplinary teamwork and communication for new learners. Team meetings have been criticized by some as an expensive and inefficient use of professional time and may indeed be extravagant for reviewing a small number of cases or relatively uncomplicated problems. The innovation of computerized charts and databases may greatly improve the efficient management of such cases. However, when the complex management of a patient requires a timely input from a variety of disciplines for a management decision, there is no substitute for the face-to-face consultation of a team meeting.

CONCLUSION

George Piersol, a renowned physiatrist, was known to have exhorted his students with the following words: "We have added years to life, let us now add life to years." This statement appropriately and succinctly poses the challenge to all involved in the health care of the elderly: to add quality to life to increased longevity. Primary preventive efforts and lifestyle changes may someday prevent or forestall the morbidity and disability of old age. However, in the foreseeable future increasing disability and functional dependence appear to be likely to accompany old age. Rehabilitation represents the most hopeful and optimistic intervention for restoring quality of life to the older years. Rehabilitation in the home setting potentiates the prospects of "adding life to years."

It is the task of those who provide care for the older person to make available all the rehabilitative options that might enhance that person's function and quality of life. It is essential to guard against the negative biases which tend to color decision making. Optimal care of the chronically ill and disabled must begin with a spirit of therapeutic optimism and strive to preserve the older person's dignity and autonomy.

REFERENCES

1. Bergman, S. (1973). Facilitating living conditions for aged in the community. *Gerontologist, 13,* 184.
2. Berry, N.J., and Evans, J.M. (1985/1986). Cost effectiveness of home health care as an alternative to inpatient care. *Home Health Care Serv. Q. 6,* 11.
3. Braun, K.L., and Rose, C.L. (1987). Geriatric patient outcomes and costs in three settings: nursing home, foster family and own home. *J. Am. Geriatr. Soc., 35,* 387.
4. Caird, F.I., Kennedy, R.D., and Williams, B.O. (1983). *Practical rehabilitation of the elderly* (pp. 22–25). London: Pitman Books.
5. Champlin, L. (1988). Long-term care: protecting the elderly from going broke. *Geriatrics 43,* 96.
6. Committee on Leadership for Academic Geriatric Medicine: Report of the Institute of Medicine. (1987). Academic geriatrics for the Year 2000. *J. Am. Geriatr. Soc., 35,* 773.
7. Congressonal Budget Office. (1977). *Long-term care for the elderly and disabled.* Washington, DC: Government Printing Office.
8. Curtiss, F.R. (1986). Recent developments in federal reimbursement for home health care. *Am. J. Hosp. Pharm. 43,* 132.
9. Dychtwald, K. (1986). The myths and realities of aging. In K. Dychtwald (Ed.), *Wellness and health promotion for the elderly* (pp. 9–17). Rockville, MD: Aspen Systems.
10. Evashwick, C. (1985). Home health care: current trends and future opportunities. *J. Ambulatory Care Med., 8,* 4.
11. Fenderson, D.A. (1986). Aging, disability, and therapeutic optimism. In S.J. Brody and G.E. Ruff (Eds.), *Aging and rehabilitation: Advances in the state of the art.* New York: Springer.
12. Haddad, A.M. (1987). *High tech home care, a practical guide* (pp. 4–15). Rockville, MD: Aspen Systems.
13. Hodgkin, J.E., Asmus, R.M., and Connors, G.A. (1987). Pulmonary rehabilitation: designing a program that works. *J. Respir. Dis., 8,* 55.

14. Jackson, B.N. (1984). Home health care and the elderly in the 1980s. *Am. J. Occup. Ther., 38,* 717.
15. Kane, R.A., and Kane, R.L. (1981). *Assessing the elderly* (pp. 1–12, 220–221). Lexington, MA: D.C. Heath.
16. Kramer, A.M., Shaughnessy, P.W., and Petigrew, M.L. (1985). Cost effectiveness implications based on a comparison of nursing home and home health care mix. *Health Serv. Res., 20,* 387.
17. Lave, J.R. (1985). Cost-containment policies in long-term care. *Inquiry 22,* 7.
18. Levine, R.E. (1984). The cultural aspects of home care delivery. *Am. J. Occup. Ther., 38,* 734.
19. Lipsman, R., et al. (1984). The Chelsea-Village program. In S. Brody, N. Persily (Eds.), *Hospitals and the aged, the new old market* (pp. 191–201). Rockville, MD: Aspen Systems.
20. Milch, R.B., and Malafronte, D. Top-down marketing for community hospitals. In S. Brody and N. Persily (Eds.), *Hospitals and the aged, the new old market* (pp. 159–164). Rockville, MD: Aspen Systems.
21. Schlag, W.A., and Piktialis, D.S. (1987). Health maintenance organizations and the elderly: The potential for vertical integration of geriatric care. *Q. Rev. Bull., 13,* 140.
22. Wilson, C.C., and Netting, F.E. (1983). Companion animals and the elderly: A state-of-the-art summary. *J. Am. Vet. Med. Assoc., 183,* 1425.
23. Wolcott, L.W. (1983). Rehabilitation and the aged. In W. Reichel (Ed.), *Clinical aspects of aging* (pp. 182–204). Baltimore: Williams & Wilkins.

CHAPTER 24

Issues in Interdisciplinary Team Care

KENNETH D. COLE
JOSEPH W. RAMSDELL

Teams often evolve from the necessity of integrating a broad array of information into a plan of action or a course of treatment. Even in the cockpits of modern aircraft, the once cherished qualities of self-reliance and machismo given way to notions of interdependence and teamwork. Because of the sheer quantity of information to be handled, cockpit crews now undergo "cockpit resource management" training in order to work together efficiently. Indeed, in several domestic airline disasters during the last decade, what was dubbed "human error" has actually been found to be "team error."[12]

In a similar fashion, health care once was typically administered by a sole provider, usually a physician. Now the "pilot-life" qualities of self-reliance and instant decision making necessary for the independent practice of medicine have given way to skills like collaborating with other professionals and coordinating care. Especially in specialties such as geriatrics and rehabilitation, the caseload is dominated by patients suffering from a multiplicity of interacting problems requiring input from several disciplines. This typically requires the team approach to patient care with all the inherent human difficulties that come with it.

Physicians caring for the elderly may be involved with a rehabilitation team in a number of ways. They may be members of a formal interdisciplinary rehabilitation team. More likely they will refer patients to such a team or will need to develop a surrogate for the classic interdisciplinary team to care effectively for their elderly patients. In each of these roles the physicians must have a clear understanding of how the team functions and the role each member should play at any given time.

This chapter is written to be a real "nuts and bolts" treatise of rehabilitation team development and maintenance. It is common to find in the literature on teams similar platitudes about team functioning. However, the reader is left with the notion that teams are somehow good, but with no firm feeling for the issues involved in interdisciplinary team care. Our intention here is to go a step or two beyond this by providing information about how teams are structured and how they function in real health care settings. First, a digression into the history of health care teams is needed to set the stage for the rest of the material to follow.

HISTORY OF TEAMWORK IN HEALTH CARE DELIVERY

Naturally, the first team was the physician and patient. Early in this narrow notion of teamwork, the emphasis was on sickness and cure rather than on any complicated wellness-illness continuum that demands more activity on the part of the patient. Surgery teams of physicians and nurses made up a rudimentary form of a team, all players performing on the same patients at the same time. Later, the team concept was broadened to include health assistants who extended the role of the physician.[15]

It is not clear whether the first establishment of true interdisciplinary teams occurred with the collaborative efforts among professionals at mission hospitals, clinics, and schools, or with the initial endeavors of Montefiore Hospital in the 1940s.[27] The Montefiore Hospital Outreach Program in New York delivered home care services with an interdisciplinary team comprised of a social worker, nurse, and physician. In the 1960s the Martin Luther King Health Care Center in the South Bronx furthered the development of the primary health care team.[36] The University of Washington gets the credit for developing a broader-based team by adding a psychologist, dietitian, medical technologist, dentist, and dental hygienist. Then in the 1970s interdisciplinary team development was encouraged when federal funding was provided to support the training of both staff and trainees in team settings.[7]

Paralleling the structural development of teams during this century was the shifting away from diagnosing patient problems from strictly parochial viewpoints.[23] The acceptance that many patient problems were nonmedical in nature,[18] coupled with the realization that illness behavior, coping strategies, and support networks often had far more impact on patient outcomes than purely physiologic indicators,[6] led to the broader interdisciplinary conception of general health status. In this more comprehensive view of the patient, it is difficult to conceive of one discipline having the expertise needed to address all of the patient's concerns, thereby reinforcing the importance of a broad team approach to patient care.[7] Now treatment teams are ubiquitous in health care settings as they function with widely different structures and in various stages of development.

DEFINITION OF TEAMS

Although the teams are often used interchangeably, multidisciplinary and interdisciplinary teams connote different degrees of team functioning. A multidisciplinary team is a mix of professionals working with the same patients and usually in the same setting. Interdisciplinary teams, really a subset of multidisciplinary teams, go further by collaborating in coordinated treatment plans for their patients and by negotiating common goals for their teams. These tasks are usually conducted during a team meeting when patients are discussed. An added feature of an interdisciplinary team often includes a commitment at least to address the conflict that inevitably arises during teamwork. The belaboring of definitions of teams is not necessary, but on the other hand the essential features of a real interdisciplinary team are worth bearing in mind. These features may be utilized by the primary care physician in establishing a multidisciplinary team in noninstitutional settings.

COMPOSITION AND ORGANIZATION OF INTERDISCIPLINARY TEAMS

The optimal time to create an interdisciplinary team is at the inception of a program or treatment unit. At that juncture careful thought can be exercised to consider issues of inclusion. The key factor in establishing a team are the needs of the patients.[25] Unfortunately for team developers, issues such as charting requirements and other extrateam demands create the rationale for adding members to a team. The focus in this chapter is on the establishment of a rehabilitation team with the caveat that there may be institutional demands competing with the more idealistic notions articulated here.

The interdisciplinary team may be viewed as the ideal model but it may not be practical or even suitable in many communities or primary care settings. In these situations the primary care physician may create a team made up of a consistent group of colleagues. The workings of such a team are in contrast to the traditional use of consultants in addressing patient's problems which cut across usual disciplinary boundaries. The key elements of the community-based team are a stable group of team members who have developed an effective method of communication and understand the roles they must play in the patient's management. The primary care physician should identify the team members prospectively, develop a system of communication among the group, and use the same group consistently. This nurtures a common approach and fosters effective communication. Once established this team can be activated on an ad hoc basis by any of the team members to deal with problems that arise. The composition of the rehabilitation team is discussed in terms of the classic institutional interdisciplinary team and the implications of this structure for primary care physicians in noninstitutional settings will be examined.

There is probably no ideal mix of professionals to include on a team. For example, Kane reviewed more than 200 health care teams and found almost as many discipline compositions as there were teams.[21] One guideline for developing teams is the smaller, the better. With the addition of each new team member, the permutations of potential interactions between team members proliferate. One method to cope with the enormity of team interactions is to conceive of an interdisciplinary team as levels of inclusion, rather than an all-or-none principle. One useful division is among core members, extended members, and consultants and resource persons.

CORE MEMBERS

Core team members are the ones that work together on the same unit every day, and they do not have patient responsibilities on other units. These professionals are teaming together day in, day out, not just for the 1-hour team meeting per week. On a rehabilitation unit, these disciplines would tend to be nursing, medicine, perhaps a physician assistant or nurse practitioner; social work; and the rehabilitation specialties of physical and occupational therapy. In a community-based multidisciplinary team, the core members should include a similar mix with the addition of a comprehensive home health service that is experienced in rehabilitation issues. Whatever the ultimate mix, this core team of professionals is responsible for developing team procedures and for deciding how to include other disciplines in the assessment and treatment of the patients.

One way in which the team can establish overall team goals, document team procedures, and define team roles is by creating an operational guide. It can outline the steps of the rehabilitation program from the initial patient contact through evaluation, daily routines, and the process of discharge. More positive clinical outcomes may be associated with a well-thought out "targeting" of the patients most able to gain from the particular interdisciplinary team assembled.[29] The guide can facilitate appropriate referrals to the program and can clarify the kinds of patient care decisions that are within the role of the interdisciplinary team.[7] This approach can also be used effectively in the community primary care setting as the physician meets with the various team members prospectively to discuss overall philosophy of care and methods of communication prior to actual referrals. By doing this initially all team members are prepared, and when referrals do begin specific individualized treatment goals and approaches can be developed collectively because each member of the team has agreed upon the importance of timely communication and on their mutual expectations.

EXTENDED MEMBERS

In many rehabilitation settings, team participation may be limited by time constraints causing staff to be assigned to multiple clinical care sites. More simply, there may not be as much work for some disciplines to do. Examples of extended team members are dietitians, psychologists, audiologists, speech pathologists, optometrists, pharmacists, and dentists. Of course, if some of these professionals are needed and are available for core team duties, then by all means they could be included. Extended team members typically interact with personnel from many varied teams, and they come to each unit's team meeting prepared to speak on the specific patients with whom they are working. However, usually they do not interact with the core team in the day-to-day exigencies of patient care.

CONSULTANTS AND RESOURCE PERSONS

The third level of team participation are the consultants and other resource persons. Consultants are involved only with those cases that the core team decides as necessary and appropriate. Consultants may be invited to team meetings to discuss their findings and recommendations, or they may merely send back reports. It is not in their purview to engage in team decision making except with the patients with whom they have clinical involvement.[7] Resource persons are either hospital or clinic personnel specializing in team development or group communications, or they may be designated outside consultants serving to help the team with tasks such as goal clarification, role negotiation, and conflict management. They are not usually a part of patient-centered team meetings. Further discussion of resource persons will appear in the team functioning section.

PATIENTS

A discussion about inclusion-exclusion is not complete without consideration of patient attendance at team meetings. Amid the quixotic ideas that surround team development, the inclusion of patients at the team meetings may sound appealing; but as Kane pointed out, this "misplaced hospitality" is easily abused.[20] Although the staff exists for the patient, their musings and conflicts do not. It is very time-consuming to translate each bit of information, and in some chronic care settings the concern about discharge can excessively frighten the patient. Of course, the patient's values, resources, and goals must be included in the planning by the treatment team and it may be helpful to appoint one team member whose explicit task is to represent the patient's viewpoint; but except in some special circumstances, patients and team meetings should be kept apart.[7,20] A more suitable setting for such discussions is patient rounds, with the interdisciplinary team needing to be ever-mindful of all patients' concerns about privacy and confidentiality.

INTERDISCIPLINARY TEAM LEADERSHIP AND FUNCTIONING

Goals and Roles

Effective team management centers around delineating team goals and negotiating roles for each team member. Commitment and performance is enhanced when team members periodically review their own goals[14] and partake in flexible, open communication, with shared responsibility for decisions and accountability for performing team tasks.[23]

Many interdisciplinary teams make the mistake of never creating clear-cut goals for their unit and for themselves as a team. One technique that can be employed to establish that sense of direction is nominal group process.[26] But any strategy that gets teams to generate overarching mission goals for the team will be useful.[26] As in marriage, conflict over basic goals can be a festering source of tension on a team for many years. With the delineation of goals, the team builds its identity and sense of purpose.[22]

Similarly, negotiation and clarification of roles are an integral part of team development.[17] One example of a role conflict involved a physician who rotated onto a geriatric assessment unit. As was her customary practice, she routinely checked and recorded the blood pressures of all the patients. The nursing staff, used to providing this function, were quietly smoldering over her presumptuous encroachment into their routine. When the physician found out about ward procedures, she agreed to nurses' checking blood pressures, as it freed her for other activities. Naturally, the nursing staff made many attributions about this physician's aggressive personality, while the physician was merely doing what she normally did on her previous rotation.

When members on a team find themselves entrenched in goal or role conflicts, it often "feels" like a personality conflict. This rigidifies each side's position. However, findings from social psychology indicate that while actors attribute their actions to situational demands, perceivers attribute the same set of behaviors to stable personal dispositions.[19] Known as the "fundamental error of attribution," this repeated tendency can lock team members into a stand-off for months or even years, instead of leading to an exploration of the differing perception of team goals and personal roles from which the members are operating.

TEAM LEADERSHIP

Traditionally, the physician or the program director is seen as the leader of the team.[23] However, a difficulty in team development is that often the person with the most power does not necessarily possess the greatest skill in team management.[14] There can be a number of different types of leadership that emerge as a team builds. There may be a program leader, but another person may lead the team meetings. Covert "socioemotional" leaders of the unit may emerge despite the power being ostensibly with the team leader. In highly functioning teams, leadership is not tightly bound to one person or discipline, but rather it resides with the team member who happens to have the most expertise for the given problem at hand.

Team chairing can be in the hands of one selected core team member, or, if the team decides, it can be shared by several of the core team members. Similarly, recording of interdisciplinary treatment plans can be routinely accomplished by one person or discipline, or the task can be rotated around the team.

In the ambulatory, primary care–oriented, multidisciplinary team the primary care physician usually initiates the team, often on an ad hoc basis, and will generally, but not necessarily always, be the team leader. This role may shift to other members depending on the nature of the patients' problems. For example, the visiting nurse or social worker may take the team leadership role in a failing elderly patient whose medical problems are stable but who requires assistance with physical conditioning, caregiver stress, accessing social support, and so forth. In such situations the team members must explicitly recognize and accept the roles they play in the patient's care and be prepared to change roles as conditions change. The sometimes fluid nature of team leadership in the role of care manager is to be contrasted with the overall administrative leadership which tends to remain fixed in both interdisciplinary and multidisciplinary teams.

The role of nursing on interdisciplinary rehabilitation teams is critical. Not only do nurses have the most observations and latest information on each patient, but also they are usually the discipline that will be implementing the treatment plan on an hour-to-hour basis.[31] Because of staff shortages and demanding schedules, critical nurses will be tempted to skip meetings. But without a good representation of nursing, the unit could have wonderful team discussions with very little of the creative input cascading down to the actual patients.

Nursing is critical in the community-based team as well. Special skills in functional assessment, assessment of the home environment, and knowledge of rehabilitation principles and community resources are especially important in an effective community-based team. Nurses with these skills may work out of the physician's office or may be connected with home health agencies. Perhaps more than with other members of the team it is important that the nurse understand the goals of the team and that her assessment be responsive to team needs. This is best accomplished by consistently using one nurse or group of nurses and prospectively discussing the goals and objectives for each patient.

TEAM FUNCTIONING

Early in the formation of the interdisciplinary team, a mechanism for making decisions and carrying out tasks should be developed. Members can become disenchanted with the team approach if initially they thought they would be consulted on all decisions. This is rarely true for practical reasons.[9] In fact, many routine tasks can be handled easily with the teaming of two or three members, leaving the more complicated, potentially creative decision making to the entire team.[10] When a task involves a simple problem of coordination, a centralized human resource network is more efficient; but decentralized networks, such as highly functioning interdisciplinary teams, are superior in solving complex tasks.[32]

Group norms on interdisciplinary teams often quickly emerge without any discussion. Norms that may develop include who is free to interrupt whom, what level of self-disclosure is within boundaries for the team, attendance and promptness issues, seating arrangements, and the pace of the meeting, just to name a few. Trainees and new staff generally adjust to the norms rather than challenge them, unless their appearance occurs at a critical point in the team's development.

CONSULTING WITH INTERDISCIPLINARY TEAMS

Even with careful efforts in developing an interdisciplinary team, no group becomes an effectively functioning team without going through some kind of developmental process akin to forming, storming, norming, and performing. Teamwork is hard work; it is not an automatic result of merely assembling a collection of health care professionals to be a geriatric rehabilitation team. Part of the initial developmental period is used for identifying and resolving the many conflicts which will emerge. During this period strengths and weaknesses are identified and changes are attempted in order to rechannel energy going into conflict toward patient care goals. Conflict is inevitable on interdisciplinary teams, and it is not necessarily destructive. Avoiding it or personalizing it can be devastating for a team.[24,34] A team consultant or facilitator can be very useful to an interdisciplinary team, especially at the beginning stages of development or during difficult transitions.[2,27,35] Consultants might look for indicators of highly functioning and poorly functional teams. On a well-functioning team there is freedom to voice divergent viewpoints and to question basic assumptions. Leadership and maintenance functions tend to be shared by all members of the team. However, on poorly functioning teams, members are late or absent, and a minority viewpoint can be pushed to the exclusion of other members' input. Decision points are demarcated in team discussion, yet definitive decisions are never reached or the responsibility for follow-through is not delineated.

A consultant engages the system of the team in a fashion similar to a family therapist, by relating to the team but not getting enmeshed in the team's system. First, the consultant helps the team assess itself in goal development and adherence, clarity of roles, level of honest communication both within the team and with those outside the team, and the sense of identity and purpose the team has created for itself.[22] Then, by attending to the group process and behavior of the team, the consultant guides the team toward successful negotiation of incomplete team issues.

Interactions between team members reflect both system issues and patient care problems. The negative interactions can serve to pull the team apart without the team's awareness of the impingements upon it.[25] However, team members can be encouraged to develop a problem-solving attitude about their group, where difficulties and conflicts are perceived as the norm rather than terrible truths that should not be unleashed. Active and forthright discussion of team problems can prevent emotions from smoldering and being played out in unproductive ways toward other members or even patients.[15]

Left to their own devices or even in concert with high-priced consultants, teams can collude in not changing. Team developers and team members may satisfy one another with modest gains in performance, but the team still will exhibit no real change. To avoid risk of failure, teams and consultants alike collude by trying to achieve a margin of success without enduring the pain and difficulty inherent in making substantial changes.[14]

To become a highly functioning team, a group of professionals needs to share some of the rewards derived from coming to team meetings. In settings like evaluation or outpatient assessment clinics, there is an air of excitement as individual disciplines successively add pieces to the puzzle of a complete interdisciplinary picture of the patient. Alternatively, team members can gain from learning the techniques and orientations of other disciplines, or they may be nourished in a more literal manner by the serving of breakfast or lunch. Unsuccessful team experiences characteristically occur in settings where the purpose of the team meeting is mainly to have perfunctory paper-signing missions. The zeal is absent as the rewards for individual disciplines are scant at best.

RESEARCH DIRECTIONS FOR INTERDISCIPLINARY TEAMS

A team is made up of professionals whose specific disciplinary techniques have rarely been empirically documented, which complicates the evaluation of their combined team efforts.[7] Empiric questions for team researchers include comparisons of different team types (i.e., interdisciplinary vs. multidisciplinary vs. tradition, consultation); concerns about what types of patients and diagnoses benefit most from team interventions; and how much start-up time is needed before the team approach becomes more effective than more traditional models. After an extensive review of the literature, Halstead found few accounts that reflect true empiric investigations.[16] Bloom and Soper also documented the dearth of research aimed at assessing the effectiveness of health services interventions.[5] Only recently have a few studies compared team care to traditional care, and this has occurred with some home health care teams, geriatric consultation teams, and geriatric evaluation teams and their follow-up endeavors.

Zimmer, Groth-Juncker, and McCuster randomized older patients into treatment by a home health care team comprised of a physician, nurse practitioner, and social worker.[38] Compared to controls the team patients had fewer hospitalizations, nursing home admissions, and outpatient visits. Patients treated by a team used more in-home services, but treatment costs were not different between the groups. Caregiver satisfaction was higher for the home health care team patients. In a recently reported home health team study,[28] 56 older adults with hip fractures were discharged early and then followed by a team made up of a nurse, occupational therapist, a physical therapist at home, and a surgeon for outpatient follow-up visits. In exploring patients over the age of 70, the authors found that control patients remained in the hospital for an average of 27 days, while the team treatment patients were discharged after 9 days and averaged about 9 days of hospital-at-home (HAH) follow-up. This level of care allowed older patients to be discharged quickly and with similar outcomes as persons who were hospitalized for almost a month.[28]

The implementation of a geriatric consultation team has been evaluated in recent years. Campion, Jette, and Berkman concluded that the introduction of a consult team in an acute care hospital promoted geriatrics and taught interdisciplinary teamwork, improved professionals' awareness of functional problems, and increased utilization of rehabilitative services without increasing length of stay.[8] However, the consult team did not lower the high rate of readmission to the hospital. Barker, Williams, and Zimmer assessed the impact of a consult team on patients in acute care settings that were deemed by their physicians as being no longer in need of such an intensive level of care.[3] Over a 6-month period there was a reduction in length of stay and a resultant decrease in the number of such patients.

In a prospective, randomized study of a geriatric consult team, Allen and her colleagues developed recommendations for almost 200 patients.[1] They placed their recommendations in the patients' charts for the treatment group and just kept them on file for the controls. Compliance with recommendations or "would-be" recommendations was markedly higher for the treatment group, with those addressing instability and falls and discharge planning being followed the most often. Caregivers of the control patients typically neglected problems like polypharmacy, sensory impairment, confusion, and depression. Unfortunately, the authors did not explore how compliance with recommendations impacted on outcome variables like length of stay, morbidity, or mortality. Also, the team had much more contact with the treatment patients than with the control patients; their almost daily interaction with the patients on the unit could have reinforced repeatedly their recommendations in the chart.

Gayton and his associates followed over 200 geriatric patients who were nonrandomly assigned to two trial wards and to control units.[13] Patients were evaluated at five time points on criteria such as survival; length of stay; disposition; physical, mental, and social functional levels; and postdischarge use of services. Although there was no randomized assignment to conditions, treatment and control groups were alike on clinical characteristics and sociodemographics at admission. At each point in the evaluation, groups were similar on the outcome measures, although there was a trend toward longer survival among the team patients.

Rubenstein argues that this almost-significant trend is noteworthy, and if geriatric services were keyed to only those patients most likely to benefit from the given interventions, better outcomes might be noted.[29] This may explain much of his success with a geriatric evaluation unit's full complement of geriatric fellows, a broadly represented interdisciplinary team, and a cohesive nursing staff impacting impressively on the outcomes of geriatric patients that were first deemed suitable for such an intervention and then randomly assigned to the treatment condition.[30]

In a more recent study, older men matched on several parameters were followed for a year after initial evaluation by either an interdisciplinary team or physicians and nurse practitioners. Although the patients followed by the interdisciplinary geriatrics clinic preferred being treated by a team, team care was not better than general medical care in the maintenance of health and functioning of stabilized elderly men. However, the interdisciplinary team was marked by multiple rotations of staff, and it even lacked a nurse for almost half of the follow-up time. The authors maintain that perhaps where interdisciplinary teams make a greater impact is in the initial evaluation of the patient's and not in their follow-up.

Targeting a specific patient group, Zeiss and Okarma compared the effects of traditional care and three team models on the outpatient treatment of arthritis patients.[37] One team model utilized a nurse as the case manager who worked individually with patients and consulted the interdisciplinary team for case formulation and treatment planning. In another model, patients met regularly with the full team to outline treatment goals and to agree on treatment plans. A third model featured these components of care coupled with the interdisciplinary team providing the requisite services. One result was that once patients worked with an interdisciplinary team, most liked it and wanted to continue with team treatment. The study also provided some support for team effectiveness, but only in psychologically oriented outcome measures like mood and life satisfaction. The case manager model, where one person has the majority of contact with the patient but the whole team contributes to treatment at least indirectly, seemed to be the most effective of the three.

As is probably clear from this discussion, there are many inherent difficulties in comparing team-delivered care to more traditional approaches. First, teams serve functions besides treatment. Especially in teaching hospitals, interdisciplinary teams have played an important part in the training of professionals who plan to practice rehabilitation or geriatrics. Sometimes teams have played a strong role in attracting young professionals to the field.

Additionally, in compiling any systematic review of team treatment outcome studies, one feels as though apples are being compared to oranges. In each successive study, there are differences in team composition and stage of development, level of involvement with the patients, and diagnoses and sociodemographics of the patients. In other studies, the interdisciplinary team is just one of an array of interventions aimed at the patients,[30] so the team effect is inextricably enmeshed in the total treatment package.

A more precise method to establish the efficacy of team interventions would be to undertake multiple site trials of teams with the same discipline composition treating patients with similar diagnoses and sociodemographic characteristics. Level of team functioning would be difficult to hold constant across sites, but at least measures of team satisfaction and functioning could be covaried with the other outcome data. Of course, patients would either be randomly assigned to team or nonteam conditions or at least be matched on key variables.

Until the time when studies like these can be conducted, interdisciplinary team supporters will have to rely on patchy empiric evidence to bolster their claims. If the question of cost-effectiveness is then entertained, the problem becomes even more difficult. If teams are more cost-effective, then, of course, the team approach would be advocated for those particular patients. But if teams are most costly, then the question becomes what degree of patient improvement or professional training must be reached in order to warrant the added expense.

CONCLUSIONS

When it comes to treating patients with functional disabilities and multiple medical problems, the rehabilitation team will probably continue to exist in one form or another. Those who work with rehabilitation teams in various settings believe that much can be gained by the thoughtful assembling and maintenance of teams. Indeed, it is hard to imagine confronting many of the problems of the elderly without a team structure. However, teams are difficult to manage and can be expensive. Because of these considerations, there is a continuing need for well-devised assessments of their impact on patient care outcomes and staff satisfaction.

REFERENCES

1. Allen, C.M., et al. (1986). A randomized, controlled clinical trial of a geriatric consultation team. *JAMA, 255,* 2617.
2. Baldwin, D.C., and Tsukuda, R.A.W. (1984). Interdisciplinary teams. In C.K. Cassell and J.R. Walsh (Eds.), *Geriatric medicine. Vol. 2: Fundamentals of geriatric care.* New York: Springer-Verlag.
3. Barker, W.H., Williams, T.F., and Zimmer J.G. (1985). Geriatric consultation teams in acute hospitals: Impact on back-up of elderly patients. *J. Am. Geriatr. Soc., 33,* 422.
4. Berkman, B., et al. (1983). Geriatric consultation team: Alternate approach to social work discharge planning. *J. Gerontol. Soc. Work, 5,* 77.
5. Bloom, B.S., and Soper, K.A. (1980). Health and medical care for the elderly and aged population: The state of the evidence. *J. Am. Geriatr. Soc., 228,* 451.
6. Campbell, L.S., and Whitenack, D.C. (1983). A interdisciplinary approach for consultation on multiproblem patients. *N.C. Med. J., 44,* 81.
7. Campbell, L.J., and Cole, K.D. (1987). Geriatric assessment teams. *Clin. Geriatr. Med., 3,* 99.
8. Campion, E.W., Jette, A., and Berkman, B. (1983). An interdisciplinary geriatric consultation service: A controlled trial. *J. Am. Geriatr. Soc., 31,* 792.
9. Charatan, F.B., Foley, C.J., and Libow, L.S. (1985). The team approach to geriatric medicine. In R. Andres, E.L. Bierman, and W.R. Hazzard (Eds.), *Principles of geriatric medicine,* New York: McGraw-Hill.
10. Cole, K.D., and Campbell, L.J. (1986). Interdisciplinary team training for occupational therapists. *Phys. Occup. Ther. Geriatr., 4,* 69.
11. De Shazer, S., and Molnar, A. (1984). Changing teams/changing families. *Fam. Process, 23,* 481.
12. Foushee, H.C. (1984). Dyads and triads at 35,000 feet: Factors affecting group process and aircrew performances. *Am. Psychol., 39,* 885.
13. Gayton, D., et al. (1987). Trial of a geriatric consultation team in an acute care hospital. *J. Am. Geriatr. Soc., 35,* 726.
14. Goren, S., and Ottaway, R. (1985). Why health-care teams don't change: Chronicity and collusion. *J. Nurs. Adm., 15,* 9.

15. Gosselin, J.Y. (1983). The team approach: For or against the patient? *Can. Ment. Health, 31,* 23.
16. Halstead, L.S. (1976). Team care in chronic illness: A critical review of the literature of the past 25 years. *Arch. Phys. Med. Rehabil., 57,* 507.
17. Halstead, L.S., et al. (1986). The innovative rehabilitation team: An experiment in team building. *Arch. Phys. Med. Rehabil., 67,* 357.
18. Johnson, R. (1983). Improving health care team work by education. *N. Z. Med. J., 96,* 660.
19. Jones, E.E., and Nisbett, R.E. (1971). *The actor and the observer: Divergent perceptions of the causes of behavior.* Morristown, NJ: General Learning Press.
20. Kane, R.A. (1982). Thoughts from the bleachers. *Health Soc. Work, 7,* 2.
21. Kane, R.A. (1975). *Interprofessional teamwork.* Manpower monograph No. 8, Syracuse University, School of Social Work, Syracuse, NY.
22. Kerski, et al. (1987). Post-geriatric evaluation unit follow-up: Team versus non-team. *J. Gerontol., 42,* 191.
23. Logan, R.L., and McKendry, M. (1982). The multi-disciplinary team: A different approach to patient management. *N. Z. Med. J., 95,* 883.
24. Lowe, J.I., and Kerranen, M. (1978). Conflict in teamwork: Understanding roles and relationships. *Soc. Work Health Care, 3,* 323.
25. Margolis, H., and Fiorelli, J.S. (1984). An applied approach to facilitating interdisciplinary teamwork. *J. Rehabil., 50,* 13.
26. Nason, F. (1983). Diagnosing the hospital team. *Soc. Work Health Care, 9,* 25.
27. Pearson, P.H. (1983). The interdisciplinary team process, or the professionals' tower of babel. *Dev. Med. Child Neurol., 25(3),* 390.
28. Pryor, G.A., et al. (1988). Team management of the elderly patient with hip fracture. *Lancet, 1,* 401.
29. Rubenstein, L.Z. (1987). Documenting impacts of geriatric consultation. *J. Am. Geriatr. Soc., 35,* 829.
30. Rubenstein, L.Z., Josephson, K., and Wieland, D.G. (1984). Effectiveness of a geriatric evaluation unit: A randomized clinical trial. *N. Engl. J. Med., 311,* 1664.
31. Saint-Yves, I.F.M. (1982). Teamwork within the primary health team. *R. Soc. Health J., 102,* 232.
32. Shaw, M.E. (1964). Communication networks. In L. Berkowitz (Ed.), *Advances in experimental social psychology, Vol. 1.* New York: Academic Press.
33. Van de Ven, A.H., and Delbecq, A.L. (1972). The nominal group as a research instrument for exploratory health studies. *Am. J. Public Health, 62,* 337.
34. Vogt, M.T., and Ducanis, A.J. (1977). Conflict and cooperation in the allied health professions: An analysis of the sources of conflict and recommendations for its management. *J. Allied Health,* Winter, 23.
35. Von Shilling, K. (1982). The consultant role in multidisciplinary team development. *Int. Nurs. Rev., 29,* 73.
36. Wise, H. (1974). *Making health teams work.* Cambridge, MA: Ballinger.
37. Zeiss, A.M., and Okarma, T.B. (1984). Effects of interdisciplinary health care teams on elderly arthritic patients. Presented at *Interdisciplinary Health Team Care: Proceedings of the Sixth Annual Conference.* Schools of Allied Health, Medicine, Nursing, and Pharmacy, University of Connecticut, Hartford.
38. Zimmer, J.G., Groth-Juncker, A., and McCuster, J. (1985). A randomized controlled study of a home health care team. *Am. J. Public Health, 75,* 134.

PART V

Special Issues in Geriatric Rehabilitation

CHAPTER 25

Rehabilitation of Persons with Dementia

HELENA CHANG CHUI
BARBARA A. SMITH

Dementia is a major cause of disability in the elderly population. In the United States it is estimated that 2.3 million persons are suffering from moderate to severe dementia. By the year 2020, this figure will reach 3.3 million.[39,44] While 10 to 15 percent of these persons have underlying conditions which may be amenable to therapy, the vast majority have neurodegenerative or vascular diseases for which there is still no adequate treatment. This includes approximately 1.4 million persons believed to have Alzheimer's disease (AD),[39] and about 700,000 persons who have vascular dementia alone or in combination with Alzheimer's. The economic and emotional burdens associated with these illnesses are staggering. In 1983, approximately $31 billion was spent for the care of persons with Alzheimer's disease alone.[15] The pain and suffering associated with insidiously progressive loss of memory, mentation, and personhood are even more difficult to measure. Research for these highly prevalent but currently irreversible diseases is critical and must be supported as a foremost national priority.

This work was supported by the State of California Department of Health Services, the Estelle Doheny Foundation, and the National Institutes of Health (KO7 NS500974).

Clearly it is important to make an accurate diagnosis of dementia, especially so as to recognize and treat reversible cases. However, even in the face of a primarily irreversible diagnosis, a nihilistic attitude is unwarranted. The absence of effective primary therapy does not preclude, but rather necessitates, a pragmatic approach to the management of persons with dementia. We agree with Reifler and Teri[34] that the principles of rehabilitation, namely, "helping someone reach his or her highest attainable level of skill and function," are relevant and essential for the satisfactory management of persons with dementia.

As with persons who have traditional "rehabilitatable" illnesses (e.g., stroke, brain injury, myocardial infarction), rehabilitation of persons with dementia requires the close interaction of a multidisciplinary team which addresses medical, social, psychologic, and functional issues. In the rehabilitation model, function is emphasized over cure. Ability and disability are just as important as reversibility and irreversibility. For prognosis, psychosocial, economic, and legal status are equally germane as the biomedical factors.

UNIQUE ASPECTS OF REHABILITATION FOR ALZHEIMER'S DISEASE

Several unique factors distinguish the rehabilitation for dementia:

1. Patients with dementia suffer cognitive and behavioral impairments which limit their participation in the formulation and implementation of the care plan. Most commonly a caregiver becomes the major architect and executor of the care plan. In these roles the caregiver needs assistance from expert and dedicated health professionals, as well as respite from the daily burden of caregiving.[5,47] It is estimated that for every American presently suffering from some degree of dementia, three close family members are deeply affected by the emotional, physical, social, and financial burdens of caregiving.[44]
2. Most dementias are not stable but produce progressive decline in function. More than in other settings, the care plan for affected persons must be reassessed and modified periodically. Different functional and ethical issues arise in various stages of dementia. Thorough familiarity with the natural course of dementing diseases is required to provide effective anticipatory guidance.
3. The concept of rehabilitation of patients with dementia is relatively new. The rehabilitative strategies discussed in this chapter have

evolved to a large extent empirically. They are based on clinical experience and the judgment of individuals and centers specializing in the management of persons with dementia. New directions and recommendations are anticipated as interventions come under more systematic evaluation.

The rehabilitative approach is appropriate for persons in all stages of dementia. However the specific content of this chapter focuses on persons with dementia who are living in the community and the dedicated caregivers who make this possible. For a discussion of management issues in long-term care facilities, the reader is referred to Schneider.[41]

SPECIAL CONSIDERATIONS IN ASSESSMENT

Accurate diagnosis of the underlying cause of dementia requires a careful history of present and past and family illnesses and a list of current medications, obtained from a reliable collateral source. The mental status examination, physical examination, and laboratory studies are equally important. This chapter assumes that an accurate differential diagnosis of dementia has been made based on a critical analysis of such information.[8,20]

The assessment described above usually suffices for the diagnosis of dementia and the institution of medical treatment. The rehabilitation of persons with dementia, however, requires considerable additional information. For the patient, cognitive and functional abilities, personality and behavior, and social and financial resources must be assessed. For the caregiver, mental and physical well-being must be evaluated. At many centers, this information is gathered by an interdisciplinary team which includes physicians, nurses, psychologists, social worker, and therapists.[36]

Rating scales, mental status questionnaires, and semistructured interviews are very helpful for the systematic assessment of the person with dementia. The *Sourcebook of Geriatric Assessment*[18] offers a list and description of most available instruments relevant to the clinical assessment of elderly persons. Instruments currently used by the Southern California Alzheimer's Disease Diagnostic and Treatment Center are listed in Table 25-1. The comprehensive assessment should identify individual areas of strength and weakness, frequency and severity of symptoms, as well as available family and community resources. This information is prerequisite to developing a practical and effective care plan.

Table 25-1. *Assessment Instruments Used at the Southern California Alzheimer's Disease Diagnostic and Treatment Center*

Dementia severity	Clinical Dementia Rating Scale (Hughes et al., 1982)[17]
Cognitive abilities	Mini-mental state examination (Folstein, et al., 1975)[9]
	Modified mini-mental state examination (Teng and Chui, 1987)[42]
	Blessed Memory Information Concentration Test (Blessed et al., 1968)[2]
	Neuropsychologic assessment battery
Activities of Daily Living	Blessed Tomlinson Roth Dementia Scale (Habits and Everyday Activities (Blessed et al., 1968)[2]
Personality and Behavior	Brief Psychiatric Rating Scale (Overall and Gorham, 1962)[30]
	Relative's Assessment of Global Symptomatology (Raskin and Crook, 1978)
Social and Financial Resources	State of California Alzheimer's Disease Diagnostic and Treatment Center intake (ADDTC)*
	Clinical Gerontology Service Home Visit

*The ADDTC Intake database was developed jointly by the Alzheimer's Disease Diagnostic and Treatment centers in the State of California, the California Department of Health Services, and the Institute of Aging and Health Policy at the University of California at San Francisco. Copies of the database and instruction manual are available from the State of California Department of Health Services, Sacramento, CA 94234.

THE CARE PLAN

After an accurate diagnosis and comprehensive assessment are completed, a care plan must be developed which addresses both the needs of the patient and those of the caregiver. For the patient, the objective is to maximize function and prevent excess disability. For the caregiver, the goal is to offer information and guidance, suggest coping strategies, and provide respite (See Table 25-2). Development and implementation of the care plan requires effort and commitment from health professionals, the caregiver, and to the extent that it is possible, the patient. At many centers which specialize in the care of patients with dementia, the initial care plan is developed in a joint conference with all interested and available family members. Arrangements are made to periodically reassess the situation and to review the care plan. This typically occurs at 3- to 6-month intervals, or more frequently as the circumstances dictate.

Table 25-2. *Elements of the Care Plan*

I. Preventing excess disability
   A. Coexistent illness
   B. Reducing medications
   C. Behavioral disturbances
   D. Ensuring safety
II. Maximizing independence and activity: Matching activities to abilities
   A. Early cognitive impairment, predementia
   B. Early stages of dementia
   C. Middle stages of dementia
   D. Late stages of dementia
III. Enabling the caregiver
   A. Providing information and support
   B. Developing coping strategies
   C. Exploring ethical and legal issues

PREVENTING EXCESS DISABILITY

Coexistent medical illness is frequently present in patients with dementia. In a study of 107 patients with dementia, Larson, Reifler, Featherstone, and English[22] identified previously unrecognized medical disease in 45 percent of patients, 23 percent of whom improved mentally with treatment. In a study of 154 patients with dementia, other investigators found 29 percent to be also depressed, 82 percent of whom responded to antidepressant treatment.[35] Thus, even in patients with "irreversible" dementia, there may often be superimposed illness or symptoms which are eminently treatable.

Patients with dementia may be less aware and communicative regarding symptoms of disease. The diagnosis of coexistent illness may depend on the recognition of sudden changes in functional abilities, rather than explicit complaints. Increased lethargy or confusion, for example, may indicate the presence of a urinary tract infection.

Reducing medications as much as possible is also important. Drugs must be used judiciously in the elderly, and even more so in older persons with cognitive impairment.[23] Medications may induce psychosis, affective or behavioral disturbance, worsen confusion, and increase the likelihood of falling.[4] Sedatives, hypnotics, antihypertensives, and major tranquilizers were the most common cause of cognitive impairment in one study.[23] Specifically, diazepam, cimetidine, digoxin (Lanoxin), propranolol, phenytoin (Dilantin), phenobarbital, levodopa, amantadine, prednisone, indomethacin, and amitriptyline are commonly implicated.[29] In managing persons with dementia, unnecessary medications should be discontinued and medications that are well indicated should be administered cautiously and in the lowest effective dose.

Behavioral disturbances are commonly associated with dementing illnesses and may be even more troublesome to caregiving than cognitive loss. Changes in personality may include passivity, dependency, suspiciousness, or egocentricity. Increased motor activity may take the form of wandering, agitation, restlessness, or aggression. The patient may express anxiety, obsessive-compulsive behaviors, tearfulness, or depression. Visual and/or auditory hallucinations and paranoid delusions are not uncommon. Disturbances in the sleep-wake cycle may also be very troublesome.[13,37,43]

Behavioral or pharmacologic interventions may alleviate many of these symptoms. Several nonpharmacologic interventions have been enumerated by Kemp.[21] These include preventing the problem if possible, modifying behaviors with rewards and consequences, improving communication with the patient, changing the environment or the activity at hand, or changing the caregiver's perception of the problem. Prevention may be a suitable way of avoiding embarrassing social interactions, catastrophic reactions, or urinary incontinence. Behavioral modification may help to reinforce or extinguish specific behaviors. If a patient is confused or aphasic, it may be more helpful to understand and respond to a person's emotional message rather than the precise word content. Change in the environment or activity may help to decrease repetitive or agitated behaviors. Finally, changing the caregiver's beliefs and perceptions of the problem may help. For example, when bathing is resisted, changing the caregiver's insistence on a daily bath to a bath twice a week may alleviate part of the problem.

Medications can also be helpful for behavioral problems, but should be selected carefully and used conservatively. It is still difficult to predict a priori which pharmacologic agent will benefit a given patient. Some patients develop paradoxical reactions and become more agitated with sedatives. Akathisia or restlessness is a common side effect of major tranquilizers.

Anxiety may be alleviated with benzodiazepines. Short- or intermediate-acting preparations (e.g., oxazepam, temazepam, alprazolam) are clearly preferred over long-acting agents (e.g., diazepam, chlorazepam, fluorazepam) whose cumulative effects may cause undue sedation, worsen confusion, and increase the likelihood of falling.[23] If benzodiazepines are taken chronically, withdrawal should be gradual. Rapid discontinuation, especially of high-potency benzodiazepines (e.g., triazolam), may be associated with withdrawal symptoms such as sleeplessness, anxiety, or confusion.

Neuroleptics may reduce agitation, delusions, and hallucinations, but may induce akathisia, parkinsonism, sedation, or hypotension. For dementia patients, relatively low doses should be used (e.g., haloperidol 0.5 to 1.0 mg orally bid or thioridazine 10 to 25 mg orally). In elderly and demented persons, anticholinergics are notorious causes of confusion and psychosis and therefore should not be prescribed to prevent neuroleptic-associated parkinsonism. Antidepressants with low anticholinergic activity (e.g., desipramine) or high anticholinergic potency should be avoided. Improvement of agitation with carbamazepine and propranolol are currently under study.

Ensuring safety is vital. Many accidents can be avoided by preventive measures. The home environment should be scrutinized for potential safety hazards. Particular attention should be paid to clutter, loose rugs, lighting, door locks, electrical appliances, hot water pipes, cigarettes, matches, firearms, power tools, knives, detergents, polishes, chemicals, medications, and the tub and shower. An emergency medical plan identifying paramedics, an emergency room, the local hospital, and their phone numbers should be established. In case of a tendency to wander, an identification bracelet or necklace which includes name, address, and indication of memory impairment should be worn, neighbors should be alerted, and identifying photographs of the patient should be available. Driving safety should be evaluated periodically. Factors to consider include visual perception, alertness and reaction time, judgment, and visual-spatial orientation both in familiar and unfamiliar settings. Once a potential hazard is identified, both family and professionals must face the issue of safety and take appropriate precautions to avert mishap.

MAXIMIZING INDEPENDENCE AND ACTIVITY

A rehabilitative approach to persons with dementia encourages maximal independence and optimal activity, as well as the prevention of excess disability. This aspect of care is summarized in the context of Alzheimer's disease by Richard Goldberg of the Massachusetts Rehabilitation Commission, who states that "management . . . should be aimed at providing the greatest amount of personal freedom in the least restrictive environment consistent with the patient's functional limitations."[12]

Allen's model of cognitive disability[1] posits that cognitive processes are maximized and behavioral responses become more effectively organized when environmental stimuli are presented to the impaired person according to the level of his or her cognitive functioning. Self-esteem and meaningfulness are also enhanced by engaging persons in activities in which they can experience some measure of success. Six levels of cognition (Allen cognitive levels of ACLs) and suitable activities for each level are described by Levy.[25]

For persons with dementia, there can be considerable heterogeneity in individual cognitive strengths and weaknesses. There can also be significant differences in the rate of progression through various stages of dementia. Given these individual differences, it is nonetheless useful to use a common measure to describe the overall severity of dementia. Two widely adopted dementia severity scales include the Clinical Dementia Rating Scale or (CDR),[17] and the Global Deterioration Scale or (GDS).[37] General guidelines for maximizing activity are suggested below for early, middle, and late stages of dementia.

EARLY COGNITIVE IMPAIRMENT, PREDEMENTIA

In the earliest stage of cognitive impairment (CDR = 0.5; GDS = 2–3; ACL = 5), when a diagnosis of dementia is premature, individuals may be forgetful and experience difficulties with higher levels of problem solving and abstraction. They may have trouble reading, writing, and solving mathematical or financial problems. However, they are still able to perform a sequence of four to five steps, can learn from mistakes, and make their own adjustments in lifestyle. These persons should be encouraged to remain actively involved and usually require no supervision.

EARLY STAGES OF DEMENTIA

In the early stages of dementia (CDR = 1–2; GDS = 4–5; ACL = 4–3), difficulties are frequently encountered with everyday activities such as planning, finances, cooking, and shopping. On the other hand, familiar, simpler, or manual tasks can be successfully realized, particularly with careful organization and planning. In these stages of dementia, memory is significantly impaired so that instructions cannot be remembered and patients are disoriented to time and sometimes to place. Clocks with the date, day, and year may assist orientation. Calendars, notes, labels, or pictures may serve as reminders of appointments, chores, and locations of objects.

Patients are able to initiate two- to three-step purposeful actions which have concrete and predictable outcomes. Activities may be disorganized and confused, as familiar gross motor patterns are sometimes used inappropriately and with poor anticipation of effect. Persons at this stage have difficulty recognizing and correcting mistakes. However, simpler and more repetitive activities which have predictable effects on the environment may provide enjoyable substitutes for more complex tasks. These include sports, dancing, household maintenance (hammering nails, sawing wood), gardening, simple kitchen and household work (mixing batter, chopping vegetables, folding laundry, sweeping floors, wiping dishes), playing a musical instrument, painting, sculpture, drawing, or needlework.

Adult cay care centers play a significant role in the care plan of persons in the early and middle stages of dementia. Day care centers provide an important source of respite to caregivers who are managing persons with dementia at home. They also provide an opportunity for ongoing assessment of a patient's abilities and disabilities and offer a varied and individualized program of activities and stimulation to maximize independence and function.

In the earlier stages of dementia, patients are often anxious and benefit from gentle reassurance and supervision. Daily routines are important. Reduction in the number of choices (such as the type and orientation of clothing) will reduce confusion. Social activities should be encouraged for as long as possible, although careful planning (such as selection of friends and degree of sensory stimulation) may be necessary to reduce unnecessary stress and embarrassment.

MIDDLE STAGES OF DEMENTIA

During the middle stages of dementia (CDR = 3–4; GDS = 5–6; ACL = 2), increasing difficulties are encountered with dressing, toileting, bathing, and other aspects of personal hygiene. Accompanying behavioral problems are frequent (such as agitation, wandering, and paranoia), which may exacerbate the situation. At this stage, caregiving can become exceedingly tedious and unrewarding. In order to foster independence and maintain existing abilities, patients should be encouraged to participate in their own care, even though tasks can be performed much more easily by others. This requires simplification of instructions into single-step commands, repetitive practice, and heretofore unknown patients. At this stage, when verbal comprehension as well as memory may be severely compromised, caregivers must be particularly sensitive to their own emotional overtones. A loud tone of voice or abrupt gestures may be threatening, while a calm tone of voice or physical signs of affection may have a positive and reassuring effect.

Patients in the middle stages of dementia may be active without clear purpose. Behavior may be highly disorganized and nonproductive (aimless pacing, constant disrobing and/or redressing), with attention limited to the person's own well-rehearsed body movements. Persons at this stage need direct visual cues (labeled, or better yet, directly visible objects). Familiar motor activities can still be performed although less accurately (folding laundry, chopping, polishing objects, catching a ball, dancing). Dressing and toileting must be reduced to single motor steps. Maintenance of a predictable daily routine and avoidance of sensory overload are important. Ambulation and simple sensory stimulation (gustatory, olfactory, tactile, visual, auditory, kinesthetic) should be encouraged.

LATE STAGES OF DEMENTIA

In the late stages of dementia (CDR = 5; GDS = 7; ACL = 1), cognition is profoundly impaired. At this stage most patients are institutionalized largely because of the increased physical burden placed on caregivers. There is loss of spontaneous purposeful activity even for ambulation, continence, and basic sustenance. Attention is not attached to any particular stimuli and patients, while conscious, appear to stare and are often unresponsive. Primitive motor reflexes such as grasping, sucking, and chewing may be preserved. The person must be fed, but usually continues to lose weight. Attempts are usually made to keep a consistent and familiar environment and to communicate at an emotional level although the effectiveness of these interventions is not clear. Assisted ambulation and later regular turning and passive range-of-motion exercises are necessary in order to forestall the secondary complications of the disease such as bed sores, contractures, osteoporosis, and infection.

ENABLING THE CAREGIVER

The caregiver becomes the "executive mind" as well as the "working hands" for the patient suffering from dementia. In order to survive and manage successfully, the caregiver must obtain accurate information, emotional support and respite, develop a sense of effectiveness as a caregiver, and become well-informed about ethical and legal issues. Health professionals can significantly help caregivers in meeting these needs. Invaluable emotional support and crisis intervention can be provided by the knowledge, commitment, and sensitivity of dedicated health professionals. Health providers should not only be prepared to provide information when specifically asked for it, but should also be able to offer "anticipatory guidance." Often caregivers are unaware of or afraid to ask the "right" questions. For example, at some point the professional may need to bring up questions of unsafe driving, sorely needed respite care, or the difficult issue of nursing home placement.

The Alzheimer's Disease and Related Disorders Association (ADRDA) is an important national resource to families. The national ADRDA publishes a newsletter and also supports scientific research and public legislation relevant to AD and other dementias. Chapters of the ADRDA help to organize local information and care networks, such as informational meetings and support groups.

A growing list of books and videotapes about AD and other dementing illnesses is available for caregivers.[7,12,16,31,47] Families need to learn about the causes and natural histry of dementing illnesses. They need to learn how to interpret and respond to specific symptoms and behaviors, to cope with stress, and to take care of themselves.[32,47] Information about respite and various care options such as in-home care, board and care, and retirement or skilled nursing homes are also needed.[3]

Beyond book learning, several instructional and intervention programs are available for caregivers.[24,47] The Southern California Alzheimer's Disease Diagnostic and Treatment Center offers an educational support group as well as a traditional support group. The educational support group is led by a member of the staff, is attended by 20 to 30 caregivers, and meets biweekly for eight sessions. The following topics are presented:

1. Introduction: the purpose of the group. What is dementia?
2. Neurologic aspects of dementia.
3. Typical problems and common family reactions.
4. Behavioral problems and management.
5. Financial and legal issues.
6. Recognition and management of other health problems. What should you know?
7. Looking at yourself: Managing stress.
8. Getting support: Where do you go from here?

Beyond the dissemination of vital information, this group provides a nucleus of emotional support to caregivers. A study comparing a group of caregivers enrolled in this educational support group with untreated caregivers showed significant improvement in knowledge as well as reductions in perceived burdens and levels of depression.[19]

Caregivers who complete the educational support group and have a common base of knowledge are invited to join a traditional ongoing support group. This group is led jointly by a social worker and nurse and is comprised mostly of children and spouses, with a few other family members or friends. This support group offers an outlet for feelings and a forum for sharing common concerns. Typical issues raised by children include hereditary risk, family dynamics and conflicts, role reversals, and the stress of caregiving with concurrent employment. Concerns of spouses frequently focus on new roles and responsibilities, sexuality, previous marital conflicts, and disagreements with adult children. Encouragement and empathy from persons dealing with similar issues can be very helpful and therapeutic to caregivers.

Family members must be urged to conserve their health and sanity by taking regular breaks from the ordeal of day-to-day caregiving. Several days each month away from caregiving responsibilities help to refresh coping mechanisms. Respite for the primary caregiver may be provided by other family members, in-home chore workers, or day care centers. Scharlach[40] found evidence that respite care programs reduced caregiver burden and decreased the likelihood of institutionalization.

It is important to emphasize that it is not the cognitive or behavioral problems associated with dementia per se, that cause caregivers to become severely stressed, depressed, or physically ill, but rather the caregiver's inability to cope with them.[21,46] This distinction emphasizes the need to address both the caregiver's ability to cope, as well as the patient's behavior. Placement in a convalescent home usually depends less on the severity of the mental impairment of the patient and more on its functional consequences to the family.[6]

Situations and coping mechanisms may differ widely among caregivers. Some family members seem to experience little stress while others become severely depressed and ill. Recent studies[4,8,10] indicate that family members who cope better with the problems associated with dementia have higher levels of "self-efficacy," namely, the belief that one is capable of performing a necessary behavior because one has the requisite skills, knowledge, talents, physical capacity, and motivation. Thus effective assistance to the caregivers requires help in developing a sense of self-efficacy, as well as education and emotional support.

EXPLORING ETHICAL AND LEGAL ISSUES

Ethical issues in patients with dementia frequently revolve around the principles of autonomy (i.e., the patient's right to self-determination) and beneficence, the overriding of a person's actions or wishes for beneficent reasons.[11] Certain dilemmas are typical in each stage of dementia. In the early stages, typical issues include telling the truth about the illness, driving, working, living arrangements, and potential suicide. In the middle stages, issues frequently relate to medications, placement, conservatorship, informed consent, and conflicts between the family's needs versus the patient's needs. Questions of withholding or withdrawing care and euthanasia may arise in the late stages of dementia.[26]

The question of whether to tell a person that he or she has an irreversible dementia has been likened to telling a patient that he or she is dying. Knowledge of the diagnosis is essential if the patient is to have the opportunity to plan for the future. Many patients with dementia may express little insight or interest in the diagnosis or prognosis, perhaps because the lack of an abstract attitude and apathy may themselves be early symptoms of the disease. On the other hand, many patients may be too frightened to seek answers or may be unable to share their feelings. Probably the best advice is to answer questions directly but sensitively and to avoid forcing explanations on patients who don't want them.[11,36]

Driving a motor vehicle frequently raises ethical and legal issues, as well as safety questions. Driving is a valued symbol of independence which may be relinquished with great reluctance. Often motor skills are relatively preserved and patients with dementia have difficulty in recognizing impairments in visual-spatial orientation, judgment, and reaction time. Sometimes it is difficult to determine whether driving is no longer safe. In other cases, driving may be clearly unsafe, but conflicts arise because the paternalistic decision to prevent driving violates an autonomous wish to continue driving. Physicians have the responsibility to inform the department of motor vehicles (DMV) if they believe a patient's capacity to drive safely is significantly impaired. The legal responsibility to determine competence belongs to the DMV.

During the early stages of dementia, patients should be encouraged to make plans for the future. Several legal instruments permit patients to retain some measure of autonomy even after they become incompetent. The durable power of attorney for health care enables patients to nominate another person to make decisions concerning their health. A living trust allows a patient to instruct how his or her assets are to be used. The living trust can protect a spouse from impoverishment due to the costs of a nursing home. After dividing their property into equal shares, dementing persons can give their share to a trustee (spouse) to hold in trust for their benefit and to use it for their care until it is exhausted. The noninstitutionalized spouse's half of the property is not considered when the patient's eligibility for Medicaid is being reviewed. If no action is taken until the patient become incompetent, the court must appoint a guardian to make decisions on his or her behalf.[11,14]

SUMMARY

Until primary therapies are developed for the highly prevalent but currently irreversible dementing illnesses, emphasis must be placed on supportive care and management. A comprehensive strategy is described to prevent excess disability, maximize function, and enable effective caregiving. This approach addresses the medical, environmen-

V. Special Issues in Geriatric Rehabilitation

tal, and psychosocial needs of both the patient and caregiver. Although a dementing disease may cause a progressive downward spiral, a commitment to the principles of rehabilitation is essential to effective coping and caregiving.

REFERENCES

1. Allen, C.K. (1982). Independence through activity: the practice of occupational therapy. *Am. J. Occup. Ther., 36,* 731.
2. Blessed, G., Tomlinson, B.E., and Martin, R. (1968). The association between quantitative measures of dementia and of senile change in the cerebral grey matter of elderly subjects. *Br. J. Psychiatry 114,* 797.
3. Blum, S.R., and Minkler, M. (1980). Toward a continuum of caring alternatives: community based care for the elderly. *J. Soc. Issues 36,* 133.
4. Buchner, D.M., and Larson, E.B. Falls and fractures in patients with Alzheimer-type dementia. *JAMA, 257,* 1492.
5. Cicerelli, V.G. (1986). Family relationships and care/management of the dementing elderly. In M.L.M. Gilhooly, S.M. Zarit, and J.E. Birren (Eds.), *The dementias: policy and management* (pp. 93–110). Englewood Cliffs, NJ: Prentice-Hall.
6. Coleric, E.J., and George, L.K. (1986). Predictors of institutionalization among caregivers of patients with Alzheimer's disease. *J. Am. Geriatr. Soc. 34,* 493.
7. Cummings, J.L., and Benson, D.F. (1983). *Dementia: A clinical approach.* Boston: Butterworths.
8. Cummings, J.L., et al. (1987). Neuropsychiatric aspects of multi-infarct dementia and dementia of the Alzheimer type. *Arch. Neurol. 44,* 389.
9. Folstein, M.F., Folstein, S.E., and McHugh, P.R. (1975). Mini-Mental State: A practical method for grading the cognitive state of patients for the clinician. *J. Psychiatr. Res., 12,* 189.
10. Gallagher, D., Lovett, S., and Zeiss, A. (1987). *Interventions with caregivers of frail elderly persons.* Palo Alto, CA: Caregiver Research Program.
11. Gilhooly, M.L.M. (1986). Legal and ethical issues in the management of the dementing elderly. In S.H. Zarit and J.E. Birren (Eds.), *The dementias: policy and management* (pp. 131–160). Englewood Cliffs, NJ: Prentice-Hall.
12. Goldberg, R.T. (1985). Alzheimer's disease: From benign neglect to community living. *Rehabil. Lit., 46,* 122.
13. Gustafson, L. (1975). Psychiatric symptoms in dementia with onset in the presenile period. *Acta Psychiatr. Scand.* Suppl., 257, 8.
14. Hankin, M. (1988). Legal and financial matters. In M. Flitterman and B. Fulmer (Eds.), *Understanding Alzheimer's disease: a specific guide for families* (pp.   –   ). Palm Springs, CA: Eisenhower Medical Center Auxiliary.
15. Hay, J.W., and Ernst, R.L. (1987). The economic costs of Alzheimer's disease. *Am. J. Public Health, 77,* 1169.
16. Heston, L.L., and White, J.A. (1983). *Dementia: a practical guide to Alzheimer's disease and related illnesses.* New York: W.H. Freeman.
17. Hughes, C.P., et al. (1982). A new clinical scale for the staging of dementia. *Br. J. Psychiatry 140,* 566.

18. Israel, L., Kozarevic, D., and Sartorius, N. (1984). *Sourcebook of geriatric assessment*, vols. 1 and 2. Basel: S. Karger.
19. Kahan, J., et al. (1985). Decreasing the burden in families caring for a relative with a dementing illness: a controlled study. *J. Am. Geriatr. Soc., 33,* 664.
20. Katzman, R. (1986). Senile dementia: Alzheimer and vascular. *N. Engl. J. Med., 314,* 964.
21. Kemp, B. (1988). Eight methods family members can use to manage behavioral problems in dementia. *Top. Geriatr. Rehabil., 4,* 50.
22. Larson, E.B., et al. (1984). Dementia in elderly outpatients. A prospective study. *Ann. Intern. Med., 100,* 417.
23. Larson, E.B., et al. (1987). Adverse drug reactions associated with global cognitive impairment in elderly persons. *Ann. Intern. Med., 107,* 169.
24. Levine, N.B., Dastoor, D.P., and Gendron, C.E. (1983). Coping with dementia: a pilot study. *J. Am. Geriatr. Soc., 31,* 12.
25. Levy, L. (1986). A practical guide to the care of the Alzheimer's disease victim: the cognitive disability perspective. *Top. Geriatr. Rehabil., 1,* 16.
26. Lo, B. (1984). Guiding the hand that feeds: caring for the demented elderly. *N. Engl. J. Med., 311,* 402.
27. Mace, N.L., and Rabins, P.V. (1981). *The 36 hour day: A family guide to caring for persons with Alzheimer's disease, related dementing illnesses, and memory loss in later life.* Baltimore: Johns Hopkins Press.
28. Mann, S.H. (1986). Practical management strategies for families with dementia victims. *Neurol. Clin., 4,* 469.
29. *Med. Lett. Drugs Ther.* (1981). *23,* 9.
30. Overall, J.E., and Gorham, D.R. (1962). The brief psychiatric rating scale. *Psychol. Rep., 10,* 799.
31. Powell, L.S., and Courtice, K. (1983). *Alzheimer's disease: a guide for families.* Menlo Park, CA: Addison-Wesley.
32. Quayhagen, M.P., and Quayhagen, M. (1988). Alzheimer's stress: coping with the caregiving role. *Gerontologist, 28,* 391.
33. Raskin, A. and Crook, T.H. (1985). Validation of a battery of tests designed to assess psychopathology in the elderly. In G.D. Burrows, T.R. Norman, and L. Dennerstein (Eds.), *Clinical and pharmacological studies in psychiatric disorders* (pp. 337–343). London: John Libbey.
34. Reifler, B.V., and Teri, L. (1986). Rehabilitation and Alzheimer's disease. In S.J. Brody and G.E. Ruff (Eds.), *Aging and rehabilitation: Advances in the state of the art* (pp. 107–121). New York, Springer.
35. Reifler, B.V., et al. (1986). Dementia of the Alzheimer's type and depression. *J. Am. Geriatr. Soc., 34,* 855.
36. Reifler, B.V., Larson, E.B., and Teri, L. (1987). An outpatient geriatric psychiatry assessment and treatment service. *Clin. Geriatr. Med., 3,* 203.
37. Reisberg, B., et al. (1982). The Global Deterioration Scale (GDS): An instrument for the assessment of primary degenerative demnetia. *Am. J. Psychiatry, 139,* 1136.
38. Reisberg, B., et al. (1986). Remediable behavioral symptomatology in Alzheimer's disease. *Hosp. Commun. Psychiatry, 37,* 1199.
39. Rocca, W.A., Amaducci, L.A., and Schoenberg, B.S. (1986). Epidemiology of clinically diagnosed Alzheimer's disease. *Ann. Neurol., 19,* 415.
40. Scharlach, A.E. (1986). An evaluation of institution-based respite care. *Gerontologist 26,* 77.

41. Schneider, E.L. (Ed). (1985). *The teaching nursing home*. New York: Beverly Foundation.
42. Teng, E.L., Chui, H.C. (1987). The modified mini-mental state (3MS) examination. *J. Clin. Psychiatry, 48*, 314.
43. Teri, L., Larson, E.B., and Reifler, B.V. (1988). Behavioral disturbance in dementia of the Alzheimer type. *J. Am. Geriatr. Soc., 36*, 1.
44. Weiler, P.G.: The public health impact of Alzheimer's disease. *Am. J. Public Health, 77*, 1157.
45. Winograd, C., and Jarvik, L. (1986). Physician management of the demented patient. *J. Am. Geriatr. Soc., 34*, 295.
46. Zarit, S.M., Reever, K.E., and Bach-Peterson, J. (1980). Relatives of impaired elderly: correlates of feelings of burden. *Gerontologist, 20*, 649.
47. Zarit, S., Orr, N., and Zarit, J. (1985). *The hidden victims of Alzheimer's disease: Families under stress*. New York, University Press.
48. Zeiss, A., et al. (1987). Self-efficacy as mediator of caregiver coping: Developing an assessment model. Presented to Association for the Advancement of Behavior Therapy, Boston, 1987.

CHAPTER 26

Ethical Issues in Rehabilitation
BERNARD LO

Rehabilitation medicine frequently raises difficult questions about what care is appropriate. Ethical dilemmas may be particularly difficult because the pathologic changes are irreversible, treatment must be chronic, and patients must participate actively in treatment. The patient's values and goals regarding rehabilitation may differ from those of the health care workers or family members. Regulations regarding reimbursement may further complicate decisions.

The following cases illustrate how ethical dilemmas can arise at each step of a rehabilitation program.

CASE 1
Mr. L., a 77-year-old man living alone, was admitted for diarrhea and dehydration. His workup was complicated by iatrogenic problems. Hypnotics prescribed in the hospital for insomnia caused confusion and agitation. Because of mistakes in scheduling barium x-rays, he was given cathartics and kept without oral intake for several days. As a result, his weakness worsened. The diarrhea eventually resolved, without any cause being found. However, Mr. L. was deconditioned by being in bed for 2 weeks and was unable to return home. He refused to work with the physical therapist; as he repeatedly said, "I need a rest." A rehabilitation facility rejected him because "he was not a good candidate for rehabilitation." Even his daughter, who visited daily, was unable to persuade him to do the recommended exercises.

The nursing and rehabilitation staff were frustrated because they felt Mr. L. was not capable of making decisions and because he would be discharged to a nursing home with little chance of returning to his own home. They felt that the attending physician did not sufficiently encourage the patient to participate in rehabilitation therapy or persuade the rehabilitation facility to accept him. The attending physician believed that aggressive rehabilitation was not indicated while he was confused, dehydrated, and hypokalemic. Indeed, she feared that until these medical problems were corrected, Mr. L. might injure himself trying to walk or exercise. However, by the time these problems resolved, the patient had exceeded the average length of stay for his diagnosis-related group (DRG), and the hospital was pressuring the attending physician to discharge the patient.

This case illustrates dilemmas that occur when patients refuse reha-bilitation, especially when it might significantly benefit the patient. The case was complicated by frustration and disagreements among the rehabilitation team, and by reimbursement pressures.

CASE 2

Mrs. T., a 72-year-old widow, suffered a left hemisphere stroke. Despite intensive speech therapy, physical therapy, and occupational therapy, she was left with significant weakness of her right arm and moderate depression and isolation. When her condition did not improve further, rehabilitation services were no longer reimbursed. She insisted on further physical therapy because she feared that her arm would get weaker. She said that she couldn't do the exercises at home as well without the encouragement of the therapists. The staff noted that visits to rehabilitation were an important social event for her and that otherwise she had little social contact except for family visits. Mrs. T. refused to attend a day care center because she was ashamed of her weakness and feared she would get more depressed seeing others who were "better" than she. She asked the attending physician to state on reimbursement forms that she was continuing to improve and that further physical therapy was needed.

HOW REHABILITATION DIFFERS FROM ACUTE CARE MEDICINE

Many discussions of medical ethics have focused on acute care medicine rather than long-term care or rehabilitation. Several important charac-teristics about rehabilitation create different problems and require dif-ferent solutions.

First, rehabilitation requires active participation of the patient, whereas many treatments in acute care medicine do not. Many high-tech procedures, such as angioplasty, are performed on passive patients. In contrast, rehabilitation requires active patient effort in doing exercises, even when those exercises may be difficult, uncomfortable, or painful.

Second, patients considered for rehabilitation may have impaired judgment or decision-making capacity. Caregivers and family members may question whether preferences expressed by the patient regarding rehabilitation reflect deeply held values, or result from temporary and reversible conditions. When professional and family caregivers believe that the capacity of the patient to make decisions is impaired, they may pressure patients to agree to and comply with rehabilitation programs.

Third, rehabilitation is carried out by a team of professionals. However, they must take orders from attending physicians, who may lack interest in rehabilitation or knowledge about it.[1] Without orders from the attending physician, rehabilitation therapists cannot carry out treatments or be reimbursed for them. Conflicts about professional authority may be exacerbated by conflicts about traditional gender roles.[1]

Fourth, family members are often more involved in rehabilitation than in other types of medical care. They may need to provide transportation, encouragement, or in-home services. They may also play a significant role in decisions about management. Patients with supportive and aggressive families may be more likely to receive rehabilitation. Conversely, conflicts of interest between patients and family members may keep patients from receiving care that might benefit them.

ETHICAL PRINCIPLES

Ethical principles which guide all clinical practice—autonomy, confidentiality, beneficence, truthtelling, and justice—should also direct decisions about rehabilitation.[2,3] We shall discuss these general principles, pointing out particular problems caused by the special nature of rehabilitation.

THE PRINCIPLE OF AUTONOMY

According to the principle of autonomy or respect for persons, individuals have a right to make decisions about their bodies and health care. They may refuse treatments recommended by their physicians, even if their refusals jeopardize their health. Furthermore, patients may stop care that they have started. Respecting patients as persons requires health care workers to obtain informed consent for medical treatments, including rehabilitation.

Respecting a patient's preferences is a crucial aspect of rehabilitation, because the patient's active cooperation is needed. Thus the patient's level of interest, preferences for scheduling, and fatigue will determine what treatment is feasible. At times such preferences by the patient may disrupt the work routine of the health care professionals or the institution. For instance, a patient may refuse treatment at a time convenient for the caregivers but agree to treatment at a different time.

Although patient autonomy is important in rehabilitation, it may be limited in several ways. Family members often play an important role in decisions about rehabilitation. If there is no family, or if family members are unwilling to assist with transportation, home care, or encouragement, rehabilitation may be impossible to arrange. The lack of concerned and active family members may cause a patient to be deemed "not a good candidate for rehabilitation."

Another restriction on autonomy is that the capacity of patients to make informed decisions about rehabilitation may be questioned. This may occur for several reasons. First, patients considered for rehabilitation generally have emotional and functional impairments that may hinder their ability to make decisions. They may feel depressed, discouraged, frustrated, dependent, or out of control. After serious illness or surgery, patients may need time to adjust to a loss of function or to a new self-image. Hence decisions about rehabilitation, particularly refusals, may appear to result from reversible aspects of the illness, rather than from deeply held values, goals, and life plans.

Second, caregivers may question whether patients who have not already experienced rehabilitation can truly appreciate what it is like and what the benefits are. Decisions about rehabilitation often must balance short-term discomfort or suffering against long-term benefits. A patient may complain about the inconvenience or discomfort of the rehabilitation program. However, health care workers may focus more attention on the long-term benefits of rehabilitation. Hence caregivers may believe that the patient is assessing the benefits and risks of rehabilitation inappropriately.

Third, patients commonly change their minds about rehabilitation. Often patients who say they want to stop rehabilitation but are persuaded to continue later are glad that they continued and thank caregivers for not accepting their refusals at face value. Such changes of mind may lead health care professionals to discount refusals of rehabilitation by patients.

Various standards have been used to determine competence to make medical decisions.[4] Strictly speaking, patients are considered competent until a court judges them to be incompetent. However, health care workers are often asked to assess whether a patient is competent and to decide how to make decisions if a patient is deemed incompetent. Although competence is generally questioned only when the patient disagrees with the recommendations of the health care professionals, disagreement per se is not tantamount to incompetence. Similarly, the ability to make a rational decision is sometimes used as a standard for judging capacity to make medical decisions. However, a competent person may make irrational decisions. Indeed, as one judge wrote,

Mr. Justice Brandeis, whose views have inspired much of the "right to be left alone" philosophy said . . .: "The makers of our Constitution . . . sought to protect Americans in their beliefs, their thoughts, their emotions and their sensations. They conferred, as against the government, the right to be left alone . . . the most comprehensive right and the right most valued by civilized man." Nothing in this utterance suggests that Justice Brandeis thought an individual possessed these rights only as to sensible beliefs, valid thoughts, reasonable emotions, or well-founded sensations. I suggest he intended to include a great many foolish, unreasonable and even absurd ideas which do not conform, such as refusing medical treatment even at great risk.[5]

In other words, the true meaning of autonomy is that we accept the decisions of others even when they seem to us to be foolish or unwise.

One recommended standard for competence is that a competent patient must appreciate the nature of recommended treatments, the benefits and risks, the likely outcomes, and the alternatives. The patient must not only comprehend information about the proposed treatment but also appreciate the implications of his decision on his life. Often the rehabilitation patient comprehends the above information, but disagrees with the physician on how to weigh the alternatives. Compared to the health care team, the patient may place more weight on the short-term side effects and give less weight to the long-term benefits of rehabilitation.

The autonomy of a patient may also be challenged when a decision appears to be inauthentic. An authentic choice is consistent with a person's character, life history, past preferences, and commitments.[6] Authentic decisions therefore reflect a coherent, integrated self. Authenticity may be a more stringent standard than competence for respecting a person's autonomy. A person's decision may be competent in that he or she appreciates the consequences of the decision, yet still be inauthentic because it contradicts prior decisions and deeply held values. At the very least, such a decision should be carefully scrutinized and discussed further before it is accepted.

Discussions of autonomy generally focus on the patient, rather than on health care professionals. However, ethical dilemmas can arise when health care workers believe that conditions of work compromise their judgment or independence. Thus rehabilitation specialists may object when patient preferences regarding scheduling or decisions by the attending physician appear to compromise care. Ideally, such disagreements should be discussed explicitly and a mutually satisfactory solution negotiated.[7]

THE PRINCIPLE OF BENEFICENCE

The principle of beneficence requires caregivers to act for the benefit of their patients, or at least not to harm them. While this principle seems clear in the abstract, applying it in particular cases may be controversial because people may disagree over what is best for the patient. All care has risks, such as discomfort, side effects, or inconvenience, as well as benefits. The exhortation to benefit patients really means acting so that the ratio of benefits to risks is favorable. People may disagree over what constitutes a benefit or risk and weigh risks and benefits differently. For example, a patient may experience a great deal of discomfort from therapy and question whether the benefits are really worth the pain. However, a health care professional may regard the discomfort of therapy as temporary and minor, particularly compared to the long-term benefits.

The principle of beneficence may conflict with the principle of autonomy when a patient declines care that caregivers consider beneficial. Allowing a patient to refuse rehabilitation may harm the patient, by leading to loss of function or independence. Caregivers may question whether it is appropriate to overrule a patient's refusal when it is in the patient's best interest.

In American culture, the principle of autonomy generally is given priority over the principle of beneficence.[8] When a competent and informed patient refuses treatment, the patient's evaluaton of the risks and benefits of treatment takes precedence over the values of the caregivers. The principle of beneficence, however, requires caregivers to do more than simply accept a patient's refusal of recommended care. Health care professionals should ascertain if the patient truly appreciates the nature and purpose of treatment, the alternatives, and the consequences of his decision.

In practice, what often occurs is a process of negotiation and accommodation. The caregiver may cajole and urge a reluctant patient, discounting the patient's complaints, or telling him that he doesn't really mean it and that it will be worth it in the long run.[5a] The scheduling, pacing, or intensity of treatments may be changed to accommodate the patient. A bargain may be struck that the patient will try the treatment for a limited period of time, perhaps a week. If there is no improvement, the treatment will stop. Paradoxically, giving the patient more control over the details of treatment often increase patient acceptance of the rehabilitation program. Family members and friends may be enlisted to help convince the patient. But caregivers should not coerce the patient. Ultimately, they must respect the refusal of informed and competent patients. Caregivers should be willing to state explicitly what the patient needs to say or do to have their refusals respected.

Conflicts between autonomy and beneficence may be particularly difficult for patients whose competence is questionable. Some writers have suggested that health care workers "initially ignore or override patient or family choices concerning the course of care for those who are suddenly or unexpectedly severely impaired in the interest of restoring or maximizing the long-term autonomy of rehabilitation candidates."[9] In other words, these writers believe that paternalism is justified in this situation. For these writers, beneficence takes priority over autonomy in this situation.

However, there are several serious difficulties with this position. First, it conflicts with the general principle that a competent, informed patient may refuse care even if such refusal harms his or her health. Second, this justification of paternalism is too broad and open-ended. Where would the limits be set? At what point would a patient's refusal of rehabilitation be accepted? What would patients have to do to convince caregivers that they would not change their minds? Giving power to professionals to determine when to accept the patient's preferences may lead to abuse. Third, such a policy of paternalism is impractical. Effective rehabilitation requires active patient participation. Caregivers must get the assent and cooperation of patients, even those who are not capable of truly informed consent. Trying to force an unwilling patient into treatment is difficult, frustrating, and counterproductive. In the long run, it may also harm caregivers by making them insensitive to patient's needs and concerns.

Another important implication of the principle of beneficence is the rule that health care professionals have no duty to treat if there is no reasonable prospect of benefit, even if the patient or family demands treatment. Thus, if rehabilitation does not achieve the desired goal of improving function, or if there is no further improvement, there is no obligation to continue treatment. In practice, once a patient's progress has plateaued, he or she is generally discharged from rehabilitation. Usually it is the health care team that first raises the issue of terminating rehabilitation.

Case 2, however, illustrates that while this rule seems clear in the abstract, it may be difficult to apply in a particular case. People may disagree over what constitutes a benefit. The usual definition by health care professionals and by reimbursement agencies is functional improvement. However, other definitions of benefit may also be reasonable. In case 2, Mrs. T. believed that prevention of dysfunction was an important benefit. Implicitly she also believed that continued rehabilitation meant that her caregivers were not giving up and had some hope for her condition. Some of her caregivers wondered whether the most significant benefit of rehabilitation was not therapy itself but the social interactions that might ameliorate her loneliness and depression. In terms of improving her ultimate quality of life and level of function, continued visits to rehabilitation might be justified if they were combined with other measures to increase social support and activities.

THE PRINCIPLE OF JUSTICE

The principle of justice requires that the benefits of health be distributed fairly. Health care resources should be allocated equitably. Such distribution is particularly important for rehabilitation because many persons considered for rehabilitation may already be vulnerable or discriminated against. In practice, the distribution of resources in rehabilitation is largely determined by reimbursement regulations and hospital policies. Because rehabilitation services will not be reimbursed for patients who show no functional improvement, caregivers will not offer them when they believe there will be no improvement. Often unilateral decisions to provide or withhold rehabilitation by the caregivers or the institution are presented as technical decisions. For example, in case 1, Mr. L. was not considered "a candidate for rehabilitation." However, such decisions are not merely technical decisions on the potential effectiveness of rehabilitation. They are also value judgments that other social goals, such as preserving the independence of Mr. L. in case 1 and improving the social isolation of Mrs. T. in case 2, and not worthwhile in comparison. Strictly speaking, these goals do not fall uniquely into the realm of rehabilitation rather than other areas of health care, such as social work. But they are consistent with the rehabilitation goal of improving functional abilities, and rehabilitation services can be the initial locus for providing services.

Reimbursement policies about rehabilitation may not reflect a coherent medical or social policy. Such policies are fragmented among Medicare, Medicaid, and private insurers. They may overlook important needs, such as assistance to enable functionally impaired elderly persons to live independently. Reimbursement policies may reflect a desire to restrain costs rather than to meet the needs of patients or society.

Reimbursement policies must be worked out through the political or judicial process, which allows competing interests to be represented. Thus regulations and budgets concerning reimbursement for rehabilitation services for the elderly will be set in administrative and legislative processes. Decisions must take into account budgetary demands for other services for the elderly, other forms of health care, and other governmental activities. But unlike in Great Britain, there is no consistent U.S. policy regarding health care for the elderly.[10] The lack of an overall policy may place caregivers in the position of acting as patient advocates in a health care system that they regard as unfair.

Caregivers who disagree with these reimbursements priorities may be tempted to misrepresent facts to obtain more care for the patient, as in case 2.

THE PRINCIPLE OF TRUTH-TELLING

The principle of truth-telling can be justified in several ways. Telling the truth to the patient has beneficial rather than harmful consequences for the patient. Serious adverse effects like severe depression, suicide, or refusal of care rarely occur. Bad news can be softened by emotional support and by reassurance about continuing care. In rehabilitation, giving accurate and thorough information is essential for gaining the patient's cooperation. In addition, not giving information may be impractical, since another member of the health care team may inadvertently disclose it.

Truthfulness can also be considered a fundamental moral duty. It shows respect for persons, patients expect it, and social interactions would be difficult without it. Honestly is particularly expected of physicians because of their special professional role. The doctor-patient relationship would suffer if patients suspected that physicians sometimes withheld information or did not tell them the truth.

Additional dilemmas about truth-telling occur when physicians act as social gatekeepers, as in case 2. Patients may ask rehabilitation physicians to give misleading or incorrect information on insurance forms, prescriptions, or applications for disability, parking permits, or transportation passes. Physicians may be inclined to misrepresent diagnoses to help individual patients, especially when a corporation or the government, rather than another person, is deceived. Some justify these practices by arguing that the benefits to the patient (and perhaps even to the insurer) outweigh the adverse effects. Such utilitarian justifications of lying, however, typically overlook long-term and indirect adverse effects. Widespread misrepresentations probably will be detected. The public, insurance companies, and the government may then lose trust in physicians. Any perception that significant amounts of fraud or unnecessary care are increasing the cost of medical care may lead to further reductions in reimbursement. In the long run, physicians may also face more administrative review and paperwork.

THE PRINCIPLE OF CONFIDENTIALITY

The principle of confidentiality of medical information respects the privacy of patients and protects them from adverse consequences that might occur if information were disclosed. It also benefits patients, by encouraging them to seek treatment and to discuss their problems frankly. Because rehabilitation requires the cooperation of family, friends, and a team of professionals, confidentiality may be difficult to maintain. When the patient agrees to disclose information, as is generally the case, there are no ethical dilemmas. But some patients may not want others to be told of their condition or treatment, even if such disclosure would help the patient gain assistance from other people. When this occurs, caregivers may be tempted to override the patient's refusal. The previous discussion of the conflict between autonomy and beneficence would apply in this situation. Although health care workers may try to persuade the patient to talk with others, ultimately they must accept the patient's decision.

RESOLVING ETHICAL DILEMMAS

The cases presented above illustrate how ethical principles may conflict. In case 1, the principle of autonomy conflicted with the principles of truth-telling and justice. No rational argument will convince everyone that one principle should supersede another. Thus, in case 1, the principle of autonomy ultimately should override the principle of beneficence. Similarly, in case 2, the principle of truth-telling should take priority.

Even though many ethical dilemmas cannot be resolved by appealing to a hierarchy of ethical principles, individual cases can generally be resolved in practical terms.[11] Caregivers, patients, and families can often agree on a plan of care in an individual case even if they cannot settle underlying philosophic debates. Good communication can often resolve disagreements. In case 1, a team meeting allowed the attending physician and the rest of the health care team to understand one another's concerns and frustrations. In a team, they were better able to listen to the concerns and frustrations of the patient and his daughter. The team made a particular effort to express its empathy for the patient's experiences and his frustration at being worse rather than better. Similarly, the team better understood his anger at being sent to different parts of the hospital, without anyone explaining what would happen or allowing him a voice in decisions. Conversely, the patient and his daughter appreciated how the caregivers wanted him to be able to live independently in his own home.

As a result of such improved communication, the caregivers tried to give the patient more control over decisions and the details of care. They were able to negotiate a schedule for care that was mutually acceptable. By asking him when he would like to have physical therapy and what pace he felt comfortable with, the team was able to get the patient to agree to a plan of care. A schedule for physical therapy was drawn up that extended his acute care hospitalization for several days but allowed him to return home with intensive home therapy and home health assistance.

In case 2, better communication and negotiation also helped the case to be resolved in a mutually satisfactory manner. The caregivers listened to the patient's fears about further disability and loss of independence and acknowledged her sadness as an natural response to her illness. The caregivers were then able to encourage her to talk about underlying psychosocial issues, rather than about the details of physical therapy. In turn, the caregivers were able to talk about their feelings for her, how they also felt sad and disappointed at the lack of improvement. By so doing, the caregivers were able to help the patient accept her neurologic limitations and to redefine the problem so that the issues were her loneliness and sense of loss. The goal then became to help her join the activities at a senior center. One therapist called a colleague at the senior center to introduce the patient. The rehabilitation team also promised to call her to see how she was doing at the senior center.

In summary, ethical dilemmas may be particularly difficult in rehabilitation medicine. The general principles of medical ethics, including autonomy, beneficence, and justice, should also apply to rehabilitation. Conflicts among ethical principles may be difficult to resolve. Disagreements over patient management, dilemmas, however, can often be resolved through improving communication and by negotiating a mutually acceptable plan of care with the patient.

REFERENCES

1. Appelbaum, P.S., Lidz, C.W., and Meisel, A. (1987). *Informed consent: Legal theory and clinical practice.* New York: Oxford University Press.
2. Application of the President and Directors of Georgetown College, Inc., a body corporate. 331 F.2d 1000 (1964).
3. Beauchamp, T.L., and Childress, J.F. (1983). *Principles of biomedical ethics.* 2nd ed. New York: Oxford University Press, 1983.
4. Brucker, J.S. (1987). Behind the curtain of silence: ethical dilemmas in rehabilitation. In D.C. Thomasma and J. Monagle (Eds.), *Medical ethics: a guide for health care professionals* (pp. 99–121). Rockville, MD: Aspen Systems.
5. Callopy, B.J. (1988). Autonomy in long-term care: some crucial distinctions. *Gerontologist, 28S,* 10.
5a. Caplan, A.L., Callahan, D., and Haas, J. (1987). Ethical and policy issues in rehabilitation medicine. *Hastings Cent. Rep., 17,* (suppl.), 1.
6. Childress, J.F. (1982). *Who should decide? Paternalism in health care.* New York: Oxford University Press.
7. Daniels, N. (1986). Why saying no to patients in the United States is so hard. *N. Engl. J. Med., 314,* 1380.
8. Fagerhaugh, S.Y., and Strauss, A. (1974). *Politics of pain management: Staff-patient interaction* (pp. 85–93). Menlo Park, CA: Addison-Wesley.

9. Jonsen, A.R., and Tolmin, S. (1988). *The abuse of casuistry.* Berkeley, CA: University of California Press.
10. Lo, B. (1988). Medical ethics. In W. Kelley (Ed.), *Textbook of internal medicine* (pp. 3–5). Philadelphia: Lippincott.
11. Quill, T.E. (1983). Partnerships in patient care: a contractual approach. *Ann. Intern. Med., 98,* 228–234.

CHAPTER 27

Public Policy and Geriatric Rehabilitation

FERNANDO TORRES-GIL
LORI L. ROSENQUIST

America is aging; and with the increasing number of older persons, we will see changing attitudes about the aging process. Conversely, America also continues to view itself as a youth-oriented nation, priding itself on its vigor and physical fitness. But the aging of the society will alter our views on aging and physical disability and will force us to confront the prospects of increased numbers of older persons with physical disabilities. Those persons will require a continuum of health care and social services unique to the problems of disease and disability (Table 27-1). Such a continuum ideally will provide choices to older persons and their families that are suited to meet their needs for independence in the community. Geriatric rehabilitation is an integral component of this continuum. Most older persons live in the community. Fewer than 5 percent live in long-term care institutions at any one time, and only about 20 percent will ever use such a service.[19] It follows that more older persons with a disability or physical impairment will likely benefit from rehabilitation services if they include community-based and home-based as well as institution-based programs.

Table 27-1. *Continuum of Care*

Institutional rehabilitation	*Community-based rehabilitation*	*Home-based rehabilitation*
Hospital	Adult day health care	Home health care
Intermediate care facilities (ICFs)	Hospice, respite	Homemaker-chore
	Residential care facilities	Personal care
Skilled nursing facilities (SNFs)		Visiting nurse

To date, a larger percent of younger disabled adults have received rehabilitation services compared to older disabled persons. In fact, according to the 1972 Survey of Disabled and Nondisabled Adults, one out of three severely disabled adults receive services, with only one out of five persons being of those 55 to 64 years of age.[17] The young and the old disabled are usually viewed as two distinct populations, requiring separate needs and programs. In reality, both groups have similar needs for health, rehabilitation, and social services. In addition, these populations are and will be affected by the aging process. Younger persons with disabilities will need more rehabilitation as they age and older persons need rehabilitation to maintain adequate functioning. Therefore, in a period of increasing interest in providing services to these populations, it becomes essential to merge their common interests and integrate rehabilitation programs and treatments in services to both the younger and older disabled.

This chapter discusses various components of existing rehabilitation and aging public policies as a set of parallel programs and funding sources requiring greater integration. The primary focus of this chapter is the elderly and the need to incorporate geriatric rehabilitation in health and long-term care services, particularly in community-based programs. A brief review of the historical development of separate public policies for younger and older persons with disabilities and their different approaches to the use of rehabilitation will provide the basis for devising strategies for promoting geriatric rehabilitation—objectives that will benefit today's elderly, as well as younger persons who will be tomorrow's elderly.

HISTORY OF HEALTH POLICY DEPARTMENT

The literature provides ample proof of the need to provide rehabilitation and long-term care services to older persons with a disability or physical impairment.[5,12] Despite this recognition, three primary barriers exist in funding and integrating services: (1) the relative absence in existing legislation of programs that promote rehabilitation and long-term care services for the elderly; (2) the overemphasis on acute care health service reimbursement to the elderly; and (3) a fragmentation of efforts between those in the rehabilitation field and those in the aging field.

A review of legislation indicates that a variety of laws and programs have been developed to promote rehabilitation and health services for persons with a disability. Interest in rehabilitation began with veterans suffering disabling injuries in the wars, with workers injured in early industrial work, and later, to assist those with childhood illnesses. For example, the poliomyelitis epidemics in the 1930s, 1940s, and 1950s provided an impetus to rehabilitate and thus mainstream people with polio.[2] Legislation authorizing development of state rehabilitation programs to provide programs for disabled persons first occurred in 1943 with the Vocational Rehabilitation Law, which was greatly expanded in 1958. The Rehabilitation Act of 1973 (P.L. 93-112) increased those services. Legislation in 1962 provided for the establishment of comprehensive rehabilitation, research, and training centers (RRTCs), now under the title of the National Institute on Disability and Rehabilitation Research (NIDRR). However, no RRTC was devoted to the problems of aging and disability until 1982. The 1973 Rehabilitation Act paved the way for passage of the Rehabilitation, Comprehensive Services, and Developmental Disabilities Amendments of 1978 (P.O. 95-602). Title VII of this act, "Comprehensive Services for Independent Living," provided for rehabilitation services for severely disabled persons without regard to vocational potential.

A White House Conference on the Handicapped and the development of the independent living center movement in the 1970s further highlighted the importance of rehabilitating persons with disabilities while allowing them to maintain independence in the community. However, those developments did not expressly include the elderly, nor have the needs of older persons with disabilities been adequately addressed since the legislation was introduced. For example, the Rehabilitation Act of 1973 did not address the issue of age as a specific criterion for service eligibility. The limited data available show that fewer than 10 percent of clients in state departments of rehabilitation are persons over age 55.[1,9]

PARALLEL APPROACHES

Legislation covering older persons developed parallel to laws covering rehabilitation services. Laws targeting the elderly were far more numerous and elaborate in both scope and funding than those for disabled persons. For example, the Social Security Act of 1935 (P.L. Aug. 14, 1935,

Ch. 531) remains the broadest and most important piece of legislation for older persons in history. It provides for a variety of income transfer programs, including old-age and survivors insurance. But it is not intended to promote health or rehabilitation programs for older persons. On the contrary, its provisions for demonstrating eligibility for disability insurance benefits were designed to prove that older persons *were not* feasible for rehabilitation, at least in the sense of returning to work. For example, those who apply for disability benefits from Social Security are routinely screened for rehabilitation potential. However, only a very small number of persons over age 50 are referred by the social security administration (SSA) to state vocational rehabilitation agencies,[16] a fact that probably reflects negative attitudes toward older persons rather than objective findings about their work potential. This view that the elderly disabled generally are not employable has clouded many opportunities for their returning to work and becoming independent of the SSA program.[6] It is evident that the provision of most services depends on the individual's perceived future productivity in particular vocations.[17]

Subsequent legislation for older persons occurred in the 1960s with the passage of the Older Americans Act of 1965 (P.L. 93-29), Medicare (Title XVIII of the Social Security Act), and Medicaid (Title XIX of the Social Security Act). The Older Americans Act (OAA), through an administrative network of state units and area agencies on aging, provides a variety of supportive social services to persons over the age of 60, including nutrition programs, senior citizen centers, counseling, homemaker chore services, ombudsmen programs, and legal assistance. However, the OAA does not address the cause or treatment of decreased functional abilities in late life.

Medicare provides health insurance benefits for most persons aged 65 and older for *acute* health problems through its Hospital Insurance Program (Part A) and Supplementary Medical Insurance Program (Part B). Medicaid is a federally aided, state-administered medical assistance program serving low-income people. Within broad federal limits, states set the scope and reimbursement rates for the medical services offered and make payments directly to providers who render the services. Supplemental Security Income (SSI) recipients are eligible for Medicaid assistance. Medicare pays for about half of most nursing home costs of older persons in institutional settings. Title XX of social security provides funding for a variety of social services, including in-home supportive services. However, Title XX is essentially a block grant program passing funds to states. The states have considerable discretion in setting eligibility criteria and determining which services will be provided. Title XX can serve any age of the population and is generally geared toward low-income people.

CURRENT POLICY STATUS

Neither the OAA, Medicare, nor Medicaid were intended to meet the needs of older persons with *chronic* health problems producing a disability. They generally do not reimburse providers for most services deemed necessary for rehabilitation of disabled persons. However, there are exceptions. Section 1115(a) of the Social Security Act (42 U.S.C. 1315a) allows the secretary of the Department of Health and Human Services to waive compliance with standard Medicaid requirements so that a state Medicaid agency can carry out significant demonstration projects that further the program's general objectives. In addition, the Health Care Financing Administration provides funds to demonstration projects that use a variety of rehabilitation techniques and services for older persons. Some of these projects offer services such as adult day care and rehabilitation-oriented programs. For example, the On Lok project in San Francisco demonstrates a successful program that attempts to move toward a continuum of care for the elderly.[14]

The On Lok Senior Health Services Program was funded by the Administration on Aging (AOA) through a research and demonstration project to develop a day center. This was followed by a Model Project on Aging Grant from the AOA for development and refinement of the day care center and the development of that program into a broader outpatient system for the frail, functionally dependent elderly. The main objectives of the On Lok program involve the following: (1) to rehabilitate a participant to the maximum extent possible through a variety of therapeutic services; (2) to maintain a participant at home by providing needed medical, supportive, nutritional, and social services; and (3) to prevent a participant from premature decline by providing health education and stimulation in a socially supportive environment.

Longer life expectancy and medical technology have brought health care issues of the older population to the attention of many in the health and rehabilitation professions. However, due to existing policies, rehabilitation services for older and frail elderly have not grown commensurate with the needs of a growing elderly population. Forty percent of all persons with a disability are now over age 60, and more than 50 percent of all persons 70 years of age and older have at least one disability that interferes with daily living.[7] The 1972 Social Security Survey of Disabled and Nondisabled Adults further demonstrates that the number of severely disabled persons sharply increases with age.[17]

An artificial dichotomy between programs for older persons and programs for persons with a disability seems to have developed in the last five decades. Existing rehabilitation services appear to be primarily geared toward younger populations—if not by law, then at least by custom and practice. Recent changes in Medicare have exacerbated those trends. The 1983 passage of a prospective payment system for the Medicare program resulted in the imposition of diagnostic-related groups (DRGs) as criteria for reimbursing hospitals through capitation payments. DRGs have created disincentives for hospitals to keep older persons any longer than necessary, resulting in further disincentives to perform in-hospital occupational and physical therapy.[4]

DRGs and prospective payment only exacerbate the present situation facing the elderly. The elderly may find that the types and degree of services offered by their local hospitals are diminished due to their attempts to lower the costs they would incur under the DRGs. A possible result of DRG implementation could be more hospitals focusing on short-term, less complicated services, which preclude a number of elderly with chronic diseases. The discharge procedure, generally known to take an extended amount of time (i.e., the time involved to transfer from the hospital to the community or nursing home), encourages hospitals to be more efficient; otherwise, those additional days could prove very costly to the hospital.[11]

However, there are some positive signs that the interests of both the young and the elderly disabled groups are being recognized. The Pepper-Roybal Long-Term Home Care bill of 1988, although defeated, would have provided a broad range of long-term home care benefits for chronically ill older Americans, disabled persons, and children under 18 unable to perform two or more normal activities of daily living (ADLs). The bill provided for an independent professional case management team with the attending physician prescribing the needed services. Those services included nursing care, homemaker chore services, therapy (e.g., physical, occupational), medical supplies, durable medical equipment, medical social services, and counseling. The financing of the bill would have been accomplished through lifting the wage ceiling for application of the Medicare hospital insurance tax rate (which is currently 1.45% on wages up to $43,500, but is scheduled to rise to $45,000 in 1988).

BARRIERS TO PROVIDING REHABILITATION SERVICES

Notwithstanding the positive approach of the Pepper-Roybal bill toward the use of rehabilitation, several questions arise: How can current resources (and any future increases in resources) be better used to promote the independence of older persons who have a disability? What barriers exist to promoting more supportive services for older persons who have a disability? The barriers in expanding geriatric rehabilitation and community-based services for the elderly are complex. The answers to these questions appear to be rooted in a variety of attitudinal, organizational, financial, political, and public policy factors.

AGEISM

Ageism is defined as negative attitudes and stereotypes concerning the elderly. These negative attitudes about older persons have been referred to repeatedly in the literature[1] as a barrier to the elderly's use of rehabilitation programs. Data developed by Benedict and Ganikos[1] shows a bias against the elderly by the Rehabilitation Services Administration, with only 2.4 percent of its clientele composed of older persons. Ageism in the operation of rehabilitation services is often based on the faulty assumption that older persons are difficult to mainstream because they cannot improve. However, ageism can also be a two-way situation, with attitudes held by patients often obstructing their own involvement in comprehensive geriatric rehabilitation programs.[10] Thus, providers require astute observation in discerning whether a patient's or family's attitude is negative or detrimental, which could preclude efficient rehabilitation treatment. Providers' negative attitudes toward older persons can also be reflected in rehabilitation departments' orientations toward younger versus older persons with disabilities. Rehabilitation departments serving younger disabled persons often concentrate on "mainstreaming" activities leading toward a return to production, "normal" lives through employment, training, and educational programs. On the other hand, older persons who require "maintenance" services that allow a minimal level of functioning receive a fewer number and variety of services.

ACUTE ILLNESS ORIENTATION

The acute illness focus of most health care services is another reason for the lack of integrated geriatric rehabilitation and community-based, long-term care services. While Medicare is designed to pay for inpatient hospital services, posthospital care in skilled nursing facilities, hospice care, care provided in the patient's home, and physician services, Medicaid remains the primary source of nursing home care. While the Medicare system pays for approximately 75 percent of hospital bills, 55 percent of physician costs, and only 2 percent of nursing home expenses, Medicaid pays for more than 50 percent of all nursing home care in the United States.[15] Medicaid has become a major cost factor for states and a majority of the estimated $15.3 billion (state and federal Medicaid expenditures in 1984) has gone for nursing home care.

According to Callahan and Wallack, most elderly persons with severe health problems or disabilities prefer to stay out of nursing homes or institutional facilities and remain at home as long as possible.[8] Efforts to encourage various types of home and community-based care have grown in recent years. However, as previously indicated, the majority of funding goes toward nursing home care, continuing the bias toward institutionalization. Callahan and Wallack list several problems facing long-term care given this bias: (1) The general quality of care is typically poor; (2) services and financing are fragmented; (3) there remain large amounts of unmet needs and a geographic maldistribution of available benefits; (4) costs have been rising rapidly, and public expenditures are not under acceptable control; (5) there is an absence of adequate case management (i.e., no centralized mechanisms for information, referral, prescription, or allocation of resources); and (6) the current situation places heavy burdens on individuals and families.[8]

The orientation toward acute care has been and continues to be a matter of major controversy within the health and social service professions and in the policy arena. That orientation is a major barrier to including geriatric rehabilitation services. Increasingly, support is growing for funding a variety of community-based, long-term care services—an approach that is more likely to allow for rehabilitation programs. Presently, what exists is a set of services and benefits that are incomplete in meeting the full range of services for existing needs and are not fully coordinated, given autonomous legislative, regulatory, and administrative structure. To better understand how alternative funding options would impact the desired goal of a comprehensive continuum of care, it is useful to place those options on a continuum that includes a full range of institutional (i.e., intermediate care facilities, skilled nursing facilities, and acute hospital services), community-based (i.e., adult day health care, respite care) and home-based (i.e., in-home support services, visiting nurse services) care. Such a continuum would also include physical and occupational therapy, respite care, case management, social services, and programs allowing older persons with a disability to remain in the community or retain mobility within an institutional setting.

COSTS

Fears about the additional costs of long-term care, the medical profession's bias against it, the federal deficit, and the continuing disagreements about whether long-term care is more cost-effective than institutional care have prevented Medicare and Medicaid from expanding into long-term care services.

On the bright side, some noninstitutional services, such as homemaker chore, visiting nurse, respite care, adult day care, and in-home supportive services have increased over the years for older persons. But their access is restricted and fragmented, and there are too few services to go around. An older person with sufficient financial resources can purchase home health care through an extensive system of companies providing those services. Some states, notably Massachusetts, provide a network of community-based home health services. However, many older persons with disabilities and chronic illnesses that require rehabilitation services and who can benefit from long-term care programs cannot afford community-based services, or are unable to find them in their area, or lack sufficient transportation to partake of the services. Lack of coordination between eligibility and financing criteria in those programs also makes it difficult to obtain a mix of services. The fragmented and sparse nature of home care services discourages or prevents many elderly persons from making arrangements to remain at home.[3] Without adequate home health and support programs, geriatric rehabilitation will not be successful.[13]

The manner in which programs for services, training, and education are funded remains a major concern, as do the assumptions underlying that funding. Funding for home health and adult day care, as well as for social services, is necessary if geriatric rehabilitation programs are to be successful. Yet with the exception of the Older Americans Act and Title XX Social Services, major aging programs do not emphasize those services. The OAA and Title XX are relatively small programs in terms of funding. Both have a full agenda of services they must provide, leaving them with limited room for major expansion of home health and community-based services. What exists is a fragmented funding stream for acute care, long-term care, and rehabilitation services. That funding stream is further reduced by legislative and regulatory policies that create disincentives for rehabilitation-oriented programs within aging services.

In summary, current policies seem to be intentionally or unintentionally biased against noninstitutional, age-related comprehensive approaches to rehabilitating older persons. If so, it affects funding, training, and the delivery of services, as well as the priority those services give to treating younger versus older persons with disabilities. The current policy and financing picture will have to change if we are to effectively address the health care needs of an aging society.

IMPLICATIONS FOR THE FUTURE

A variety of approaches for developing better home support and other community-based services are possible and some are available. For example, there have been scores of demonstration studies done through-out the country examining community-based long-term care. Unfor-tunately, these have not yet been analyzed from a rehabilitation point of view. That is, how can geriatric rehabilitation be an integral part of those programs? Other efforts include Medicare reforms that have expanded Medicare reimbursement for long-term care services; Medicaid reforms that have altered benefit requirements to cover a broader range of home care services; social insurance programs that require long-term care insurance or fund long-term care systems; private financing such as reverse annuity mortgages and increased family contributions; and private insurance and organization changes that promote coordination from existing services.[3,18]

The need to change or adapt the present policy and financing system is apparent if we are to effectively offer services to the disabled. Health care professionals, whether serving younger or older disabled persons, are key players in removing the attitudinal barriers that preclude optimal service allocation to both groups. Knowing about and working with elderly persons requires education and training in gerontology and geriatrics. Professional organizations and advocacy groups representing the health and social services are important players in influencing public policy to minimize the dichotomy in rehabilitation services to the young and to the old. Researchers are important in devising the best strategies, program approaches, and treatments to a growing disabled population.

The need to provide these strategies and the resulting benefits are quite clear. For example, geriatric rehabilitation is cost-effective by keeping older persons out of hospitals and skilled nursing facilities and allowing them a greater measure of independence and mobility. The psychologic benefit to the elderly and their families is self-evident. The importance to merge and expand the existing two systems involves the following factors:

1. Cost benefits—keeping the elderly out of costly institutions and in their communities may save money.
2. Political benefits—incorporating rehabilitation programs for the elderly as well as younger persons is an intergenerational approach and demonstrates to policymakers that public dollars are being used well.
3. Efficiency of operations—greater opportunity to merge programs and agencies.
4. Ethical concerns—provides frail elderly with greater choices.

There is cause for optimism when one looks to the future in the field of rehabilitation. The younger disabled groups are increasingly recognizing that the aging process will no doubt include them and will lead them toward the types of services that are available for older persons. For example, postpolio syndrome and the need for rehabilitation is showing up in older persons who had polio when they were younger. Recent hearings by the House Select Committee on Aging on postpolio demonstrated the importance of developing long-term care services that include rehabilitation programs. Public attitudes and public policy evidenced by the Pepper-Roybal bill is recognizing the similarity of concerns. The similarities of needed services is becoming more evident among persons working in the field. But the continued effort to educate the public and key public officials about the ongoing needs and services of disabled persons is crucial for the future. Unless we recognize and merge such systems, it is possible that we may find both groups, young and old, losing services and benefits presently available, particularly with the ever-present fiscal problems and budget deficits.

In recent years, "generational conflict" has become a popular phrase, implying that young persons and old persons are competing for scarce public resources. In actuality, that implication is spurious; polls consistently show that young persons support public programs and benefits for the elderly. However, there is a chance that intergenerational tension might develop if separate programs for young and old persist when they can be brought together. Rehabilitation programs are one such area that benefits both groups. In the final analysis, old and young persons have the same goals: equal opportunities for social integration and independence. Comprehensive rehabilitation services for young and old alike are one means that can assist persons in meeting these goals.

REFERENCES

1. Benedict, R.C., and Ganikos, M.L. (1981). Coming to terms with ageism in rehabilitation. *J. Rehabil., 47*, 10.
2. Berkowitz, M., et al. (1975). *An evaluation of policy-related rehabilitation research.* New York: Praeger.
3. Brecher, C., and Kinickman, J. (1985). A reconsideration of long-term care policy. *J. Health Polit. Policy Law, 2*, 245.
4. Brody, S.J., and Nagel, J.S. (1985). Diagnosis related groups. *Center Stud. Aging Newslett., 6*, 6.
5. Brody, S.J., and Ruff, G.E. (Eds.). (1986). *Aging and rehabilitation: Advances in the state of the art.* New York: Springer.
6. Baumann, N.J., Anderson, J.C., and Morrison, M.H. (1985). Employment of the older disabled person: Environment outlook and research needs. In S.J. Brody, and G.E. Ruff (Eds.), *Aging and rehabilitation: Advances in the state of the art* (pp. 329–342). New York: Springer.
7. Blake, R. (1984). What disables the American elderly? *Generations, 8*, 6.

8. Callahan, J.J., and Wallack, S.S. (1981). *Reforming the long term care system.* Lexington, MA: Lexington Books.
9. Cromar, E. (1984). Research and the disabled elderly. *Generations, 8,* 55.
10. Hesse, K.A., Campion, E.W., and Karamouz, N. (1984). Attitudinal stumbling blocks to geriatric rehabilitation. *J. Am. Geriatr. Soc., 32,* 747.
11. Jones, A.A. (1984). Prospective payment: Curbing Medicare costs at patient's expense? *Generations, 9,* 19.
12. Kane, R., Ouslander, J.G., and Abrass, I. (1984). *Essentials of clinical geriatrics.* New York: McGraw-Hill.
13. Kornblatt, S. (1984). Social support systems. *Generations, 8,* 40.
14. On Lok Senior Health Services (1979). *Toward a continuum of care. Final report: Model project on aging.* San Francisco: U.S. Dept. of Health, Education and Welfare.
15. Schulz, J.H. (1985). *The economics of aging,* 3rd ed. Belmont, CA: Wadsworth.
16. Treitel, R. (1973). *Identifying disabled workers who may return to work. Research and Statistics Note No. 5.* Social Security Administration, Office of Research and Statistics, Washington; D.C.: Government Printing Office.
17. U.S. Department of Health and Human Services and the Social Security Administration. (1981). *Disabled and nondisabled adults: A monograph.* Disability Survey 72, Research Report No. 56.
18. Weissert, W. (1985). The cost-effectiveness trap. *Generations, 9,* 47.
19. Williams, T.F. (1986). The aging process: Biological and psychological considerations. In S.J. Brody and G.E. Ruff (Eds.), *Aging and rehabilitation: Advances in the state of the art* (pp. 13–17). New York: Springer.

CHAPTER 28

Measuring the Effectiveness of Rehabilitation Programs
ROBERT L. KANE

A good program in rehabilitation must often meet two separate sets of criteria to prove its worth and survivability. One set addresses the effectiveness of the program. The second is a test of professional orthodoxy. The former looks for objective evidence of merit. The latter generally involves intense and subjective (i.e., political) discussions about how many of which disciplines need be represented. I suggest that it is more useful to look at *what* works rather than *who* works. Indeed, the tension between these factors and methodologic constraints make identifying what really makes a difference in rehabilitation a very difficult task.

Many of the problems of assessing rehabilitation are similar to those faced in addressing any clinical issue. The interested reader should refer to one of the several volumes on clinical research and clinical epidemiology.[1-3] However, there are also some special aspects that are particularly pertinent to rehabilitation.

EFFICACY, EFFECTIVENESS, AND EFFICIENCY

A useful point of departure is the distinction among efficacy, effectiveness, and efficiency. Although many health analysts are quick to ask whether you are efficient, they fail to realize that you cannot be efficient until you are first effective. Doing things at very little cost that make no difference in outcome is not efficient. In examining new ways of doing something the first challenge is to determine whether or not that approach is efficacious. By efficacious we mean that, when done properly, it does make a real difference. To test if something makes a real difference it is not adequate to simply measure improvement over time.

Because the natural course of many problems is recovery, control groups are essential and randomized clinical trials are highly desirable. Rehabilitation is a field that cries out for good studies to establish the efficacy of interventions, but one has first to be very clear about what those interventions are and then spend the time to develop tight experimental designs which will allow them to be tested.

Particularly in the area of rehabilitation, we encounter several major common errors. One is not defining precisely what is being tested. If you are going to go to the trouble of testing whether something is efficacious, that is, whether it really works when it is done properly, then you must be very careful to ensure that the intervention is what you believe it to be. Ironically, we spend much time worrying about measuring the effect of treatments, but we never bother to see whether we have a legitimate treatment in the first place. Much time has been given over to debates on the merits of a five-point scale versus a seven-point scale to measure the impact of a treatment on patient functioning without bothering to ask whether something significant was actually done. In the final analysis, this type of research must focus on whether we were really measuring important effects of a substantial intervention.

It is difficult to do exhaustive studies of efficacy. Such studies are very expensive in terms of time, resources, and energy. Therefore, it is reasonable to move through a progression. If something proves to be efficacious, that is, if it has been shown that at its best it really makes a difference, then we usually go on to ask the more pragmatic question, "Is it effective?"

For example, in testing a new drug you want to find the dose that is most potent while having the fewest side effects. Clinical trials require a lot of effort in making sure that patients being studied really take the drug. Both the compliance and the outcomes are measured. However, once the drug is put on the market, patients will undoubtedly take it at various times and at al sorts of dosages. The social question, "Does the drug work in common practice?," is an issue of effectiveness. Although the drug may be efficacious under very tightly controlled situations, prescribed by the common physician and taken by the common patient it may be much less effective than it was efficacious.

Having looked at the question of effectiveness, the next question is, "How much does effectiveness cost?" Efficiency is equal to effectiveness-cost. Therefore, relative efficiency can be achieved either by being more effective for the same cost or by costing less to achieve the same effect.

In selecting targets for study one must also determine who is a candidate for rehabilitation. Any efforts to assess effectiveness must begin from a common starting point. Criteria for candidates should be clearly specified in terms of clinical characteristics and, perhaps, social and other relevant factors. One useful approach to developing a common starting pint is to rely on clinical judgment prior to randomization. This may be as simple as beginning from the point of referral and screening. In this case potential clients are referred by primary physicians because they were judged to be in need of and likely to benefit from rehabilitation. Subjects are then reviewed by a common panel using specific criteria. Those accepted into the study may be treated as a single group or further divided into classes on the basis of their expected course. In the latter case, these classes form strata which can be used as the basis for random assignment, in what Alvan Feinstein has called "prognostic stratification."[1]

Once a subject has been entered into the trial, he or she is charged to the group assigned for the duration of the study. Failure to receive the full measure of treatment or less than an ideal course should not lead to dropping the case from analysis. Although this is common practice, it results in retention in treatment of only those cases that show progress and will greatly bias the results of any trial.

Although rehabilitation specialists are ready to attest that indeed they know a good response when they see it, this remains a difficult problem to approach scientifically. Witness the difficulty in trying to define when rehabilitation begins. Many of those in rehabilitation insist that it begins, or should begin, as soon as the event occurs, that is, at the first sign of a stroke. Certainly there is great pressure to start rehabilitation very early in the process. We hear assertions of evidence to suggest that differences in outcome depend on when the rehabilitation process begins. Practically, however, it is very dificult to know when rehabilitation begins or even when it ought to begin. In some cases the patient may not be stable enough to really tolerate rehabilitation. Some people would argue that rehabilitation is more an environmental concern and an attitudinal concern rather than a specific list of disciplines and skills, in which case it can begin very early. If it does, then probably one of the worst things we do to geriatric patients is put them into hospitals, because hospitals are about as antirehabilitative a set of environments as one could design. Then one might argue that the most important rehabilitation begins in the ambulance with the key decision on whether to bring the patient to the hospital! Nonetheless, a careful definition of the rehabilitation process to be studied, prior to data collection, can clarify some of these issues.

In the face of the difficulty of defining when rehabilitation begins, we do not want to fall victim to the funding argument that rehabilitation under Medicare begins when the patient is transferred from his diagnosis-related group (DRG) category to a prospective payment system (PPS)–exempt category. In this country form follows funding. We have a health care system created by accountants. It is important to distinguish between accounting and accountability. We have imposed on our system a perversity by virtue of what gets paid for and what does not. The problem is, if we do it long enough we tend to believe it, we begin to accept it, and then we begin to incorporate it, and even worse, we begin to defend it. If we look at the patient rather than the system that has perversely grown up around the various funding incentives, then it is often very hard to know when rehabilitation begins, and it is very hard to know what constitutes a case or rehabilitation.

DEFINING GOALS

The other issue about rehabilitation is when does it end. This becomes a very important question in terms of measuring the effectiveness of rehabilitation. Because it aims at improving function, its end points are more difficult to establish. It is critical, for example, to decide in advance what is the most appropriate functional measure of success. Is functioning best measured in terms of performance (measured in terms of activities of daily living [ADLs], ergonomics, or whatever) under ideal or simulated conditions, or should it be established by performance under conditions of community living? The former provides a more standardized measure but the latter is a more socially useful one. However, the latter also depends on the availability of conditions and support systems that may extend beyond the usual capabilities of a rehabilitation unit. At the same time, one can argue that rehabilitation that does not address the issue of community function has limited social value.

On the one hand, the goal of rehabilitation is sometimes viewed as getting the patient to a higher level of functioning; a process that is completed when the patient crosses some kind of a threshold. This can lead to a patient being "fully rehabilitated" with nowhere to go. He may be stuck back in the nursing home and allowed to dwindle. The patient may be perfectly rehabilitated but the process is of no final benefit to the quality of that patient's life.

The contrary argument is that it is reasonable to expect rehabilitation to return the patient to the community where he can function at the highest possible level of autonomy. In this case can one hold the rehabilitation unit accountable if the patient does not have a decent family to support him, or cannot mobilize a set of community services? The line between clinical rehabilitation and social policy is a fine one. Rehabilitation as an organized group must struggle with this major issue much more than it has. It must be very clear about what kinds of signals it sends to the public and for what it is willing to take responsibility. Until we can get over that hump, we will not have many useful studies of rehabilitation.

It is my position that if in the end patients are not at a level where they can function at maximum autonomy in their natural settings then you have not achieved meaningful rehabilitation. On that basis one needs to measure many fewer things, because that type of achievement is easy to see. The best test of measurement in rehabilitation is what kind of evidence one would be comfortable presenting to a congressional committee. When asked, "How did you know the patient was better?," it will not suffice to say he moved up two decimal points on the XYZ scale. The congressman is likely to ask, "Could that patient walk? Could that patient stand? Could that patient get out of bed himself?" "Well, we don't measure simple things like that. We have these very sophisticated measurements. We have ergonomic data that provides thirty-three data points on his ergonomic functioning on all body systems." In a commonsense setting, that kind of response will not go over well.

Basically, the kinds of things that we want from an evaluation system are very simple, basic holistic constructs. We are interested in the effectiveness of rehabilitation as reflected in people's ability to do large-scale tasks, which allow them to function independently. It is true that for some purposes one may want to be able to detect small increments of change; this level of detail may play an important role in clinical rehabilitation, but it is too fine to demonstrate the effectiveness of rehabilitation. We need major outcomes that show major changes to justify the extra effort and cost associated with different forms of rehabilitation.

At the same time, we must acknowledge the difficulty involved in mounting research studies in the midst of enormous pressures coming from regulation and reimbursement policies. These forces have created an orthodoxy which impacts on every aspect of geriatric rehabilitation research. For every innovative idea in rehabilitation there are at least five rules against it. Innovations provoke disciplinary protectionism. Each professional union has put into the books some regulation that require that its discipline be represented, so we wind up with organizations that are essentially staffed very inefficiently, with the equivalent of a fireman on a diesel locomotive. There are incredible redundancies, because nobody has demanded evidence of what needs to be done to make a difference. Finally, we must acknowledge that the system is shaped by reimbursement policies. For example, the PPS exemption requires 3 hours a day of therapy. This interesting regulation essentially stipulates an orthodoxy apparently arbitrarily determined but actively enforced. Such orthodoxy will influence the goals and the aliquots of rehabilitation.

EXPECTATIONS

Does the site of care really make a difference? One can develop very elaborate, architecturally exciting, flashy, and flamboyant inpatient situations. One can do many of the same things on outpatient situations. But the important aspects may not be architectural. Probably even more important than the physical environment is the social environment.

Almost axiomatic in geriatrics is the centrality of geriatric teams. It is considered heretical to be against teamwork in geriatrics; but teamwork in geriatrics is very uneconomical. When eight people meet for an hour, it represents one person-day. Few geriatric teams are efficient enough to make up for that loss. Opposing teams does not mean being against having different disciplines involved, but the disciplines need to come together to function in a systematic way, each contributing its unique set of skills. Most teamwork is incredibly redundant. Too much teamwork tends to serve the team, not the patient, providing "team-building" skills that reinforce people and get them to feel good about what they are doing.

When studying the effectiveness of geriatric rehabilitation and geriatric rehabilitation teams or units, it is important to distinguish what a team does from what happens in the milieu that is developed. As we examine the treatments in geriatric rehabilitation, more attention should be given to separating the effects of geriatric rehabilitation attributable to staffing by true believers from that produced by competent practice. Certainly the two are not mutually exclusive, but as one looks at the variety of geriatric interventions performed under the name of geriatric assessment, and the similarity of results despite wide variations in input, one must consider that at least part of the effect is due less to the particular mix of services than to a self-fulfilling positive prophecy. An important step in rehabilitation, and particularly in geriatric rehabilitation, is a belief that one can make a difference. If the caregiver believes that and if that belief is transmitted to the patient, 90 percent of the goal may have been achieved. Motivating the patient by motivating the caregivers, rather than simply accepting the traditional negative stereotype about the potential of older people, is a key to improving function.

Using placebos is not bad, but it is important to know what is being done. A famous colonial public health physician in Philadelphia went every morning to Chestnut Hill to fire a cannon to ward off yellow fever; most days it worked! We have picked up all sorts of orthodoxies in medicine that have not been examined. As we address what defines true treatment in rehabilitation, distinguishing the psychologic component, the positive self-fulfilling prophecy becomes very important.

A pertinent study applicable to the field of geriatric rehabilitation comes from psychology. Two groups of college students were randomly assigned to witness an experiment. The subject was strapped into a chair behind a glass booth, she was asked to learn nonsense words, and every time she missed one of the words, the instructor administered a shock. As they watched the experiment, the students described their feelings about the anonymous subject using a discriminant adjective check list. Half the class simply watched and each of the other half had a button he or she could push that could change the intensity of the shock the subject was going to receive. In truth, the "experiment" was a sham, no shock was administered, but there was a dramatic difference in the ratings by the two groups. The students who perceived that they could intervene to change the intensity of the shock were much more positive about this totally anonymous subject than were the students in the other group.

This finding, which is called the "innocent victim syndrome,"[6] provides important insight about geriatric rehabilitation, because it explains a great deal about the behavior of caregivers. If the caregiver feels important enough to make a difference, he or she will feel very negative toward the patient. But if that person is imbued with a sense of power to make a difference, this may explain a great deal of what is involved in the milieu of rehabilitation. One may be able to change that person's attitude toward that patient and hence be able to change his or her effectiveness in working with that patient.

PROGNOSIS

Some have said that diagnoses make no difference. In fact, diagnoses make a lot of difference. One of the most important concepts in evaluating any kind of a trial of therapies is prognostic stratification. When comparing cases, one wants to compare those believed to have similar kinds of outcomes without special attention. We have generally put a great deal of trust in the principle of random allocation. But even within randomized control trials there may be subgroups with differences that interact with the treatments. These are important distinctions to make.

In comparing the effectiveness of an intervention, one wants to be sure to compare apples to apples on the basis of whatever clinical insight says ought to make a difference. The treatment of a stroke victim who is also a diabetic is different from a stroke victim who is not only a diabetic but has congestive heart failure, or arthritis, or is blind. Age is certainly important; one would not want to accept a study in which the control group was made up of 60-year-olds and the treatment group of 90-year-olds. One needs to be sensitive to variations in duration of the problem; the length of time since onset becomes a very important predictive variable for a number of these things, both for better and for worse.

Often, particularly under the conditions of modern rehabilitation, one has to be able to somehow make a judgment on the basis of inadequate information. Many of the patients being discharged from hospitals today are discharged before they have even begun to stabilize, let alone peak. In such cases, one of the most important variables may be the prognosis at the time of allocation to the treatment or control group. In using such clinical prognoses, it is critical to make them all first and then randomize within prognostically controlled groups.

OUTCOMES

Having looked at interventions, it is important to consider which outcomes are of greatest importance. Some interesting distinctions are familiar but bear close scrutiny. We have alluded earlier to the question of defining goals in terms of site of function. Specific measurement of function must distinguish between measuring demonstrated and regular performance. In any of the measurement issues with regard to rehabilitation motivation is an important factor. If you put somebody on a treadmill, the level and type of encouragement make a big difference in whether or not they go for their maximum effort. Similarly, when you seek to inspire patients to do things independently, motivation makes a great deal of difference.

Likewise, it is important to appreciate the difference in measuring performance under standardized test situations from simply observing functioning under the patient's natural situation. It is not a matter of right or wrong, but of knowing what one is doing and how to interpret it. One gets two different kinds of information. The first is a very standardized measurement of how the patient would do in a controlled situation, but patients rarely live in a controlled situation. The relevant question is whether one is interested in bringing people up to a standard level of performance that is equivalent across different patient groups, or whether one is interested in devising a measure that looks at the patient's performance in his natural environment.

Measures also need to be sensitive to the variation in treatment levels. Ideally, one would like to plot a dose-response curve for the treatments provided for a problem in rehabilitation with a good distribution of variables at all levels of functioning, especially the higher levels. Most of the variables currently used distinguish between bad and worse, but not between good and better. Ideally, one wants to get a spread across all levels of function, but one is often working in a very narrow band of the distribution. This means one can miss different parts of the distribution for different kinds of interventions. One of the challenges in looking for standardization of measures across different conditions is the consequent difficulty in detecting dose responses for particular kinds of conditions. Choosing appropriate variables for a given situation represents a fundamental trade-off question, for which there is no right or wrong answer, but which must be appreciated when choosing measures.

Another pertinent issue for rehabilitation is the way benefits are calculated. The standard approach uses "utiles," or measures of utility based on the worth of different kinds of outcomes. People have developed measures like quality-adjusted life-years (QALYs). Others simply measure survival. Katz and colleagues[5] have introduced "active life expectancy," based on functional years of survival. All of those measures are very closely tied to survival. Despite their modifiers, they all have life-years at their core. Those concerned about the elderly must pay close attention to inherent biases in the system with regard to the kinds of measures used to sum the value-preference weights that are assigned to different components of functioning. The more the functioning is measured in large units, for example, autonomy, rather than small units, for example, joint movement, the less that is a problem and the more one is dealing with meaningful concepts that are more easily valued across different parts of the society.

Rehabilitation today faces a problem that comes under the general area of what might be called "ethical concerns." Although there are scarce data to establish the effectiveness of rehabilitation, it is considered unethical not to do it. Thus, conducting randomized studies is hard, because few institutions are comfortable giving the control group no rehabilitation. Therefore, most studies are comparing new forms of rehabilitation to so-called standard care. The problem, of course, is to define standard care, which turns out to be a rather mixed bag. Planning studies, one has to be very careful to vary the amount of rehabilitation enough by withholding sufficient care to establish the marginal difference. For example, just comparing 2 hours a day instead of 3 hours a day, or substituting one type of therapist for another, is not likely to show much.

THE NEED FOR RESEARCH IN GERIATRIC REHABILITATION

There are thus two key questions in geriatric rehabilitation research: (1) Do you have enough of an intervention to reasonably expect a difference?, and (2), How big a difference need you find to say that you have something interesting?

The major challenge to rehabilitation today is to justify its existence. Ironically, most of the people now interested in funding rehabilitation are not interested in showing a difference. If they find no difference, they can urge using cheaper alternatives that are available. Gornick and Hall[4] have shown much higher costs associated with rehabilitation compared with home care and nursing home care for Medicare patients with the same DRGs. They suggest that the burden of proof of better results lies with those who charge tenfold more for potentially equally effective care. Thus, the pragmatic question asked most often is not whether we can do more but whether we can do less. Can the same outcomes be achieved for less money?

This difference in emphasis has important design implications. The statistics involved in measuring no difference are more complicated than statistics to show a difference. It is a harder calculation to decide that you have enough observations to show that it is meaningful to say there is no difference, than it is to calculate the sample size you need for sufficient observations to show a statistically significant difference. Of course, the sample size needed depends on the size of that difference. With enough observations, one can show that even very minute differences are statistically significant, but they will not likely be clinically significant. This distinction between statistical and clinical significance has important implications.

POST–ACUTE CARE STUDY

An example of a study with substantial implications for rehabilitation is the study of post–acute care (PAC) currently being conducted by the University of Minnesota. The introduction of PPS has created great interest in what happens to patients discharged from the acute hospital. Simply looking at patterns of discharges grouped by DRG, there appears to be great variation in the post–acute care given to persons with the same DRG, with great variations in price.

Because certain kinds of care, including rehabilitation in hospitals, is exempted from the DRG system, there was great concern that there might be a market response to using such care. The observation that people with the same diagnoses, for example, strokes, had markedly different utilization patterns, some going to nursing homes, some to rehabilitation, and some to home care, raised eyebrows. Clinicians quickly pointed out that a stroke is not a stroke; different kinds of strokes need different kinds of care. But the government correctly demanded evidence that these folks (a) are different and (b) have different outcomes.

The PAC study thus addresses the distribution and effects of services covered under Medicare, namely, skilled nursing care, rehabilitation, and home health care, plus no care. Of course people do not get one kind of care; many have what we would call long-term care careers, in which they move from one kind of service to another. We are trying to answer four basic questions: The first is what kinds of patients get what kinds of PAC; in this regard, we are interested in the clinical and socio-demographic parameters that can distinguish a truly random event from those developed in response to certain events or situations. The second question is, what are the careers of these people; "career" here is not used in the occupational sense, but is a word used in lieu of the term "episode" referring to the way people move from one kind of a system to the other. Therefore, much of the payoff for PAC may derive from reducing the rate of rehospitalizations. Merged data sets from 1984 developed by the Rand Corporation indicate that over 30 percent of the patients with the most common DRGs associated with PAC are rehospitalized within 9 months.[7] Although a major rationale for the concept of PAC lies in its potential for reducing the subsequent use of expensive services, preliminary results suggest that this may not be happening. No major differences in the rates of readmission are seen between users and nonusers of PAC.

The critical question then is whether there is a difference in the outcomes of care, adjusted for the differences in the case mix of the people going into these different streams. Here, outcomes include patients' functioning as well as the costs of care. The outcomes are measured in terms of ADLs, affect, and cognition. The measures were chosen to be applicable across the range of treatments. The change in each parameter from predischarge to follow-up will be adjusted for case mix. In addition, we will also look at such basic issues as whether the person has survived and is living independently in the community.

We will be following a group of these patients from the time just prior to discharge until 6 weeks and 6 months after discharge to see what happens to them, what kind of services they use, and whether it makes any difference.

We will also use the national Medicare data to see whether in patterns of PAC there is evidence of substitution. For example, do places with less rehabilitation show greater use of other PAC modalities to compensate?

SUMMARY

Rehabilitation represents an important potential component of geriatric care. Its worth will be better established by careful trials of intervention with well-defined groups of elderly patients than by simply arguing that more is better or professional training is essential. At present it is hard to distinguish rehabilitation from those who provide it. Circular arguments suggest that rehabilitation is care provided by rehabilitative specialists. We have to do better.

A second critical point is deciding where to look for benefits and how to measure them. Successful rehabilitation cannot leave a patient unable to function more independently in his or her usual daily life. If functioning is the evidence of success, it should be assessed in the context of the patient's natural environment. Ability to function in a sheltered environment is different from ability to function in an unsupported environment. Rehabilitation's commitment to functioning implies an obligation to address both the client and his living environment. The measures of functioning should be readily understood by those outside rehabilitation if the benefits are to be appreciated.

REFERENCES

1. Feinstein, A.R. (1977). *Clinical Biostatistics*. St. Louis, Mosby.
2. Feinstein, A.R. (1987). *Clinimetrics*. New Haven; Yale University Press.
3. Fletcher, R.H., and Wagner, E.H. (1988). *Clinical epidemiology*, 2nd edi. Baltimore; Williams & Wilkins.
4. Gornick, M., and Hall, M.J. (1988). Trends in medicare utilization of SNFs, HHAs, and rehabilitation hospitals. *Health Care Financing Review, Special Supplement on Post-Hospital Care*. Pp. 27–38.
5. Katz, S., et al. (1983). Active life expectancy. *N. Engl. J. Med., 309,* 1218.
6. Lerner, M.J., and Simmons, C.H. (1966). Observer's reaction to the "innocent victim": Compassion or rejection? *J. Pers. Soc. Psychol., 4,* 203.
7. Neu, C.R., and Harrison, S.C. (1988). *Posthospital care before and after the medicare prospective payment system.* Rand/R-3590-HCFA, Santa Monica, CA, 1988.

INDEX

Index

Osteoporosis
History, medical, personal, and
    functionally oriented, 63–
    65, 110, 268, 269, 282, 340.
    *See also under assessment, di-
    agnosis, evaluation, and his-
    tory for specific impairments*
Holter monitor, 204
Home health aides and home-
    makers, 27, 217
Home rehabilitation program, 17,
    27. *See also* In-home geria-
    tric rehabilitation
Homeostatic reserve capacity, 62–
    63
Homonymous hemianopia, 70
Hospital. *See* Acute illness and
    care settings
Hospital-at-home (HAH), 381
Humor, 262
Huntington's disease, 122
Hydroxychloroquine, 101
Hypertension, 67, 85
Hypertrophic cardiomyopathy,
    200
Hyperuricemia, 98
Hypnotics, 264, 393
Hypochondriasis, 170, 276
Hypotension, 63, 79, 231. *See also*
    Orthostatic hypotension
Hypotonia, 71
Hypoxemia, 79, 111, 113, 115, 116,
    118

"Identified patient," 313–314
Immobilization, 179, 184, 195,
    340, 341, 342. *See also* Bed
    rest; Chronic inactivity;
    Deconditioning
Immunosuppressive drugs, 97
Impairment, 4, 28, 30, 31, 33, 35,
    36, 38, 46, 137, 138. *See also*
    Cognitive impairment;

Hearing impairments; Sen-
    sory impairment; Vision
    impairments
Incontinence, 82, 83, 204
Independence-dependence, 42–
    43, 51. *See also* Activities of
    daily living; Autonomy
Indomethacin, 393
In-home geriatric rehabilitation,
    17, 27, 357–359
    application for, 360–365
    definition and rationale for,
    359–360
    limitations of, 365–367
    team approach to, 367
"Innocent victim syndrome," 435
Innovation, 433
Inspiratory resistance loading,
    116
Intervention, 4–5, 8, 146–151
Interview, patient and family, 35,
    110, 268, 282–283
Isocapnic hyperventilation, 116

Joint function, 158, 159, 160, 161,
    166, 167
    and deconditioning, 184
Joint surgery, 94, 97
Justice, 412–413

Katz index, 65, 204, 340
Kenny self-care index, 65

Lawton IADL scale, 64, 160
Laser card, 213, 221
Learning and memory, 11, 32–33,
    53, 113, 150–151, 165, 300,
    301. *See also* Cognitive im-
    pairment
Legislation, 418–422
Leisure, as ADL, 140
Levadopa, 125, 126, 127–128, 129,
    130, 393

DATE DUE

JUL 1 2 1995	AUG 2 2 1995		